# ACSM's
# Certification Review

## FOURTH EDITION

# EDITORS*

## SENIOR EDITOR

**Gregory B. Dwyer, PhD, FACSM, ACSM-ETT, ACSM-CES, ACSM-RCEP, ACSM-PD**
East Stroudsburg University
East Stroudsburg, Pennsylvania

## ASSOCIATE EDITORS

**Nancy J. Belli, MA, ACSM-HFS**
Asphalt Green
New York, New York

**Meir Magal, PhD, FACSM, ACSM-CES**
North Carolina Wesleyan College
Rocky Mount, North Carolina

**Paul Sorace, MS, ACSM-RCEP**
Hackensack University Medical Center
Hackensack, New Jersey

*See Appendix B for a list of editors for the previous two editions.*

# ACSM's
# Certification Review

## FOURTH EDITION

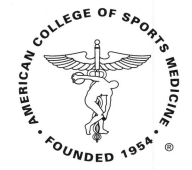

**AMERICAN COLLEGE
OF SPORTS MEDICINE**

Wolters Kluwer | Lippincott Williams & Wilkins
Health

Philadelphia · Baltimore · New York · London
Buenos Aires · Hong Kong · Sydney · Tokyo

*Acquisitions Editor*: Emily Lupash
*Managing Editor*: Meredith L. Brittain
*Marketing Manager*: Sarah Schuessler
*Manufacturing Coordinator*: Margie Orzech
*Creative Director*: Doug Smock
*Compositor*: Absolute Service, Inc.

*ACSM Publication Committee Chair*: Walter R. Thompson, PhD, FACSM, FAACVPR
*ACSM Group Publisher*: Kerry O'Rourke
*Umbrella Editor*: Jonathan K. Ehrman, PhD, FACSM

4th Edition

351 West Camden Street          Two Commerce Square / 2001 Market Street
Baltimore, MD 21201             Philadelphia, PA 19103

Printed in China

9  8  7  6  5  4  3  2  1

Library of Congress Cataloging-in-Publication Data

ACSM's certification review. — 4th ed. / senior editor, Gregory B. Dwyer ; associate editors, Nancy J. Belli, Meir Magal, Paul Sorace.
      p. ; cm.
  Includes index.
  ISBN 978-1-60913-954-4
  I. Dwyer, Gregory Byron, 1959- II. American College of Sports Medicine.
  [DNLM: 1. Sports Medicine—Case Reports. 2. Sports Medicine—Examination Questions. 3. Exercise—Case Reports. 4. Exercise—Examination Questions. 5. Physical Fitness—Case Reports. 6. Physical Fitness—Examination Questions. QT 18.2]

  617.1'027076—dc23

2012037317

### DISCLAIMER

To purchase additional copies of this book, call our customer service department at (800) 638-3030 or fax orders to (301) 223-2320. International customers should call (301) 223-2300.

Visit Lippincott Williams & Wilkins on the Internet: http://www.lww.com. Lippincott Williams & Wilkins customer service representatives are available from 8:30 am to 6:00 pm, EST.

**Nancy J. Belli, MA, ACSM-HFS**
Asphalt Green
New York, New York
Cases: Domain of Legal, Professional, Business, and
Marketing for CPT

**Clinton Brawner, MS, FACSM, ACSM-RCEP,
ACSM-CES**
Henry Ford Hospital
Detroit, Michigan
Cases: Domain of Patient/Client Assessment for CES
(Electrocardiograms)

**Nikki Carosone Russo, MS, ACSM-CPT**
Long Island University
Brooklyn, New York
Cases: Domain of Exercise Programming and
Implementation for CPT

**Brian Coyne, MEd, ACSM-RCEP,
ACSM/NCPAD-CIFT**
Duke University Health System
Durham, North Carolina
Cases: Domain of Exercise Counseling and Behavioral
Strategies for HFS

**Donald M. Cummings, PhD, ACSM-CES**
East Stroudsburg University
East Stroudsburg, Pennsylvania
Cases: Domain of Exercise Prescription for CES

**Shala E. Davis, PhD, FACSM, ACSM-ETT,
ACSM-CES, ACSM-PD**
East Stroudsburg University
East Stroudsburg, Pennsylvania
Cases: Domain of Leadership and Counseling for CES

**Kimberly DeLeo, BS, PTA, ACSM-CPT**
Health and Exercise Connections, LLC
Middleboro, Massachusetts
Cases: Domain of Legal, Professional, Business, and
Marketing for CPT

**Julie J. Downing, PhD, FACSM, ACSM-CPT,
ACSM-HFD**
Central Oregon Community College
Bend, Oregon
Cases: Domain of Health and Fitness Assessment
for HFS

**Shawn Drake, PT, PhD, ACSM-RCEP, ACSM-PD**
Arkansas State University
Jonesboro, Arkansas
Cases: Domain of Exercise Prescription and
Implementation for HFS

**Trent A. Hargens, PhD, ACSM-CES**
James Madison University
Harrisonburg, Virginia
Cases: Domain of Patient/Client Assessment for CES

**Dennis Kerrigan, PhD, ACSM-CES**
Henry Ford Hospital
Detroit, Michigan
Cases: Domain of Patient/Client Assessment for CES
(Electrocardiograms)

**Frederick Klinge, MBA, ACSM-HFS**
Ochsner Health System / Varsity Sports
New Orleans, Louisiana
Cases: Domain of Management for HFS

**Timothy S. Maynard, MS, ACSM-PD**
Providence Hospital
Mobile, Alabama
Cases: Domain of Legal and Professional Considerations
for CES

**Matthew W. Parrott, PhD, ACSM-HFD**
H-P Fitness, LLC
Kansas City, Missouri
Cases: Domain of Legal/Professional for HFS

**James H. Ross, MS, ACSM-RCEP, ACSM-CES**
Wake Forest University
Winston-Salem, North Carolina
Cases: Domain of Exercise Prescription for CES

*See Appendix C for a list of contributors to the previous two editions.*

**Tom Spring, MS, FAACVPR, ACSM-CPT, ACSM-HFS, ACSM-CES**
WebMD Health Services
Detroit, Michigan
Cases: Domain of Initial Client Consultation and Assessment for CPT

**David E. Verrill, MS, FAACVPR, ACSM-RCEP, ACSM-CES**
University of North Carolina at Charlotte
Charlotte, North Carolina
Cases: Domain of Program Implementation and Ongoing Support for CES

**Janet P. Wallace, PhD, FACSM, ACSM-CES, ACSM-PD**
Indiana University
Bloomington, Indiana
Cases: Domain of Exercise Prescription for CES

**Michael J. Webster, PhD, FACSM, ACSM-CES**
University of Southern Mississippi
Hattiesburg, Mississippi
Cases: Domain of Exercise Leadership and Client Education for CPT

**Christopher G. Berger, PhD**
The George Washington University
Washington, District of Columbia
HFS Case Studies

**Andy Bosak, PhD**
Georgia Southwestern State University
Americus, Georgia
HFS Job Task Analysis

**Mindy Caplan, ACSM-HFS**
Lake Austin Spa Resort
Austin, Texas
HFS Practice Examination

**Teresa Fitts, DPE, FACSM**
Westfield State College
Westfield, Massachussetts
HFS Case Studies

**Julie Hansen, MPH, ACSM-CPT**
Montage Hotels and Resorts
Park City, Utah
CPT Case Studies

**Tarra L. Hodge, MS**
Purdue University
West Lafayette, Indiana
HFS Job Task Analysis and CPT Practice Examination

**Dennis J. Kerrigan, PhD**
Henry Ford Hospital
Detroit, Michigan
CES Case Studies and CES Practice Examination

**Tom LaFontaine, PhD, FACSM, FAACVPR**
Optimus: The Center for Health
Columbia, Missouri
CES Case Studies

**Tony Musto, PhD**
University of Miami
Miami, Florida
CES Job Task Analysis

**Neal I. Pire, MA, FACSM**
InsPIRE Training Systems
Ridgewood, New Jersey
CPT Job Task Analysis

**Nikki Carosone Russo, MS**
Long Island University
Brooklyn, New York
CPT Job Task Analysis

**Mitchel Whaley, PhD, FACSM**
Ball State University
Muncie, Indiana
CES Case Studies (Electrocardiograms)

**Mary Yoke, MS**
Indiana University
Bloomington, Indiana
CPT Case Studies

**Mark Zaleskiewicz, MS, FAACVPR**
Shore Medical Center
Mays Landing, New Jersey
CES Job Task Analysis

As an undergraduate student at Wake Forest University, I took my first American College of Sports Medicines (ACSM) certification examination in 1978 (which I had to retake in 1979!). The experience of being certified by ACSM was one of the great accomplishments of my young career and helped me get my first job with Dr. Noel Nequin at Swedish Covenant Hospital in Chicago. Under Noel's guidance and urging, I became certified as an ACSM program director for Preventive and Rehabilitative Exercise Programs (which is no longer an ACSM certification) in 1983. At about that same time (1981), I was invited to sit on the ACSM Certification and Education Committee (now known as the Committee on Certification and Registry Boards [CCRB]), and I have held various positions on that committee for more than 30 years. For six of those years, I served as the chair. During those 30 years, there has been an exponential growth in the number of certification candidates and in the resources being provided to certification candidates.

In 2009, CCRB decided to simultaneously publish *ACSM's Guidelines for Exercise Testing and Prescription* (8th edition), *ACSM's Resource Manual for Guidelines for Exercise Testing and Prescription* (6th edition), *ACSM's Resources for Clinical Exercise Physiology* (2nd edition), and *ACSM's Certification Review* (3rd edition). This was an amazing accomplishment as the books were written by four sets of writers and editors. It proved to be such a great success that the plan was implemented for the next editions of the books, including this one (except for *ACSM's Resources for Clinical Exercise Physiology*, which did not need revision).

This fourth edition of *ACSM's Certification Review* is by far the most comprehensive edition of this title. Senior Editor Gregory Dwyer and his talented team of associate editors (Nancy Belli, Meir Magal, and Paul Sorace) and writers have developed the quintessential review for ACSM Certified Personal Trainer (CPT), ACSM Certified Health Fitness Specialist (HFS), and ACSM Certified Clinical Exercise Specialist (CES). Although the scope of this fourth edition targets these three certifications, the ACSM Certified Group Exercise Instructor, ACSM Registered Clinical Exercise Physiologist, and those preparing for the Exercise is Medicine Credential will also find this book to be very useful.

The fourth edition was developed strategically into three parts for each certification — cases for each certification, a detailed breakdown of the knowledge and skills for each certification, and sample questions that are similar to those found on each certification examination. One of the more unique features of this edition is the cases, which are organized within the text according to the domains, a result of the recent job task analysis. The four domains include health and fitness assessment (initial client consultation and assessment for CPT, health and fitness assessment for HFS, and patient/client assessment for CES); exercise programming (exercise programming and implementation for CPT, exercise prescription and implementation for HFS, and exercise prescription for CES); exercise counseling and behavioral strategies (exercise leadership and client education for CPT, exercise counseling and behavioral strategies for HFS, and program implementation for CES); program administration (legal/professional/business/marketing for CPT, management for HFS, and leadership and counseling for CES); and legal and professional considerations for all three certifications.

Greg, Nancy, Meir, and Paul will receive much praise for the contents of this book and their professional approach to providing for certification candidates the very best resource to prepare for their examinations. For me, it is a simple "thank you" to them for their dedication and their friendship. To present and future certification candidates — this book will be your guide to success.

Walter R. Thompson, PhD, FACSM
Regents Professor
Department of Kinesiology and Health
(College of Education) and
Division of Nutrition
(Byrdine F. Lewis School of Nursing and
Health Professions)
Georgia State University
Atlanta, Georgia

This fourth edition of the *ACSM's Certification Review* has been extensively revised from previous editions of this text. This edition covers all the current knowledge, skills, and abilities (KSAs) for the certifications of the Certified Personal Trainer (CPT), the Certified Health Fitness Specialist (HFS), and the Certified Clinical Exercise Specialist (CES).

## TEXT ORGANIZATION

This text is organized into parts by certification level and is further subdivided into three main sections in each part as follows:

- **Case studies** that involve both multiple-choice questions as well as open-ended discussion questions are divided by certification level and domain. There are 30 case studies (and 10 accompanying ECGs) in the book.
- **Job task analysis (JTA) tables** that contain a detailed breakdown of all the KSAs by certification level and domain. In this section, there is a further breakdown of what each KSA statement refers to as well as helpful study resources for each KSA. The KSA section was extensively impacted by the recent ACSM JTA that was performed on all certification levels.
- **Practice examinations**, one for each certification, contain 100 multiple-choice practice questions with answers and explanations. At the end of each exam, a table indicates which questions in that practice test correspond to which domain(s).

## STUDYING FOR A CERTIFICATION EXAM

The many individuals involved in the preparation of this text intend that it be used as a review aid for the certification exams and assume that the reader is actively preparing to sit for one of the three ACSM certifications covered. This text represents one of many study tools available and should not be viewed as the sole source of information to use in preparing to take one of these three certification exams.

As a study or review tool, this text may help you clarify areas of strengths and weaknesses. Your individual weaknesses should be eliminated by further study. This text should be viewed as part of a study kit that each of you needs to identify for yourself. Certainly, *ACSM's Guidelines for Exercise Testing and Prescription*, Ninth Edition (*GETP9*) must be considered as part of that package. The ACSM has also written *ACSM's Resource Manual for Guidelines for Exercise Testing and Prescription*, Seventh Edition (*RM7*). As a commitment to the certification field, ACSM is coordinating the updating of these texts, which are publishing at the same time this book publishes.

ACSM certification levels build upon one another. For instance, the CES certification encompasses all HFS and CPT KSAs. Thus, individuals who intend to use this book to review for the CES certification are responsible for all KSAs covered in the HFS and CPT sections as well as all KSAs covered in the CES section. Similarly, individuals preparing for the HFS certification are responsible for all KSAs covered in the CPT section.

We are aware that facts, standards, and guidelines change on a regular basis in this ever growing field of knowledge. Hence, in the event that conflict may be noted between this book and the *GETP9*, the latter text should be used as the **definitive and final resource**. In such cases, where an update is needed or where a conflict or error is identified, I will make every effort to provide further explanations or corrections online. The web address for any corrections is http://certification.acsm.org/cr4updates.

If I can play a small role in your ACSM certification success, I would feel truly happy that all the hard work put into this project has paid off.

Gregory B. Dwyer, PhD, FACSM, ACSM-ETT,
ACSM-CES, ACSM-RCEP, ACSM-PD
*Senior Editor*

## ADDITIONAL RESOURCES

*ACSM's Certification Review, Fourth Edition* includes additional resources for instructors that are available on the book's companion Web site at http://thepoint.lww.com/ACSMCR4e.

### INSTRUCTORS

Approved adopting instructors will be given access to the following additional resource:

- Image bank

In addition, purchasers of the text can access the searchable Full Text Online by going to the *ACSM's Certification Review, Fourth Edition* Web site at http://thepoint.lww.com/ACSMCR4e. See the inside front cover of this text for more details, including the passcode you will need to gain access to the Web site.

I fear to mention specific names as I might exclude those who deserve so much of my acknowledgment. Many have mentored me in my more than 30-year ACSM certification career (I was first certified in 1982). To all those who added so much to my career, I give my heartfelt thanks (I have thought of these many individuals often during this textbook writing/editing process, *in a good way!*). To those who have been involved in this project who have added much, especially my associate editors, I give you thanks for allowing me to stand on your shoulders. The ACSM certification staff, the ACSM Committee on Certification and Registry Boards, as well as Lippincott Williams & Wilkins have fully supported this project, and a great debt of gratitude is owed to them all. I would like to thank Dr. Jon Ehrman, the umbrella editor of this project, who made it his mission to ensure congruency between the ninth edition of the *Guidelines* and seventh edition of *ACSM's Resource Manual for Guidelines for Exercise Testing and Prescription* as well as this text. Dr. Ehrman is also the umbrella editor for *ACSM's Resources for the Personal Trainer*, Fourth Edition and the new *ACSM's Resources for the Health Fitness Specialist*.

Finally, my wonderful family — Beth, Kevin, and Eric — have provided me much grounding, nourishment, and encouragement throughout the years.

— Gregory B. Dwyer

I am grateful to the many individuals with whom I have worked and collaborated, but there are a few that need special acknowledgement. First of all, to Greg Dwyer for having the confidence in me to be such an integral part of this project. Second, to Neal Pire for his belief in me and recommending that I contribute my talents to ACSM on a national level. On a personal level, to my sister, Mary Lou, who is an inspiration at what can be accomplished over the course of a day. Most importantly, to my family, who love and support me to do the work that fulfills my soul.

— Nancy J. Belli

I would like to thank all the contributors and reviewers; without their dedicated work, this project would not have been possible. I would also like to thank my parents, Esther and Dani Magal, for the values and ethics they have instilled in me, and my wife Dana and my children, Yuval and Amit, for giving me the inspiration, support, and patience needed to complete this work.

— Meir Magal

A special thanks to the ACSM Committee on Certification and Registry Boards for their diligent reviews of this textbook. Their commitment to ACSM and the exercise profession is invaluable.

— Paul Sorace

Contributing Authors to the Fourth Edition ................................................................................ v
Reviewers for the Fourth Edition................................................................................................ vii
Foreword ...................................................................................................................................... ix
Preface .......................................................................................................................................... xi
Acknowledgments ....................................................................................................................... xiii


**PART 1 ACSM CERTIFIED PERSONAL TRAINER (CPT)**.................................................................. 1

*Associate Editor: Nancy J. Belli, MA, ACSM-HFS*

**Section 1    CPT Case Studies** ................................................................................................... 3
Case Study CPT.I................................................................................................................ 3
Case Study CPT.II............................................................................................................... 4
Case Study CPT.III ............................................................................................................. 6
Case Study CPT.IV(1) ........................................................................................................ 8
Case Study CPT.IV(2) ........................................................................................................ 9
CPT Case Studies Answers and Explanations.................................................................... 10

**Section 2    CPT Job Task Analysis**......................................................................................... 15
Domain I: Initial Client Consultation and Assessment....................................................... 15
Domain II: Exercise Programming and Implementation ..................................................... 24
Domain III: Leadership and Education Implementation ..................................................... 35
Domain IV: Legal, Professional, Business, and Marketing .................................................. 40

**Section 3    CPT Examination** .................................................................................................. 55
CPT Examination Answers and Explanations .................................................................... 63
CPT Examination Questions by Domain ............................................................................ 74


**PART 2 ACSM CERTIFIED HEALTH FITNESS SPECIALIST (HFS)** ............................................... 75

*Associate Editor: Meir Magal, PhD, FACSM, ACSM-CES*

**Section 4    HFS Case Studies** ................................................................................................. 77
Case Study HFS.I................................................................................................................ 77
Case Study HFS.II............................................................................................................... 79
Case Study HFS.III ............................................................................................................. 80
Case Study HFS.IV ............................................................................................................. 82
Case Study HFS.V............................................................................................................... 83
HFS Case Studies Answers and Explanations.................................................................... 86

**Section 5    HFS Job Task Analysis** ........................................................................................ 93
Domain I: Health and Fitness Assessment ......................................................................... 93
Domain II: Exercise Prescription and Implementation....................................................... 101
Domain III: Exercise Counseling and Behavioral Strategies .............................................. 117
Domain IV: Legal/Professional ......................................................................................... 122
Domain V: Management ..................................................................................................... 126

**Section 6    HFS Examination** .................................................................................................. 131
HFS Examination Answers and Explanations.................................................................... 139
HFS Examination Questions by Domain ............................................................................ 150

**PART 3 ACSM CERTIFIED CLINICAL EXERCISE SPECIALIST (CES)** ........................................... 151
*Associate Editor: Paul Sorace, MS, ACSM-RCEP*

**Section 7     CES Case Studies** ............................................................................................................ 153
Case Study CES.I ...................................................................................................................... 153
Case Study CES.II(1) ............................................................................................................... 154
Case Study CES.II(2) ............................................................................................................... 157
Case Study CES.II(3) ............................................................................................................... 158
Case Study CES.II(4) ............................................................................................................... 160
Case Study CES.II(5) ............................................................................................................... 161
Case Study CES.III .................................................................................................................. 163
Case Study CES.IV .................................................................................................................. 165
Case Study CES.V(1) ............................................................................................................... 166
Case Study CES.V(2) ............................................................................................................... 168
Case Study CES.V(3) ............................................................................................................... 168
ECG Case Studies ................................................................................................................... 171
   CES.ECG(1) ....................................................................................................................... 171
   CES.ECG(2) ....................................................................................................................... 172
   CES.ECG(3) ....................................................................................................................... 173
   CES.ECG(4) ....................................................................................................................... 174
   CES.ECG(5) ....................................................................................................................... 174
   CES.ECG(6) ....................................................................................................................... 175
   CES.ECG(7) ....................................................................................................................... 176
   CES.ECG(8) ....................................................................................................................... 176
   CES.ECG(9) ....................................................................................................................... 177
   CES.ECG(10) ..................................................................................................................... 178
CES Case Studies Answers and Explanations ........................................................................ 179
ECG Case Studies Answers and Explanations ....................................................................... 190

**Section 8     CES Job Task Analysis** .................................................................................................... 195
Domain I: Patient/Client Assessment ..................................................................................... 195
Domain II: Exercise Prescription ............................................................................................ 200
Domain III: Program Implementation and Ongoing Support ................................................ 205
Domain IV: Leadership and Counseling ................................................................................. 211
Domain V: Legal and Professional Considerations ................................................................ 216

**Section 9     CES Examination** ............................................................................................................. 219
CES Examination Answers and Explanations ......................................................................... 228
CES Examination Questions by Domain ................................................................................. 237

**Appendix A Supplementary Figures, Tables, and Boxes from Other ACSM Certification Texts** ............. 239

**Appendix B Editors for the Previous Two Editions** ............................................................................. 285

**Appendix C Contributors to the Previous Two Editions** ..................................................................... 287

Index ........................................................................................................................................ 291

PART

# 1

# ACSM Certified Personal Trainer (CPT)

NANCY J. BELLI, MA, ACSM-HFS, *Associate Editor*

# SECTION

# 1

## CPT Case Studies

## DOMAIN I: INITIAL CLIENT CONSULTATION AND ASSESSMENT

**CASE STUDY
CPT.I**

Author: **Tom Spring, MS, FAACVPR**
Author's Certifications: **ACSM-CPT, ACSM-HFS, ACSM-CES**

Your fitness manager has assigned a new client to you, Beth (54 yr old), who would like to start an exercise program with you as soon as possible. Prior to your initial visit, your manager tells you that Beth called to begin a weight loss program and may also want to work with your club's staff dietician. Upon meeting Beth, you do your club's routine health assessment revealing the following information:

| | |
|---|---|
| Height | 5 ft 6 in |
| Weight | 195 lb |
| Body mass index (BMI) | 31 kg · m$^{-2}$ |
| Resting blood pressure at assessment | 138/88 mm Hg |
| Resting heart rate (HR$_{rest}$) | 88 bpm |
| Lipids | High-density lipoprotein (HDL): 56; low-density lipoprotein (LDL): 122; triglycerides (TG): 111 (all mg · dL$^{-1}$) |
| Fasting blood glucose | 102 mg · dL$^{-1}$ |
| Family history | Mother had a heart attack at about the age of 58 yr, father died from cancer at age 66 yr, and siblings (two younger sisters) are in good health as far as she knows |
| Medications | Aleve, occasional Advil for knee pain, vitamins designed for women |
| Exercise history | None to speak of in the past 20 yr or so; was a high school basketball player |
| Surgeries | None since appendix was removed 10 yr ago; no orthopedic surgeries or injuries |

As mentioned, Beth would like to begin an intense exercise regimen after hearing about high-intensity training from a friend and fitness enthusiast. She will manage her diet as you see fit and would like advice from a dietician to begin her quest to lose at least 20 lb. After discussing her preferences for exercise, you think she would be well suited for resistance training using free weights and body weight exercises as well as aerobic exercise on the treadmill and elliptical trainers. You also suggest starting a stretching program to help with some lower back pain she reports when sitting at work for prolonged periods of time.

## MULTIPLE-CHOICE QUESTIONS FOR CASE STUDY CPT.I

1. Beth should be risk classified as
   A) High risk
   B) Low risk
   C) Moderate risk
   D) Indeterminate

2. Beth should be characterized as meeting all the American College of Sports Medicine (ACSM) Risk Factor Thresholds for cardiovascular disease, except
   A) Hypertension
   B) Obesity
   C) Sedentary lifestyle
   D) Family history

3. According to her history and goals, your next session would occur when?
   A) Immediately, including high-intensity exercise
   B) Immediately, only for resistance training
   C) After meeting with the dietician
   D) After physician clearance has been obtained

4. Based on Beth's fasting glucose level, she would be classified as
   A) Normal
   B) Prediabetic
   C) Hypoglycemic
   D) Diabetic

5. What would you expect Beth's maximum heart rate to be (approximately) (using formula 220-age)?
   A) 145 bpm
   B) 166 bpm
   C) 186 bpm
   D) Cannot be determined

6. Based on Beth's lipid profile, she would be considered
   A) Normal
   B) Hyperlipidemic
   C) Dyslipidemic
   D) At risk for atherosclerosis

## DISCUSSION QUESTIONS FOR CASE STUDY CPT.I

1. After Beth's initial history and required clearance have been obtained, you decide to perform an initial fitness assessment. Discuss which fitness field tests would be appropriate for you to perform and why they might be selected.

2. Beth's desire to lose weight lead to significant discussion regarding her dietary habits. She solicits your advice to avoid the cost associated with the club's dietician. You decide to provide some advice and tips for her to help out where you can. Discuss the limitations and scope of practice for the certified personal trainer (CPT) as it relates to providing dietary information.

3. Using the Karvonen heart rate reserve formula, calculate an appropriate training heart rate for Beth that she may use in her initial training phase for cardiovascular exercise. Discuss the rationale for choosing the training range used in the calculations.

# DOMAIN II: EXERCISE PROGRAMMING AND IMPLEMENTATION

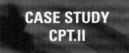

**CASE STUDY CPT.II**

Author: **Nikki Carosone Russo, MS**
Author's Certifications: **ACSM-CPT**

You are a CPT at a corporate fitness center. Stan, a new client, has joined your facility and is seeking his initial fitness evaluation and first workout session. Stan is a 39-yr-old male, who is 5 ft 9 in tall. He currently weighs 165 lb. Upon completing a body composition and fitness evaluation using the Jackson-Pollock 3-site skinfold method, you record his measurements as follows:

| | |
|---|---|
| Weight: | 165 lb |
| Triceps skinfold: | 12 mm |
| Subscapular skinfold: | 14 mm |
| Chest skinfold: | 16 mm |
| Waist circumference: | 33 in |
| Hip circumference: | 39 in |

Based on the results of the skinfold test, you predict his body fat to be 23.3%. His strength assessment reveals he is within normal ranges for strength and his sit and reach test shows he falls slightly below the flexibility parameters and has slight low back and hamstring tightness. During the initial evaluation, resting heart rate and blood pressure were measured at 66 bpm and 118/70 mm Hg, respectively.

When discussing his medical history, Stan reports that he is not a smoker and is not currently taking any medications. Stan does take an allergy suppressant during the spring and summer months and is prone to allergy-related symptoms such as headaches, sinus infections, and general lethargy during that time. He does not have any orthopedic contra-indications to exercise but reports that 5 yr ago, his doctor found a "slight bulging disc" in his "lower back" area. Stan does not currently have any low back pain and hopes that a structured, full-body routine will keep him strong and pain free.

During the goals review portion of the evaluation, Stan reported that he is a sporadic exerciser who would like to become a regular exerciser. He lacks the proper motivation and feels that working with a CPT will help him overcome this hurdle. His primary goals are to stay active enough to keep up with his two young children, lose 5 lb, and gain muscle in his upper body. Stan states that his lower body is very strong because he used to play competitive basketball and was on the track team in college. Currently, Stan is an avid golfer. He tells you that historically, his lower body has always appeared stronger and he would like to primarily work on increasing tone his upper body, specifically his chest and biceps. Stan also states that he usually sticks to select equipment and weight machines and would like to start doing more free weight and sport-specific exercises to increase strength, definition, and his golf swing. Optimally, he prefers to work his full body at least 3 d · wk$^{-1}$.

## MULTIPLE-CHOICE QUESTIONS FOR CASE STUDY CPT.II

1. According to the most recent edition of the *ACSM's Guidelines for Exercise Testing and Prescription* (*GETP*), this client would be classified as
   A) Low risk
   B) Moderate risk
   C) High risk

2. Design an exercise program for Stan based on the *ACSM's GETP* standards as well as Stan's goals of exercising at least 3 d · wk$^{-1}$.
   A) Full-body strength training program once per week: muscular strength and endurance, resistance exercises, calisthenics, balance and agility training
   B) Moderate intensity (40%–60% oxygen uptake reserve [$\dot{V}O_2R$]) aerobic activities, weight-bearing and flexibility exercises
   C) A combination of moderate-to-vigorous aerobic activities, weight-bearing and flexibility exercises
   D) Vigorous intensity (≥60% $\dot{V}O_2R$) aerobic activities, weight-bearing and flexibility exercises

3. Based on the rates of progression when initially working with Stan, what would your rate of progression look like?
   A) An increase of 5–10 min every 1–2 wk over the first 4–6 wk
   B) An increase of 2–5 min every 1–2 wk over the first 4–6 wk
   C) An increase of 10–15 min every week over the first 4 wk
   D) An increase of 10–15 min every 2 wk over the first 4–6 wk

4. In order to address Stan's goals for building muscle mass and improving strength, how many repetitions (reps) per set would you recommend?
   A) 6–8
   B) 12–15
   C) 8–12
   D) 10–15

5. According to the *ACSM's GETP*, all of the following are resistance training guidelines for healthy adults **except**
   A) Each major muscle group should be trained 2–3 d · wk$^{-1}$.
   B) The resistance training program should feature exercises that are multijoint, or compound exercises that involve more than one muscle group at a time.
   C) The resistance training program should feature exercises that are single joint and involve only one specific muscle group at a time.
   D) While performing repetitions, the individual should maintain a regular breathing pattern that typically involves exhaling during the "lift" and inhaling during the "lowering" phase of each exercise.

## DISCUSSION QUESTIONS FOR CASE STUDY CPT.II

1.  Based on what you know about Stan from his initial assessment, what are the various modalities of resistance training that you think he might be most inclined to adhere to?

2.  Given Stan's occasional back pain, what recommendations would you make regarding flexibility training to help keep him limber and pain free?

## DOMAIN III: EXERCISE LEADERSHIP AND CLIENT EDUCATION

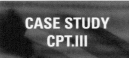

**CASE STUDY CPT.III**

Author: **Michael J. Webster, PhD, FACSM**
Author's Certifications: **ACSM-CES**

Bob is a relatively sedentary, 37-yr-old, Caucasian male. He has been married for 9 yr and has two daughters ages 7 and 5 yr. He has a Master's degree in Chemistry and worked in laboratory research for 5 yr before beginning his current position as a sales representative for a major pharmaceutical company, which he has been with for the past 7 yr. Bob's clients are hospital physicians in a major metropolitan city with a population of approximately 5 million. He finds the job to be enjoyable yet stressful. A typical work day involves approximately 2 hr of driving, meeting with physicians 3–4 hr, and 3–4 hr of work on the computer. He entertains clients at restaurant lunch and dinner meetings approximately four times per week. Weekends typically require another 5–6 hr of computer work at home. He typically gets no more than 6 hr of sleep each night. When Bob was in college, his height and weight were 5 ft 10 in (178 cm) and 154 lb (70 kg), respectively. He was a recreationally competitive runner, training 30–40 miles $\cdot$ wk$^{-1}$, with a best 5-km race time of 18:30. His body fat was 10%. Since his graduation from college, he has not been involved in any regular physical activity and has gradually put on weight. On the urging of his wife, Bob had a physical exam and it revealed the following:

Anthropometric measures
  Height: 5 ft 10 in (178 cm)
  Weight: 198 lb (90 kg)
  Body fat: 28%
Resting blood pressure (measured on two separate occasions): 142/78 mm Hg
Fasting blood glucose and lipids
  Blood glucose (measured on two separate occasions): 112 mg $\cdot$ dL$^{-1}$
  Total cholesterol: 198 mg $\cdot$ dL$^{-1}$
  LDL cholesterol: 136 mg $\cdot$ dL$^{-1}$
  HDL cholesterol: 29 mg $\cdot$ dL$^{-1}$
3-d dietary recall and nutritional analyses
  Daily caloric intake: 2,500 cal
  Daily carbohydrate (CHO) intake: 350 g
  — 60% simple or refined carbohydrates
  — 40% complex carbohydrates
  Daily protein intake: 100 g
  Daily fat intake: 55.5 g
  — 70% saturated fats
  Caffeine intake: 500 mg (five cups of coffee)
  Alcohol intake: 16 oz of regular beer (28.5 g)
Submaximal treadmill exercise test
  Predicted maximal oxygen uptake ($\dot{V}O_{2max}$): 35.6 mL $O_2$ $\cdot$ kg$^{-1}$ $\cdot$ min$^{-1}$
  Predicted final treadmill velocity corresponding with 100% of age predicted maximal heart rate: 6.0 mph (160.8 m $\cdot$ min$^{-1}$)

Flexibility (category based on gender and age)
   Sit and reach test: Poor
Muscular strength, endurance (percentile rating based on gender and age)
   one repetition maximum (1-RM) bench press: 30th percentile
   Sit-ups: 20th percentile
   Push-ups: 20th percentile

Bob's physician strongly recommended that he begin an exercise program, lose weight, and start eating better. Although hating to admit it, Bob knows that the physician's recommendation is what he needs and he is committed to making some changes to improve his overall health. Bob comes to you for guidance.

## MULTIPLE-CHOICE QUESTIONS FOR CASE STUDY CPT.III

1. Calculate Bob's current BMI.
   A) 25.2 kg · m$^{-2}$
   B) 26.3 kg · m$^{-2}$
   C) 28.0 kg · m$^{-2}$
   D) 28.4 kg · m$^{-2}$

2. Determine Bob's current classification based on his BMI.
   A) Normal weight
   B) Overweight
   C) Class 1 obesity
   D) Class 2 obesity

3. To address Bob's weight and body composition, he is advised to diet and exercise. Bob wants to decrease his daily energy intake by 200 cal, with the balance coming from an increase in exercise energy expenditure (EE). What should his daily exercise energy expenditure be to achieve a target BMI of 24.9 kg · m$^{-2}$ in 12 wk? You can assume that he is presently in energy balance and that all weight loss is from fat.
   A) 48 cal
   B) 200 cal
   C) 483 cal
   D) 683 cal

4. How many pounds would Bob need to lose to achieve a target body weight of 20% body fat?
   A) 19.8
   B) 23.2
   C) 26.9
   D) 39.6

5. In order to best help Bob with necessary behavioral changes, you evaluate his readiness to change. You find that he is in the _____ stage of change.
   A) Precontemplation
   B) Contemplation
   C) Preparation
   D) Action

6. What is Bob's daily energy intake of carbohydrate, protein, and fat calories?
   A) Carbohydrate: 1,400; protein: 400; fat: 500
   B) Carbohydrate: 1,750; protein: 400; fat: 250
   C) Carbohydrate: 1,400; protein: 510; fat: 390
   D) Carbohydrate: 1,400; protein: 700; fat: 200

## DISCUSSION QUESTIONS FOR CASE STUDY CPT.III

1. Bob understands how his BMI is calculated; however, he questions its validity. His argument is that it doesn't take into account the muscle mass and overall body composition. Is Bob's argument valid? How would you address Bob's concern?

2. Bob has done some reading on the Internet about diets and considers his diet to be "fairly" good. What aspects of Bob's diet are good and what areas need to be addressed?

CPT

# DOMAIN IV: LEGAL, PROFESSIONAL, BUSINESS, AND MARKETING

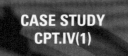

**CASE STUDY CPT.IV(1)**

Author: **Kimberly DeLeo, BS, PTA**
Author's Certifications: **ACSM-CPT**

You have recently started working in a very busy health club as a full-time fitness specialist. Your job responsibilities include supervising the fitness floor, new member orientations, general exercise programming, assisting members with the proper use and safety of the exercise equipment, and maintenance of the fitness equipment.

The facility also offers personal training packages to their members, and you are able to personal train clients "off hours." You are responsible for getting your own personal training clients and are paid as an independent contractor. Your regular work hours are Monday to Friday, 8 a.m. to 5 p.m.

## TRUE OR FALSE AND MULTIPLE-CHOICE QUESTIONS FOR CASE STUDY CPT.IV(1)

1. Your personal training client, Joe, is going through a difficult time and has confided in you that he is having difficulties with his marriage and has started drinking excessively. As an ACSM CPT, it is appropriate to
   A) Give him advice on what he should do with his marriage.
   B) Explain to him about the risk factors of excessive alcohol intake and how it can affect his training program.
   C) Refer him to local professionals that specialize in counseling and behavior change.
   D) Just listen and do nothing.

2. While running on the treadmill, a member stops abruptly and grabs his chest. The very first thing you should do is
   A) Activate emergency medical services (EMS).
   B) Start chest compressions.
   C) Have the member sit down and tell him to rest.
   D) Immediately attend to the member and ask him if he is having chest pain. If he says yes, activate EMS and monitor him until help arrives.

3. Medical emergency plans must be written and easily available to all staff. Review of the emergency plan should also be done. How often should emergency drills be conducted?
   A) Once per year
   B) Twice per year
   C) Quarterly
   D) Once per month

4. While personal training your client in the fitness center, the cable on the lat pull-down machine broke. The weights dropped and your client lost his grip on the bar. He is now complaining of pain in his shoulder. The first thing you do is
   A) Try to fix the machine so your client can finish his exercise.
   B) Fill out an incident report and put a "do not use" sign on the equipment.
   C) Get ice for your client.
   D) None of the above.

5. True or False: A CPT does not need professional liability insurance when he or she is personal training in a fitness center.

## DISCUSSION QUESTION FOR CASE STUDY CPT.IV(1)

1. Why is it important to keep your clients'/members' files in a secure place?

# DOMAIN IV: LEGAL, PROFESSIONAL, BUSINESS, AND MARKETING

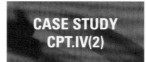

**CASE STUDY CPT.IV(2)**

Author: **Nancy J. Belli, MA**
Author's Certifications: **ACSM-HFS**

You are a personal trainer at a health/fitness facility. You have been working with your client, Tom, for approximately 3 months to enhance his overall tennis stamina and performance. While playing doubles this past weekend, Tom reached for a forehand volley and felt his right ankle roll over (inverted). Tom immediately got up and walked around and stretched the surrounding musculature and continued to play for the next 90 min, slightly favoring the right leg/ankle. As a precaution, Tom iced his ankle when he got home after the match.

Tom comes in for his training session 2 days later and relays the series of events to you and says that his ankle feels weak. He tells you that he has not had any pain or swelling but he lacks confidence in his ability to fully use the right ankle.

## MULTIPLE-CHOICE QUESTIONS FOR CASE STUDY CPT.IV(2)

1.  According to *ACSM's Guidelines*, what are the signs/symptoms of mild ankle sprain?
    A)  Light edema, pain, point tenderness, strength loss
    B)  Moderate edema, light pain, hemorrhage, measurable laxity
    C)  Excessive edema, moderate pain, hemorrhage, measurable laxity
    D)  Excessive edema, excessive pain, hemorrhage, palpable or observable defect

2.  According to *ACSM's Guidelines*, what does the acronym RICES stand for?
    A)  Rehab, ice, compression, elevation, sterilization
    B)  Rest, inactivity, compression, elevation, stabilization
    C)  Rest, ice, compression, elevation, stabilization
    D)  Rehab, immobilize, cold, elevate, support

3.  According to the most recent *American Heart Association and American Red Cross Guidelines for First Aid* (2010), which of the following cold applications is recommended concerning the management of Tom's soft-tissue injury?
    A)  Ice the ankle for 10 min using a gel pack directly on the skin
    B)  Ice the ankle for 15 min placing the ice directly on the skin
    C)  Ice the ankle for 20 min using a mixture of ice and water
    D)  Ice the ankle for 25 min using a gel pack

4.  According to the most recent *ACSM's Guidelines*, which of the following actions is required by Tom prior to resuming training after an injury?
    A)  The client should be referred to a physician before resuming training.
    B)  The client should be referred to a physical therapist before resuming training.
    C)  The client should immobilize the ankle and be immediately referred to a physician before resuming training.
    D)  The client does not require clearance before resuming training.

5.  What assessments would you perform to address Tom's lack of confidence in fully using his leg/ankle?
    A)  Muscular endurance assessment for the quads and hamstrings
    B)  Flexibility assessment for the quads and hamstring
    C)  One-legged balance assessment
    D)  40-yd dash to test speed

6.  What adjustments will you make to Tom's program?
    A)  Add exercises that strengthen the medial aspect of the lower leg and ankle.
    B)  Add unilateral dynamic leg balance, eversion exercises, and proprioception exercises to the program.
    C)  Add exercises that strengthen the quads and hamstrings.
    D)  Add flexibility exercises for his quads and hamstrings.

## DISCUSSION QUESTION FOR CASE STUDY CPT.IV(2)

1.  What additional adjustments and progressions will you make to Tom's program to get him back to playing with confidence?

# CPT CASE STUDIES ANSWERS AND EXPLANATIONS

## CASE STUDY CPT.I

### Multiple-Choice Answers for Case Study CPT.I

**1—C.** Moderate risk

**2—A.** Hypertension

**3—D.** After physician clearance has been obtained

**4—B.** Prediabetic

**5—B.** 166 bpm

**6—A.** Normal

> *Resource:* Pescatello LS, senior editor. *ACSM's Guidelines for Exercise Testing and Prescription.* 9th ed. Baltimore (MD): Lippincott Williams and Wilkins; 2014.

### Discussion Question Answers for Case Study CPT.I

1. Submaximal tests are appropriate, including the Young Men's Christian Association (YMCA) bike test, various step tests (depending upon knee pain), submaximal treadmill protocols, track tests (*e.g.*, 6 min walk, Rockport), muscular endurance tests (*e.g.*, push-up, curl-up) (depending on back pain). Maximal testing would not be appropriate in a gym setting due to her moderate risk stratification.

   > *Resource:* Bushman BA, senior editor. *ACSM's Resources for the Personal Trainer.* 4th ed. Baltimore (MD): Lippincott Williams and Wilkins; 2014.

2. Avoid overstepping the CPT's scope of practice by avoiding direct dietary advice; specific recommendations, particularly for a person who is pre-diabetic, should never be given. Referral and deferral to trained dietary professionals should be the course of action. MyPyramid.gov and ChooseMyPlate.gov are acceptable resources for clients with general questions.

3. Calculation
   $220 - 54 = 166$
   $166 - 88 = 78$
   Low end: $(78 \times 0.5) + 88 = 127$
   High end: $(78 \times 0.7) + 88 = 143$

   Fifty percent to 70% should be chosen for Beth as a new exerciser with moderate risk stratification. This range will maintain a moderate intensity and promote weight loss if maintained for a significant duration.

## CASE STUDY CPT.II

### Multiple-Choice Answers for Case Study CPT.II

**1—A.** Low risk

> *Resource:* Pescatello LS, senior editor. *ACSM's Guidelines for Exercise Testing and Prescription.* 9th ed. Baltimore: Lippincott Williams and Wilkins; 2014.

**2—D.** Vigorous intensity ($\geq 60\%$ $\dot{V}O_2R$) aerobic activities, weight-bearing and flexibility exercises

> *Resource: ACSM's GETP*, Chapter 7, Table 7.1 General Exercise Recommendations for Healthy Adults. These are general recommendations provided in the *GETP* for designing a health/fitness training program for apparently healthy adults.

**3—A.** An increase of 5–10 min every 1–2 wk over the first 4–6 wk

> *Resource: ACSM's GETP*, Chapter 7, General Principles of Exercise Prescription.

An increase of 5–10 min every 1–2 wk over the first 4–6 wk of exercise; after the individual has been exercising for 1 mo or more, the frequency, intensity, and/or time of exercise is gradually adjusted upward over the next 4–8 mo.

**4—C.** 8–12

> *Resource: ACSM's GETP*, Chapter 7, General Principles of Exercise Prescription.

To improve muscular strength, mass, and to some extent — endurance, a resistance exercise that allows a person to complete 8–12 repetitions per set should be selected. This translates to a resistance that is ~60%–80% of the individual's 1-RM.

**5—B.** The resistance training program should feature exercises that are multijoint or compound exercises that involve more than one muscle group at a time.

> *Resource: ACSM's GETP*, Chapter 7, General Principles of Exercise Prescription. Box 7.3. This table indicates the Resistance Training Guidelines for Healthy Adults.

## Discussion Question Answers for Case Study CPT.II

1.  Weight machines are a great starting point for Stan. Although Stan is relatively young, he has a significant low back issue. Thus, you will want to be careful with resistance exercise (all exercises) that his lower back is well supported and light resistance is applied to the area (as opposed to heavy resistance).

2.  Once again, be careful of his low back by demonstrating correct posture and flexibility exercises. There are some "popular" stretches that may not be appropriate for low back issues. If you are unsure, there are many great resources that can be consulted.

## CASE STUDY CPT.III

### Multiple-Choice Answers for Case Study CPT.III

**1—D.** $28.4 \text{ kg} \cdot \text{m}^{-2}$

BMI is an index used to assess weight relative to height and is calculated by dividing the body mass (kg) by the height (m) squared ($kg/m^2$).

*Resource:* Pescatello LS, senior editor. *ACSM's Guidelines for Exercise Testing and Prescription.* 9th ed. Baltimore (MD): Lippincott Williams and Wilkins; 2014.

**2—B.** Overweight

Based on BMI, calculated as $\text{kg} \cdot \text{m}^{-2}$, individuals are classified as follows:

-   Underweight ($<18.5$)
-   Normal weight (18.5–24.9)
-   Overweight (25.0–29.9)
-   Class 1 obesity (30.0–34.9)
-   Class 2 obesity (35.0–39.9)
-   Class 3 obesity ($>39.9$)

Bob's calculated BMI = 28.4, which classifies him as overweight.

*Resource:* Pescatello LS, senior editor. *ACSM's Guidelines for Exercise Testing and Prescription.* 9th ed. Baltimore (MD): Lippincott Williams and Wilkins; 2014.

**3—C.** 483 cal

To correctly answer this question requires multiple steps:

a.  Determine the goal body weight corresponding with a BMI of 24.9.

$$24.9 = x/1.78 \text{ m}^2 \qquad 78.9 \text{ kg} = x$$

b.  Determine the current amount of weight that needs to be lost.

$$198 \text{ lb} - 173.6 \text{ lb} = 16.4 \text{ lb}$$

c.  Determine the caloric content of the amount of weight need to be lost. 16.4 lb of fat $\times$ $3,500 \text{ kcal} \cdot \text{lb}^{-1}$ of fat = 57,400 kcal of fat

d.  Determine the number of days to obtain his target. 12 wk $\times$ $7 \text{ d} \cdot \text{wk}^{-1}$ = 84 d

e.  Determine the daily energy deficit necessary to achieve the target weight. 57,400 cal divided by 84 d = $\sim 683 \text{ cal} \cdot \text{d}^{-1}$

f.  Determine the daily exercise energy expenditure. 683 cal deficit needed $-$ 200 cal dietary energy deficit = 483 cal daily exercise energy expenditure.

*Resource:* Pescatello LS, senior editor. *ACSM's Guidelines for Exercise Testing and Prescription.* 9th ed. Baltimore (MD): Lippincott Williams and Wilkins; 2014.

**4—A.** 19.8

To correctly answer this question requires multiple steps:

a.  Determine current fat mass (FM).

198 lb (body weight [BW]) $\times$ 28% body fat = 55.44 lb FM

b.  Determine current lean body mass (LBM).

198 lb $-$ 55.44 lb FM = 142.56 lb LBM

c.  Determine target BW (TBW) at 20% body fat.

142.56 (LBM)/(1$-$ 0.2) = 178.2 lb TBW

d.  Determine amount of weight loss needed to achieve target weight at 20% body fat.

198 lb (BW) $-$ 178.2 lb (TBW) = 19.8 lb fat loss

**5—B.** Contemplation

The stages of motivational readiness for change (SOC), or transtheoretical model (TTM), include the stages of change and the processes of change. The SOC postulates that

CPT

individuals move through a series of stages and face common barriers when making behavior changes and that intervention approaches many vary by the client's identified stage of change. The different SOC include the following:

a. Precontemplation: An individual that is not active and is not thinking about becoming active.

b. Contemplation: An individual that is not physically active but is thinking about becoming active.

c. Preparation: An individual that is currently engaging in some physical activity but not at the recommended level.

d. Action: An individual that is physically active at the recommended level but for fewer than 6 mo.

e. Maintenance: An individual that has been physically active at the recommended level for six or more months.

Bob is not presently active; however, he indicates that he is committed to becoming active. This indicates that he is at the "contemplation stage of readiness for change."

*Resource:* Pescatello LS, senior editor. *ACSM's Guidelines for Exercise Testing and Prescription.* 9th ed. Baltimore (MD): Lippincott Williams and Wilkins; 2014.

**6—A.**   Carbohydrate: 1,400; protein: 400; fat: 500

The energy content of each gram of carbohydrate, protein and fat is 4, 4, and 9 cal, respectively. Bob's daily

carbohydrate intake

$$350 \text{ g} \times 4 \text{ cal} \cdot \text{g}^{-1} = 1,400 \text{ cal}$$

protein intake

$$100 \text{ g} \times 4 \text{ cal} \cdot \text{g}^{-1} = 400 \text{ cal}$$

fat intake

$$55.5 \text{ g} \times 9 \text{ cal} \cdot \text{g}^{-1} = 499.5 \text{ (500) cal}$$

*Resource:* Nieman D. *Exercise Testing and Prescription: A Health-Related Approach.* 7th ed. New York (NY): McGraw-Hill Companies, Inc; 2011. p. 223.

## Discussion Question Answers for Case Study CPT.III

1. Bob's argument is valid. Specifically, the BMI does not take into consideration an individual's body composition. Muscular individuals as well as small-framed sedentary individuals are quite likely to be classified incorrectly. The BMI assesses the "average individual's" statistical risk of developing chronic disease. It is a much better indicator for determining the prevalence of overweight and obesity in a large population than for an individual. For the "average individual," BMI generally works well.

   *Resource:* Pescatello LS, senior editor. *ACSM's Guidelines for Exercise Testing and Prescription.* 9th ed. Baltimore (MD): Lippincott Williams and Wilkins; 2014.

2. Bob's overall caloric intake is quite likely higher than his daily need, hence his gradual weight gain over the years. His daily carbohydrate intake is adequate and amounts to 56% of his total daily energy intake. This is approximately at the recommended intake of 55%. However, he has an excessive consumption of simple/refined carbohydrates. He should emphasize the intake of whole grain products followed by fruits and vegetables. His protein intake accounts for 16% of his daily energy intake, which is within the recommended range. Bob's fat intake is at the lower end of the recommended range (20%–35%); however, his intake of saturated fats is 14%, which is 40% higher than the recommended range of <10%. He needs to decrease his intake of saturated fats (typically animal fats) and replace this with unsaturated fats. His alcohol consumption accounts for 8% of his daily energy intake. Each gram of alcohol contains 7 cal but does not provide essential nutrients. Its use should be in moderation (less than two drinks per day). Caffeine intake for adults ranges from 106 to 170 mg · d$^{-1}$, and the 90th percentile is 227–382 mg · d$^{-1}$. Bob's intake is well in excess of the 90th percentile; however, there is little evidence of health risk with excessive intake.

   *Resource:* Nieman D. *Exercise Testing and Prescription: a health-related approach.* 7th ed. New York (NY): McGraw-Hill Companies, Inc; 2011. p. 223–33.

   Knight CA, Knight I, Mitchell DC, Zepp JE. Beverage caffeine intake in US consumers and subpopulations of interest: Estimates from the Share of Intake Panel survey. *Food Chem Toxicol.* 2004;42:1923–30.

## CASE STUDY CPT.IV(1)

### Multiple-Choice Answers to Case Study CPT.IV(1)

**1—C.** Refer him to local professionals that specialize in counseling and behavior change.

It is beyond the scope of practice for a CPT to give advice and/or counsel clients on their marriage, alcohol consumption, or any other personal issue. You can counsel/coach clients on making positive lifestyle changes but need to be very careful to draw the line and to keep all recommendations professional. A CPT needs to know when it is appropriate to refer their clients/members to the appropriate health care professional.

*Resource:* Pescatello LS, senior editor. *ACSM's Guidelines for Exercise Testing and Prescription.* 9th ed. Baltimore (MD): Lippincott Williams and Wilkins; 2014.

**2—D.** Immediately attend to the member and ask him if he is having chest pain. If he says yes, activate EMS and monitor him until help arrives.

You will need to attend to the member to see what is wrong. If he is having chest pain, it is important that you activate EMS immediately. It is always better to be safe. If possible, ask another person to make the call so that you can stay with the member and monitor him until help arrives. You should also make sure that you have the automated external defibrillator(AED) available just in case. If he becomes unconscious and does not have a pulse, you will need to start cardiopulmonary resuscitation (CPR). If an AED is available, then that should be used first.

**3—C.** Quarterly

Accidents and emergencies can happen at any time. It is important that all staff know the emergency plan of the facility. Regular drills should be conducted at least quarterly for all staff, including part-time staff.

*Resource:* American College of Sports Medicine. *ACSM Health/Fitness Facility Standards and Guidelines.* 3rd ed. Champaign (IL): Human Kinetics; 2007. p. 20.

**4—B.** Fill out an incident report and put a "do not use" sign on the equipment.

It is important to fill out an incident report immediately after an incident and while it is fresh in the victim's mind. Putting a sign on the damaged equipment is also very important for the safety of other members.

*Resource:* American College of Sports Medicine. *ACSM Health/Fitness Facility Standards and Guidelines.* 3rd ed. Champaign (IL): Human Kinetics; 2007. p. 23.

**5—False**

Personal trainers should always carry their own professional liability insurance. Most fitness centers do not cover trainers, especially when they are training "off" their regular paid hours.

### Discussion Question Answer to Case Study CPT.IV(1)

1. Personal trainers must follow the guidelines set by the Family Educational Rights and Privacy Act (FERPA) and Health Insurance Portability and Accountability Act (HIPPA) laws depending on the setting and state that business resides in. The personal information that your client/member shares with you is just that: "personal." CPTs must have systems in place to safeguard client confidentiality. Any information that you collect must be kept confidential. It is not "ok" to talk about anything your client has shared with you, unless you obtain written permission for specific information and keep that paper on file for 6 yr.

## CASE STUDY CPT.IV(2)

**Multiple-Choice Answers to Case Study CPT.IV(2)**

**1—A.** Light edema, pain, point tenderness, strength loss

**2—C.** Rest, ice, compression, elevation, stabilization

**3—C.** Ice the ankle for 20 min using a mixture of ice and water.

*2010 American Heart Association and American Red Cross Guidelines* recommend a mixture of ice and water be applied for <20 min using a barrier between the bag and skin.

*Resource*: Part 17, First Aid: 2010 American Heart Association and American Red Cross Guidelines for First Aid. *Circulation.* 2010;122:S934–46.

**4—D.** The client does not require clearance before resuming training.

Tom does not appear to have sustained an injury. No signs/symptoms are present with a first degree sprain. Medical clearance or referral is required if the person needs to be transported to the hospital and/or a second or third degree sprain occurs as stability would then be compromised.

**5—C.** One-legged balance assessment

**6—B.** Add unilateral dynamic leg balance, eversion exercises, and proprioception exercises to the program. Eversion strengthening exercises may also be appropriate.

**Discussion Question Answer to Case Study CPT.IV(2)**

1. Additional adjustments and progressions include the following:

   I. Review Tom's injury history concerning his leg.
      a. Inversion ankle sprains account for about 90% of all ankle sprains. The goal should be to prevent reinjuring the ankle.

   II. Look at his mechanics — especially above and below the "injury." Observe the operation of the kinetic chain during his movements.
      a. Observe his ability to move efficiently to both sides and push off both feet. See if he favors either side and/or if there is a dominant muscular pattern. Is there compensation for muscular imbalances?

   III. Assess ankle joint strength, flexibility, and motion while performing exercises and movement.

   IV. Based on assessments, add exercises with progressions (both as homework and during sessions) to increase strength and mobility as needed, such as the following:

      a. Towel scrunches for plantar foot muscles
      b. Marble pickup and release for plantar foot muscles
      c. Eversion exercises with an elastic band for peroneals
      d. One-legged balance exercises — static then dynamic
      e. Lateral movement exercises on the floor, then a towel, and then a balance pad to wobble board
      f. Hopping and jumping
      g. Lateral movement and change of direction drills such as figure eight drills and box runs
      h. Slide board activities

# 2

# CPT Job Task Analysis

## DOMAIN I: INITIAL CLIENT CONSULTATION AND ASSESSMENT

### A. Provide instructions and initial documents to the client in order to proceed to the interview.

| Knowledge or Skill Statement | Explanation/Examples | Resources |
|---|---|---|
| **Knowledge** of components and preparation for the initial client consultation | • Use new Client Intake form to qualify client.<br>• Assess compatibility, goals, scope, style, and schedule.<br>• Exchange contact information (including emergency contact) and identify schedule preferences.<br>• Discuss medical considerations and limitations; assess risk and need for medical doctor (MD) release form.<br>• Schedule initial client consultation.<br>• Provide service intro package. | *ACSM's Resources for the Personal Trainer*, 4th edition (10)<br>• Chapter 10<br>• Figures 10.1 and 10.3 |
| **Knowledge** of the necessary paperwork to be completed by client prior to initial client interview | • American Heart Association/American College of Sports and Medicine (AHA/ACSM) Health/Fitness Facility Preparticipation Screening Questionnaire, Physical Activity Readiness Questionnaire (PAR-Q), informed consent, waiver<br>• Medical clearance form (be sure to include Health Insurance Portability and Accountability Act [HIPAA] Release of Information Authorization Form)<br>• Trainer–client contract<br>• Organizational policies and procedures | *ACSM's Resources for the Personal Trainer*, 4th edition (10)<br>• Chapters 10 and 11<br>• Figures 10.4, 11.1, and 11.2<br>*ACSM's Guidelines for Exercise Testing and Prescription* (GETP), 9th edition (15)<br>• Chapter 2<br>U.S. Department of Health and Human Services, Health Insurance Portability and Accountability Act (42,43) |
| **Skill** in effective communication and in using multimedia resources (*i.e.*, e-mail, phone, text messaging) and/or in-person resources | • Provide information on the club's Web site dedicated to service introduction.<br>• Verbal and nonverbal communication skills<br>• Trainer contact information<br>• Verbally explain process and preparation to client, such as attire, equipment, hydration, etc.<br>• Remind client of day and time of next meeting and length of appointment.<br>• Remind client to complete and return forms.<br>• Give the opportunity to ask questions and/or to contact if concerns arise. | *ACSM's Resources for the Personal Trainer*, 4th edition (10)<br>• Chapter 10 |

## B.  Interview client in order to gather and provide pertinent information to proceed to the fitness testing and program design.

| Knowledge or Skill Statement | Explanation/Examples | Resources |
|---|---|---|
| **Knowledge** of the components and limitations of a health/medical history, preparticipation screening tools, informed consent, trainer–client contract, and organizational policies and procedures<br>**Skill** in obtaining a health/medical history, medical clearance, and informed consent<br>**Knowledge** of the use of medical clearance for exercise testing and program participation<br>**Knowledge** of health behavior modification theories and strategies in order to determine client goals and expectations<br>**Knowledge** of orientation procedures, including equipment use and facility layout | • Purpose, current health status, legal concerns, consent, administration, client commitment<br>• Operational information concerning billing, cancellation, hours of operation, all policies and procedures<br>• Review medical history form; stratify and establish trust and confidentiality; ask questions to clarify; document responses in a clear and concise manner.<br>• Refer client to physician if warranted.<br>• Review health/medical history for known disease, signs/symptoms, American College of Sports Medicine (ACSM) Risk Stratification or coronary artery disease (CAD) risk factors and stratify into low, moderate, or high risk.<br>• Identify stage of change; use motivational interviewing; connect goal to core values plan for lapses in behavior, track changes, and progress.<br>• Group or personal orientation session, which provides general guidelines on physical activity; personalized exercise regime; proper setup, usage, and safety of equipment; hands-on walk through of facility; identification of emergency exits and *phones with emergency numbers on them*, location of "public access" automated external defibrillator (AED) (in the cases of unstaffed facilities), or literature or Web site with available resources and services | *ACSM's Resources for the Personal Trainer*, 4th edition (10)<br>• Chapters 7, 10, and 11<br>• Figures 11.3, 11.4, 11.5, and 11.6<br>*ACSM's Resource Manual for Guidelines for Exercise Testing and Prescription*, 7th edition (18)<br>• Chapters 11, 44, and 45<br>*ACSM's Health/Fitness Facility Standards and Guidelines*, 3rd edition (10)<br>• Chapter 3 |

## C.  Review and analyze client data (*i.e.*, classify risk) to formulate a plan of action and/or conduct physical assessments.

| Knowledge or Skill Statement | Explanation/Examples | Resources |
|---|---|---|
| **Knowledge** in ACSM risk factors and associated risk thresholds<br>**Knowledge** of signs and symptoms suggestive of chronic cardiovascular, metabolic, and/or pulmonary disease | • Determine number of risk factors based on medical and family history using Table 13.1.<br>• Distinguish between positive and negative risk factors.<br>• Determine number of signs and symptoms based on Table 13.2. | *ACSM's Resources for the Personal Trainer*, 4th edition (10)<br>• Chapter 11<br>• Tables 11.1 and 11.2<br>*ACSM's Guidelines for Exercise Testing and Prescription* (GETP), 9th edition (15)<br>• Chapter 2<br>• Tables 2.2 and 2.3 |

## C. Review and analyze client data (*i.e.*, classify risk) to formulate a plan of action and/or conduct physical assessments. (cont.)

| Knowledge or Skill Statement | Explanation/Examples | Resources |
|---|---|---|
| **Skill** in determining appropriate physical assessments based on summary of initial client consultation, risk stratification, and medical clearance or physician recommendations | • Classify risk based on health/medical history for known disease, signs/symptoms, or coronary artery disease (CAD) risk factors; stratify into low, moderate, or high risk; physician referral.<br>• Choice of assessments based on risk, limiting orthopedic or metabolic conditions, goals, equipment availability, physician recommendations | *ACSM's Guidelines for Exercise Testing and Prescription* (GETP), 9th edition (15)<br>• Chapter 2<br>• Figures 2.1–2.4<br>*ACSM's Resources for the Personal Trainer*, 4th edition (10)<br>• Chapter 12 |

## D. Evaluate behavioral readiness to optimize exercise adherence.

| Knowledge or Skill Statement | Explanation/Examples | Resources |
|---|---|---|
| **Knowledge** of behavioral strategies to enhance exercise and health behavior change (*e.g.*, reinforcement; specific, measurable, attainable, realistic and relevant, and time-bound [SMART] goal setting, social support) | • Help client create specific SMART goals.<br>• Connect goals to deep motivation.<br>• Determine between client-centered and behavior-oriented goals.<br>• Create weekly manageable goals schedule.<br>• Concentrate on what client is willing and able to do and works for them. | *ACSM's Resources for the Personal Trainer*, 4th edition (10)<br>• Chapters 8 and 9<br>*ACSM's Guidelines for Exercise Testing and Prescription* (GETP), 9th edition (15)<br>• Chapter 11 |
| **Knowledge** of applications of health behavior change models (socioecologic model, readiness to change model, social cognitive theory, and theory of planned behavior, etc.) and effective strategies that support and facilitate behavioral change | • Raise consciousness through education.<br>• Establish positive self-image.<br>• Make formal commitment.<br>• Create a structure of accountability.<br>• Identify and eliminate cause of problem behavior from environment.<br>• Substitute healthy behaviors for unhealthy ones.<br>• Establish support and reinforcement.<br>• Provide feedback. | *ACSM's Resources for the Personal Trainer*, 4th edition (10)<br>• Chapters 7 and 8<br>*ACSM's Resource Manual for Guidelines for Exercise Testing and Prescription*, 7th edition (18)<br>• Chapters 44 and 45<br>*ACSM's Guidelines for Exercise Testing and Prescription* (GETP), 9th edition (15)<br>• Chapter 11 |
| **Skill** in setting effective client-oriented behavioral goals (*i.e.*, SMART goals) | • Coach clients to set achievable goals and overcome potential obstacles. | *ACSM's Resources for the Personal Trainer*, 4th edition (10)<br>• Chapters 8 and 9<br>*ACSM's Resource Manual for Guidelines for Exercise Testing and Prescription*, 7th edition (18)<br>• Chapter 46<br>*ACSM's Guidelines for Exercise Testing and Prescription* (GETP), 9th edition (15)<br>• Chapter 11 |

| | | |
|---|---|---|
| **E.  Assess physical fitness, including cardiorespiratory fitness, muscular strength, muscular endurance, flexibility, and anthropometric measures in order to set goals and establish a baseline for program development.** | | |
| **Knowledge or Skill Statement** | **Explanation/Examples** | **Resources** |
| **Knowledge** of the basic structures of bone, skeletal muscle, and connective tissue | • Identify types and classification of bone; structure and function; components of skeletal system; axial and appendicular skeletons, origins, and insertions of muscles. | *ACSM's Resources for the Personal Trainer*, 4th edition (10)<br>• Chapter 3<br>• Figures 3.5 and 3.6 |
| **Knowledge** of the basic anatomy of the cardiovascular (CV) and respiratory systems | • Location of and relationship between heart and lungs<br>• Identify the structures of the heart.<br>• Identify the structures of the upper and lower respiratory tract. | *ACSM's Resources for the Personal Trainer*, 4th edition (10)<br>• Chapter 5<br>*ACSM's Resource Manual for Guidelines for Exercise Testing and Prescription*, 7th edition (18)<br>• Chapter 1 |
| **Knowledge** of the definition of the following terms: inferior, superior, medial, lateral, supination, pronation, flexion, extension, adduction, abduction, hyperextension, rotation, circumduction, agonist, antagonist, and stabilizer | • Anatomical locations and positions contained within Table 3.1<br>• Joint movements and lever systems | *ACSM's Resources for the Personal Trainer*, 4th edition (10)<br>• Chapter 3<br>• Table 3.1 |
| **Knowledge** of the plane in which each muscle action occurs | • Anatomical planes — Figure 3.2<br>• Joint motions and planes of motion — Table 3.3 | *ACSM's Resources for the Personal Trainer*, 4th edition (10)<br>• Chapter 3<br>• Figure 3.2<br>• Table 3.3 |
| **Knowledge** of the interrelationships among center of gravity, base of support, balance, stability, and proper spinal alignment | • Line of gravity: defines proper body alignment and posture<br>• Center of gravity: location of a theoretical point that can be used to represent the total weight of an object<br>• Base of support: the area of the supporting surface of an object such as the feet standing<br>• Balance: ability to maintain a position for a given period of time without moving — control center of mass with respect to base of support<br>• Stability: ability to lean without changing the base of support<br>• Spinal alignment and movements | *ACSM's Resources for the Personal Trainer*, 4th edition (10)<br>• Chapter 3<br>• Figure 3.4<br>*ACSM Resource Manual for Guidelines for Exercise Testing and Prescription*, 7th edition (18)<br>• Chapter 2 |
| **Knowledge** of the following curvatures of the spine: lordosis, scoliosis, and kyphosis | • Identify normal spinal curvatures and deviations from normal | *ACSM's Resources for the Personal Trainer*, 4th edition (10)<br>• Chapter 3<br>• Figures 3.48 and 3.49 |
| **Knowledge** of differences between aerobic and anaerobic energy systems and the effects of acute and chronic exercise on each | • Energy production with and without oxygen<br>• Adaptations to exercise capacity and physiological systems | *ACSM's Resources for the Personal Trainer*, 4th edition (10)<br>• Chapter 5<br>• Tables 5.1 and 5.2<br>• Figure 5.4 |

**E. Assess physical fitness, including cardiorespiratory fitness, muscular strength, muscular endurance, flexibility, and anthropometric measures in order to set goals and establish a baseline for program development. (cont.)**

| Knowledge or Skill Statement | Explanation/Examples | Resources |
|---|---|---|
| **Knowledge** of the normal acute responses to CV exercise and resistance training | • Supply oxygenated blood to active tissues: effects on heart rate (HR), stroke volume (SV), cardiac output ($\dot{Q}$), blood flow and pressure, arteriovenous oxygen (a-v $O_2$) difference<br>• Static and dynamic resistance training effects on muscle fibers and physiological systems | *ACSM's Resources for the Personal Trainer*, 4th edition (10)<br>• Chapter 5<br>• Figure 5.3 |
| **Knowledge** of the normal chronic physiologic adaptations associated with CV exercise and resistance training | • Benefits of CV training<br>• Benefits of resistance training<br>• Muscular hypertrophy, adaptations to muscle fibers, aerobic enzyme systems, nervous system | *ACSM's Resources for the Personal Trainer*, 4th edition (10)<br>• Chapter 5<br>• Table 5.2 |
| **Knowledge** of the physiologic responses related to warm-up and cool-down | • Periods of metabolic and CV adjustments from rest to exercise and exercise to rest, respectively | *ACSM's Resources for the Personal Trainer*, 4th edition (10)<br>• Chapters 15 and 17 |
| **Knowledge** of the physiological basis of acute muscle fatigue and delayed onset muscle soreness (DOMS) vs. musculoskeletal injury or overtraining | • Use of Likert-type chart to determine appropriate muscle soreness ranges<br>• Signs of muscle damage: swelling, pain, soreness, discoloration | *ACSM's Resources for the Personal Trainer*, 4th edition (10)<br>• Chapter 14<br>• Box 14.1 |
| **Knowledge** of the physiological adaptations that occur at rest and during submaximal and maximal exercise following chronic aerobic and anaerobic exercise training | • CV benefits of exercise: improvement in CV and respiratory function, decreased risk from premature death, reduction in death, increased health benefits | *ACSM's Resources for the Personal Trainer*, 4th edition (10)<br>• Chapter 15<br>• Box 15.1<br>*ACSM's Guidelines for Exercise Testing and Prescription* (GETP), 9th edition (15)<br>• Chapter 1<br>• Box 1.2 |
| **Knowledge** of the physiological basis for improvements in muscular strength and endurance | • Adaptations to muscle fibers and contractile proteins, aerobic enzyme systems, capillary supply, and nervous system | *ACSM's Resources for the Personal Trainer*, 4th edition (10)<br>• Chapter 5 |
| **Knowledge** of blood pressure (BP) responses associated with acute, chronic exercise, and postural changes | • Acute: linear increase in systolic BP (SBP) with increased levels of exercise; diastolic BP (DBP) may decrease slightly or remain unchanged.<br>• Chronic: resting SBP and DBP may decrease; lower BP at fixed submaximal work rate.<br>• Postural changes can produce hypotensive response. | *ACSM's Resources for the Personal Trainer*, 4th edition (10)<br>• Chapters 5 and 12 |

**E.  Assess physical fitness, including cardiorespiratory fitness, muscular strength, muscular endurance, flexibility, and anthropometric measures in order to set goals and establish a baseline for program development. (cont.)**

| Knowledge or Skill Statement | Explanation/Examples | Resources |
|---|---|---|
| **Knowledge** of muscle actions, such as isotonic, isometric (static), isokinetic, concentric, and eccentric | • Isotonic: muscle contraction, which exerts a constant tension<br>• Isometric (static): no change in muscle length<br>• Isokinetic: muscle resistance throughout the range of motion (ROM) by controlling speed of movement<br>• Concentric: muscle shortening (contraction)<br>• Eccentric: muscle lengthening | *ACSM's Resources for the Personal Trainer*, 4th edition (10)<br>• Chapter 14 |
| **Knowledge** of major muscles including but are not limited to the following: trapezius, pectoralis major, latissimus dorsi, biceps, triceps, rectus abdominis, internal and external obliques, erector spinae, gluteus maximus, quadriceps, hamstrings, adductors, abductors, and gastrocnemius | • Upper and lower extremity joints, movements, muscles, and resistance exercises — Tables 3.4 and 3.5 | *ACSM's Resources for the Personal Trainer*, 4th edition (10)<br>• Chapter 3<br>• Figures 3.1–3.19, 3.22–3.23, 3.26–3.27, 3.33–3.36, and 3.43–3.45<br>• Tables 3.4–3.5 |
| **Knowledge** of the identification of major bones including but are not limited to the clavicle, scapula, sternum, humerus, carpals, ulna, radius, femur, fibula, tibia, and tarsals | • Figure 3.5 | *ACSM's Resources for the Personal Trainer*, 4th edition (10)<br>• Chapter 3<br>• Figure 3.5 |
| **Knowledge** of joint classifications (*e.g.*, hinge, ball and socket) | • Describe characteristics that comprise different types of joints. | *ACSM's Resources for the Personal Trainer*, 4th edition (10)<br>• Chapter 3<br>• Table 3.2 |
| **Knowledge** of the primary action and joint ROM for each major muscle group. | • Table 3.3 | *ACSM's Resources for the Personal Trainer*, 4th edition (10)<br>• Chapter 3<br>• Table 3.3 |
| **Knowledge** of the following terms related to muscles: hypertrophy, atrophy, and hyperplasia | • Hypertrophy: increase in muscular size<br>• Atrophy: wasting away or loss of a part — usually muscle<br>• Hyperplasia: increased cell production in a normal tissue | *ACSM's Resources for the Personal Trainer*, 4th edition (10)<br>• Chapter 3 |
| **Knowledge** of the ability to discuss the physiologic basis of the components of health-related physical fitness — CV fitness, muscular strength, muscular endurance, body composition, and flexibility | • CV fitness: the ability of the circulatory and respiratory systems to supply oxygen during sustained physical activity<br>• Muscular strength: the ability of muscle to exert force<br>• Muscular endurance: the ability of muscle to continue to perform without fatigue<br>• Body composition: the relative amounts of muscle, fat, bone, and other vital parts of the body<br>• Flexibility: the range of motion around a joint | *ACSM's Resources for the Personal Trainer*, 4th edition (10)<br>• Chapters 5 and 15<br>• Box 15.1<br>• Table 5.2<br>*ACSM's Guidelines for Exercise Testing and Prescription* (GETP), 9th edition (15)<br>• Chapter 1<br>• Box 1.1 |

**E.  Assess physical fitness, including cardiorespiratory fitness, muscular strength, muscular endurance, flexibility, and anthropometric measures in order to set goals and establish a baseline for program development. (cont.)**

| Knowledge or Skill Statement | Explanation/Examples | Resources |
|---|---|---|
| **Knowledge** of the normal chronic physiologic adaptations associated with CV, resistance, and flexibility training | • Benefits of CV training<br>• Muscular hypertrophy, adaptations to muscle fibers, aerobic enzyme systems, nervous system<br>• Flex: improve ROM and joint mobility | *ACSM's Resources for the Personal Trainer*, 4th edition (10)<br>• Chapter 5<br>• Table 5.2 |
| **Knowledge** of relative and absolute contraindications to exercise testing, test termination criteria, and proper procedures to be followed after discontinuing an exercise test | • Relative contraindications — Box 3.5; may be tested only after careful evaluation of the risk/benefit ratio<br>• Absolute contraindications — Box 3.5; should not perform exercise tests until conditions are stabilized or adequately treated<br>• Test termination criteria — Box 4.5; volitional fatigue, predetermined endpoint, or general indications<br>• Postexercise procedures includes passive cool-down, physiological observations continued for at least 5 min or longer of recovery, low level exercise until HR and BP stabilize. | *ACSM's Guidelines for Exercise Testing and Prescription* (GETP), 9th edition (15)<br>• Chapters 3 and 4<br>• Boxes 3.5, 4.4, and 4.5 |
| **Knowledge** of the advantages, disadvantages, and limitations of the various body composition techniques including but not limited to skinfolds, plethysmography (BOD POD), bioelectrical impedance, infrared, dual-energy X-ray absorptiometry (DEXA), and circumference measurements | • Discuss basis of technique; reliability; sources of error; ease in administering, measuring, and calculating; pretest preparation; and client comfort. | *ACSM's Resources for the Personal Trainer*, 4th edition (10)<br>• Chapter 12<br>• Box 12.2 |
| **Knowledge** of preactivity fitness testing including assessments of flexibility, CV fitness, muscular strength, muscular endurance, and body composition | • Selection of test dependent on population, mass testing vs. individual testing, ease and reliability in administering, orthopedic or metabolic restrictions, equipment availability | *ACSM's Resources for the Personal Trainer*, 4th edition (10)<br>• Chapter 12 |
| **Knowledge** of interpretation of fitness test results (*i.e.*, favorable vs. unfavorable results) | • Use norm charts to classify results, application of knowledge of acute responses to exercise. | *ACSM's Resources for the Personal Trainer*, 4th edition (10)<br>• Chapters 5 and 12 |
| **Knowledge** of the recommended order of fitness assessments (*e.g.*, CV test prior to strength assessment) | • HR<br>• BP<br>• Body composition<br>• CV assessment<br>• Muscular fitness<br>• Flexibility | *ACSM's Resources for the Personal Trainer*, 4th edition (10)<br>• Chapter 12 |
| **Knowledge** of appropriate documentation of abnormal signs or symptoms during an exercise session and subsequent referral to a physician | • Formal and informal means of evaluating health status<br>• Recognizing situations, signs, symptoms, and injuries (shortness of breath, abnormal response to increase in intensity, etc.)<br>• Stop training session and refer to physician. | *ACSM's Resources for the Personal Trainer*, 4th edition (10)<br>• Chapter 11 |

**E.  Assess physical fitness, including cardiorespiratory fitness, muscular strength, muscular endurance, flexibility, and anthropometric measures in order to set goals and establish a baseline for program development. (cont.)**

| Knowledge or Skill Statement | Explanation/Examples | Resources |
|---|---|---|
| **Knowledge** of various mechanisms for appropriate referral to a physician | • Significant change in frequency, intensity, or nature of existing signs and symptoms<br>• Onset of new signs and symptoms associated with CV or metabolic disease (Table 11.2)<br>• Serious joint injuries that do not resolve quickly; clients reporting muscular or joint problems, dizziness or nausea | *ACSM's Resources for the Personal Trainer*, 4th edition (10)<br>• Chapter 11<br>• Table 11.2 |
| **Skill** in locating/palpating pulse landmarks, accurately measuring HR, and obtaining rating of perceived exertion (RPE) | • Three common sites are radial, brachial, and carotid.<br>• Start counting exercise HR with zero as reference.<br>• Measure for 30 s and multiply by 2 to convert to minute value.<br>• RPE: two scales used as a subjective measure to rate overall feelings of exertion instead of specific areas. Obtain rating during steady state. | *ACSM's Resources for the Personal Trainer*, 4th edition (10)<br>• Chapter 12<br>• Figure 12.1<br>• Chapter 15<br>• Table 15.10 |
| **Skill** in selecting and administering safe and appropriate CV assessments according to established guidelines and determining normal acute responses to CV exercise | • Selection of test dependent on population, mass testing vs. individual testing, ease and reliability in administering, orthopedic or metabolic restrictions, equipment availability<br>• Ability to recognize signs of poor circulation and perfusion, failure for HR and SBP to increase with workload | *ACSM's Resources for the Personal Trainer*, 4th edition (10)<br>• Chapters 12 and 15<br>*ACSM's Guidelines for Exercise Testing and Prescription* (GETP), 9th edition (15)<br>• Chapter 4<br>• Box 4.5 |
| **Skill** in locating anatomical sites for circumference (girth) measurements and associated risk | • Anatomical sites are located within the description of each site.<br>• Waist-to-hip ratio identifies fat distribution; higher amount of abdominal fat associated with increased risk for CAD | *ACSM's Guidelines for Exercise Testing and Prescription* (GETP), 9th edition (15)<br>• Chapter 4<br>• Box 4.1 |
| **Skill** in locating anatomical sites for skinfold measurement to estimate body fat percentage | • Anatomical landmarks and type of fold are located within the description of the skinfold site. | *ACSM's Resources for the Personal Trainer*, 4th edition (10)<br>• Chapter 12<br>• Box 12.1<br>• Figure 12.6 |
| **Skill** in selecting/administering safe muscular strength and muscular endurance assessments and determining normal acute responses to resistance training | • Selection of test dependent on population, mass testing vs. individual testing, ease and reliability in administering, orthopedic or metabolic restrictions, equipment availability, participant's skill level/limitations.<br>• Ability to recognize volitional fatigue, poor form, muscle compensation, poor alignment, incomplete ROM | *ACSM's Resources for the Personal Trainer*, 4th edition (10)<br>• Chapters 12 and 14 |

## E.  Assess physical fitness, including cardiorespiratory fitness, muscular strength, muscular endurance, flexibility, and anthropometric measures in order to set goals and establish a baseline for program development. (cont.)

| Knowledge or Skill Statement | Explanation/Examples | Resources |
|---|---|---|
| **Skill** in selecting/administering safe flexibility assessments for various muscle groups and determining normal acute responses to flexibility training | • Selection of test dependent on population, mass testing vs. individual testing, ease and reliability in administering, orthopedic or metabolic restrictions, equipment availability<br>• Knowledge of normal joint ROM<br>• Ability to detect muscle tightness, breath and holding patterns | *ACSM's Resources for the Personal Trainer*, 4th edition (10)<br>• Chapters 12 and 16 |
| **Skill** in recognizing postural abnormalities that may affect exercise performance and body alignment | • Knowledge of deviations from normal spinal curvatures | *ACSM's Resources for the Personal Trainer*, 4th edition (10)<br>• Chapter 3<br>• Figures 3.48 and 3.49 |
| **Skill** in delivering test and assessment results in a positive manner and not negatively impact client self-esteem (*e.g.*, use information to encourage client, not discourage or embarrass) | • Make client feel comfortable; be respectful; demonstrate professionalism, trust, and competence; maintain confidentiality, use as a baseline; accept client where they are; develop a plan for improvement; be empathetic, and nonjudgmental | *ACSM's Resources for the Personal Trainer*, 4th edition (10)<br>• Chapters 9 and 12 |

## F.  Develop a comprehensive (*i.e.*, physical fitness, goals, behavior) reassessment plan/timeline.

| Knowledge or Skill Statement | Explanation/Examples | Resources |
|---|---|---|
| **Knowledge** of development of fitness plans based on client interview, risk stratification, and physical fitness assessments | • Use frequency, intensity, time, and type, volume and progress (FITT-VP) framework for each component based on risk stratification, test results, goals, client availability, and commitment level. | *ACSM's Resources for the Personal Trainer*, 4th edition (10)<br>• Chapter 13<br>• Box 13.1 |
| **Knowledge** of effective and applicable health behavior modification strategies to meet client goals | • Use short-term goals based on specific, measurable, attainable, realistic and relevant, and time-bound (SMART) goals.<br>• Behavior change pyramid | *ACSM's Resources for the Personal Trainer*, 4th edition (10)<br>• Chapters 7, 8, and 9 |
| **Knowledge** of the purpose and appropriate time line for reassessing (*i.e.*, 6 wk, 12 wk) each component of physical fitness (cardiovascular, muscular strength and endurance, flexibility, and body composition measures) | • Fitness changes dependent on time, frequency and intensity of training efforts, behavioral change status, physiological changes being measured<br>• Standard follow-up 4 wk to 3 mo | *ACSM's Resources for the Personal Trainer*, 4th edition (10)<br>• Chapters 5 and 12 |

# DOMAIN II: EXERCISE PROGRAMMING AND IMPLEMENTATION

## A. Review assessment results, medical history, and goals to determine appropriate training program.

| Knowledge or Skill Statement | Explanation/Examples | Resources |
|---|---|---|
| **Knowledge** of the risks and benefits associated with guidelines for exercise training and programming for healthy adults, seniors, children and adolescents, and pregnant women | • Understanding of physiological changes of aging and growth<br>• Effects of chronic exercise on physiological systems | *ACSM's Resources for the Personal Trainer*, 4th edition (10)<br>• Chapter 19<br>*ACSM's Guidelines for Exercise Testing and Prescription* (GETP), 9th edition (15)<br>• Chapters 7 and 8 |
| **Knowledge** of the benefits and risks associated with exercise training and guidelines for exercise programming for individuals medically cleared to exercise with chronic disease (*e.g.,* stable coronary artery disease, other cardiovascular diseases, diabetes mellitus, obesity, metabolic syndrome, hypertension, arthritis, chronic back pain, osteoporosis, chronic obstructive pulmonary disease (COPD), and those with chronic pain) | • American Heart Association (AHA) risk classification for exercise training (Class B)<br>• Recognize abnormal responses to exercise and medication effects on exercise capacity.<br>• Dose-response relationship between exercise and health outcomes<br>• Activity needs to be individualized, with exercise prescription provided by qualified individuals and approved by primary health care provider.<br>• Program modifications based on condition<br>• Exercise capacity <6 metabolic equivalents (METs)<br>• Target energy expenditure of 150–400 kcal · d$^{-1}$ | *ACSM's Resources for the Personal Trainer*, 4th edition (10)<br>• Chapter 19<br>*ACSM's Guidelines for Exercise Testing and Prescription* (GETP), 9th edition (15)<br>• Chapters 8–10 |
| **Knowledge** of cardiovascular risk factors or conditions that may require consultations with medical personnel prior to initiating physical activity (*e.g.,* inappropriate changes of resting or exercise heart rate and blood pressure; new-onset discomfort in chest, neck, shoulder, or arm; changes in the pattern of discomfort during rest or exercise; shortness of breath at rest or with light exertion; fainting or dizzy spells; and claudication). | • Risks of exercise testing that outweigh the benefits need to be evaluated by a physician.<br>• Review of preexercise test evaluation and careful review of medical history helps to identify potential contraindications and safety of testing and participation.<br>• Absolute and relative contraindications of exercise | *ACSM's Guidelines for Exercise Testing and Prescription* (GETP), 9th edition (15)<br>• Chapter 3<br>• Box 3.5 |
| **Knowledge** of components of physical fitness including cardiovascular endurance, muscular strength and endurance, flexibility, and body composition | • Physical fitness components defined as a set of attributes or characteristics that people have or achieve that relates to the ability to perform physical activity.<br>• Health-related and/or skill-related components | *ACSM's Guidelines for Exercise Testing and Prescription* (GETP), 9th edition (15)<br>• Chapter 1<br>• Box 1.1 |

## A. Review assessment results, medical history, and goals to determine appropriate training program. (cont.)

| Knowledge or Skill Statement | Explanation/Examples | Resources |
|---|---|---|
| **Knowledge** of program development for specific client needs (*i.e.*, specific sports, performance, lifestyle, functional, balance, agility, aerobic, and anaerobic) | • Program development based on the following:<br>  • Needs assessment — screening and risk stratification<br>  • Review of goals, motivation, and level of commitment<br>  • Assessment results<br>  • Client interview | *ACSM's Resources for the Personal Trainer*, 4th edition (10)<br>• Chapters 10–13<br>• American College of Sports Medicine position stand. Quantity and quality of exercise for developing and maintaining cardiorespiratory, musculoskeletal, and neuromotor fitness in apparently healthy adults: guidance for prescribing exercise (12) |
| **Knowledge** of special precautions and modifications of exercise programming for participation in various environmental conditions (altitude, different ambient temperatures, humidity, and environmental pollution) | • Basic understanding of how environmental conditions affect physiological systems during exercise<br>• Tools used to evaluate environmental conditions<br>• May need to adjust length of time exposed to the environment, decrease intensity, proper hydration, proper clothing, and adjust rest periods | *ACSM's Guidelines for Exercise Testing and Prescription* (GETP), 9th edition (15)<br>• Chapter 8<br>• Tables 8.5 and 8.6<br>• Box 8.5<br>• Figure 8.3<br>*American Red Cross First Aid/CPR/AED Participant Manual* (21)<br>• Chapter 6 |
| **Knowledge** of the importance and ability to record exercise sessions and perform periodic reevaluations to assess changes in fitness status | • Accurately track workouts and training sessions. Include observations (*i.e.*, holding breath, form deviations, reported pain) and performance parameters (*i.e.*, load, repetitions [reps])<br>• Accurately chart effects of exercise.<br>• Reassessments 4 wk to 3 mo<br>• Compare to baseline. | *ACSM's Resources for the Personal Trainer*, 4th edition (10)<br>• Chapters 13 and 17 |

## B. Select exercise modalities to achieve desired adaptations based on goals, medical history, and assessment results.

| Knowledge or Skill Statement | Explanation/Examples | Resources |
|---|---|---|
| **Knowledge** of selecting appropriate exercises and training modalities based on age, functional capacity, and exercise test results | • Selection of modalities dependent on availability, client ability to perform specific exercise, client preference, client goal, medical and physical limitations, skill and fitness levels, and client commitment level | *ACSM's Resources for the Personal Trainer*, 4th Edition (10)<br>• Chapters 13–16 |
| **Knowledge** of the principles of specificity and program progression | • Specificity: only muscles that are trained will adapt and change in response to resistance or stimulus.<br>• Progressive overload: as a body adapts to a given stimulus, an increase in stimulus is required for further adaptations or improvements<br>• Specific Adaptations to Imposed Demands (SAID), variation, and periodization | *ACSM's Resources for the Personal Trainer*, 4th edition (10)<br>• Chapters 13 and 14 |

## B. Select exercise modalities to achieve desired adaptations based on goals, medical history, and assessment results. (cont.)

| Knowledge or Skill Statement | Explanation/Examples | Resources |
|---|---|---|
| **Knowledge** of the advantages, disadvantages, and applications of interval, continuous, and circuit training programs for cardiovascular fitness improvements. | • Cardiovascular modes of training — selection of modalities dependent on availability, client ability to perform specific exercise, client preference, client goal, medical and physical limitations, skill and fitness levels, and client commitment level | *ACSM's Resources for the Personal Trainer*, 4th edition (10)<br>• Chapter 15<br>*ACSM's Guidelines for Exercise Testing and Prescription* (GETP), 9th edition (15)<br>• Chapter 8 |
| **Knowledge** of activities of daily living (ADL) and their role in the overall health and fitness of the individual | • Ability to perform daily task such as self-care and essential household chores or essential work-related physical tasks<br>• Exercises and activities that improve a person's overall physical functionality can enhance the ability to live independently. | *ACSM's Resources for the Personal Trainer*, 4th edition (10)<br>• Chapters 13 and 17 |
| **Knowledge** of differences between physical activity recommendations and training principles for general health benefits, weight management, fitness improvements, and athletic performance enhancement | • Adjustments in FITT-VP for different goals with greatest variation in intensity, time, and total number of kilocalorie per week; as goal along continuum increases, so does intensity.<br>• Mode of training and variety are important factors. | *ACSM's Resources for the Personal Trainer*, 4th edition (10)<br>• Chapters 13 and 17<br>• Table 13.5<br>*ACSM's Guidelines for Exercise Testing and Prescription* (GETP), 9th edition (15)<br>• Chapter 7<br>• Tables 7.5–7.8 |
| **Knowledge** of advanced resistance training exercises (*e.g.*, super setting, Olympic lifting, plyometric exercises, pyramid training) and when such techniques are contraindicated | • Advanced exercises are highly technical and intensive.<br>• Exercises must not be completed with client if there are any preexisting conditions that may require medical clearance.<br>• Client must be evaluated on form, technique, kinesthetic awareness, body alignment, skill, and experience. | *ACSM's Resources for the Personal Trainer*, 4th edition (10)<br>• Chapters 14 and 18 |
| **Knowledge** of the six motor skill–related physical fitness components and agility, balance, coordination, reaction time, speed and power | • Performance training based on core strength, conditioning level, functional training, and sport specifics<br>• Use of plyometric exercises for upper and lower body to enhance ability to generate force | *ACSM's Resources for the Personal Trainer*, 4th edition (10)<br>• Chapters 13 and 18 |
| **Knowledge** of the benefits, risks, and contraindications for a wide variety of resistance training exercises specific to individual muscle groups (*e.g.*, for rectus abdominis performing crunches, supine leg raises, and plank exercises) | • Evaluate exercise based on the following:<br>• Biomechanical characteristics of the movement<br>• Exercise is designed to be primary or assistive.<br>• Single joint vs. multijoint exercises<br>• Bilateral vs. unilateral<br>• Client's goal, fitness and skill level, and experience | *ACSM's Resources for the Personal Trainer*, 4th edition (10)<br>• Chapters 3, 4, and 14 |

## B. Select exercise modalities to achieve desired adaptations based on goals, medical history, and assessment results. (cont.)

| Knowledge or Skill Statement | Explanation/Examples | Resources |
|---|---|---|
| **Knowledge** of the benefits, risks, and contraindications for a wide variety of range of motion (ROM) exercises (*e.g.*, dynamic and passive stretching, tai chi, Pilates, yoga, proprioceptive neuromuscular facilitation, partner stretching) | • Benefits: improved ROM and improved performance of ADL<br>• Risks: joint hypermobility, decreased strength, ineffectiveness<br>• Evaluate based on the following:<br>• Anatomy and physical limitations<br>• Biomechanical characteristics<br>• Physical and psychological qualities of the client<br>• Client's goal, fitness and skill level, and experience | *ACSM's Resources for the Personal Trainer*, 4th edition (10)<br>• Chapter 16 |
| **Knowledge** of the benefits, risks, and contraindications for a wide variety of cardiovascular training exercises and applications based on client experience, skill level, current fitness level, and goals (*e.g.*, progression example: walking, jogging, cross-country skiing, and racquet sports) | • Benefits: decreased risk from premature death, reduction in death, increased health benefits<br>• Evaluate based on the following:<br>• Anatomy and physical limitations<br>• Biomechanical characteristics<br>• Physical and psychological qualities of the client<br>• Client's goal, fitness and skill level, and experience | *ACSM's Resources for the Personal Trainer*, 4th edition (10)<br>• Chapter 15<br>• Box 15.1 |

## C. Determine initial frequency, intensity, time (duration), and type (*i.e.*, the FITT principle of exercise prescription) of exercise based on goals, medical history, and assessment results.

| Knowledge or Skill Statement | Explanation/Examples | Resources |
|---|---|---|
| **Knowledge** of the recommended frequency (F), intensity (I), and duration (T) of physical activity necessary for development of cardiovascular (CV) and musculoskeletal fitness in healthy adults, seniors, children/adolescents, and pregnant women | • Recommendations for healthy adults: Tables 7.5–7.8<br>• Seniors CV: F = minimum (min) 5 times a week moderate (mod), 3 times a week vigorous (vig), or combo; I = 5–6 times a week mod; 7–8 times a week vig (1–10 scale); T = 30–60 min mod, 20–30 min vig; T = any that does not impose excessive orthopedic stress<br>• Senior resistance: F = 2 times a week min; I = mod to vig; T = progressive weight-training or weight-bearing calisthenics + balance<br>• Children/Adolescents: F = at least 3–4 times a week preferably all; I = mod to vig; T = 30 mod + 30 vig; T = variety<br>• Pregnancy: adjust for symptoms, discomforts, and abilities; contraindications and considerations<br>• F = at least 3 times a week, preferably 4 times; I = mod, RPE 12–14; T = 15–30 min (150 total per week); T = dynamic, rhythmic that use large muscle groups | *ACSM's Guidelines for Exercise Testing and Prescription* (GETP), 9th edition (15)<br>• Chapter 7<br>• Tables 7.5–7.8<br>*ACSM's Guidelines for Exercise Testing and Prescription* (GETP), 9th edition (15)<br>• Chapter 8<br>*ACSM's Resources for the Personal Trainer*, 4th Edition (10)<br>• Chapters 13 and 19<br>*ACSM's Resource Manual for Guidelines for Exercise Testing and Prescription*, 7th edition (18)<br>• Chapter 36 |

## C. Determine initial frequency, intensity, time (duration), and type (*i.e.*, the FITT principle of exercise prescription) of exercise based on goals, medical history, and assessment results. (cont.)

| Knowledge or Skill Statement | Explanation/Examples | Resources |
|---|---|---|
| **Knowledge** of the recommended frequency, intensity, and duration of physical activity necessary for development of CV and musculoskeletal fitness in clients with stable chronic diseases who are medically cleared for exercise, including stable coronary artery disease, other CV diseases, diabetes mellitus (DM), obesity, metabolic syndrome, hypertension (HTN), arthritis, chronic back pain, osteoporosis, chronic obstructive pulmonary disease (COPD), and chronic pain | • CV disease: Chapter 9, *ACSM's GETP* <br> • Arthritis: Chapter 10, *ACSM's GETP*; use Borg CR 10 for pain management (Figure 10.1) and special considerations <br> • DM: Chapter 10, *ACSM's GETP*; use Table 10.2 diagnostic criteria and special considerations <br> • HTN: Chapter 10, *ACSM's GETP*; use exercise prescription (Ex R$_x$) + special considerations <br> • Metabolic syndrome: Chapter 10, *ACSM's GETP*; use Table 10.3 clinical criteria and special considerations <br> • Obesity: Chapter 10, *ACSM's GETP*; use Ex R$_x$, special considerations, and behavioral programs <br> • Osteoporosis: Chapter 10, *ACSM's GETP*; use Ex R$_x$ + special considerations <br> • COPD: Chapter 10, *ACSM's GETP*; use Box 10.1 for classification, Ex R$_x$ + special considerations | *ACSM's Guidelines for Exercise Testing and Prescription* (GETP), 9th edition (15) <br> • Chapters 7–10 <br> *ACSM's Resources for the Personal Trainer*, 4th edition (10) <br> • Chapter 19 <br> *ACSM's Resource Manual for Guidelines for Exercise Testing and Prescription*, 7th edition (18) <br> • Chapters 37–43 |
| **Knowledge** of appropriate exercise modifications based on individual abilities, physical limitations, and other special considerations (*e.g.*, injury rehabilitation, neuromuscular and postural limitations, and scoliosis) | • Research condition through physical therapy and medical networks; use reputable sources for information. <br> • Proper alignment and posture <br> • Do not aggravate condition; avoid exercises that are contraindicated. <br> • Train surrounding musculature to enhance strength and function of joint. <br> • Injury rehabilitation: determine primary site of injury and prior injury profile. | *ACSM's Resources for the Personal Trainer*, 4th edition (10) <br> • Chapters 3 and 13 <br> *ACSM's Resource Manual for Guidelines for Exercise Testing and Prescription*, 7th edition (18) <br> • Chapters 27 and 31 |
| **Knowledge** of implementation of the components of an exercise program including warm-up, training stimulus, cool-down, and stretching | • Warm-up: 5–10 min of low- to moderate-intensity CV exercise and ms endurance exercises <br> • Training stimulus: 20–60 min of aerobic, resistance, neuromuscular, and/or sport activities <br> • Cool-down: 5–10 min of low- to moderate-intensity CV and ms endurance exercises <br> • Stretching: at least 10 min after warm-up and cool-down | *ACSM's Guidelines for Exercise Testing and Prescription* (GETP), 9th edition (15) <br> • Chapter 7 <br> • Box 7.1 <br> *ACSM's Resources for the Personal Trainer*, 4th edition (10) <br> • Chapters 13 and 17 |
| **Knowledge** of applied biomechanics and exercises associated with movements of the major muscle groups (*e.g.*, seated knee extension — quadriceps) | • Evaluate muscle length, movement arm and resistance arm distances, exercise type, movement direction, and speed of movement for specific joint associated with exercise. | *ACSM's Resources for the Personal Trainer*, 4th edition (10) <br> • Chapters 4 and 14 |

## C. Determine initial frequency, intensity, time (duration), and type (*i.e.*, the FITT principle of exercise prescription) of exercise based on goals, medical history, and assessment results. (cont.)

| Knowledge or Skill Statement | Explanation/Examples | Resources |
|---|---|---|
| **Knowledge** of the application of various methods for establishing and monitoring levels of exercise intensity, including heart rate, rating of perceived exertion (RPE), pace, oxygen consumption and/or metabolic equivalents (METs) | • Determine appropriate method based on conditioning level, medications, information available (maximal volume of oxygen per unit of time [$\dot{V}O_{2max}$], etc.), and shortcomings of each method.<br>• Use metabolic equations (*ACSM's GETP*) to estimate work rate for various modes of training. | *ACSM's Resources for the Personal Trainer*, 4th edition (10)<br>• Chapter 15<br>• Table 15.2<br>*ACSM's Resource Manual for Guidelines for Exercise Testing and Prescription*, 7th edition (18)<br>• Chapter 21<br>*ACSM's Guidelines for Exercise Testing and Prescription* (GETP), 9th edition (15)<br>• Chapter 7<br>• Table 7.3<br>• Box 7.2 |
| **Knowledge** of the determination of target/training heart rates (THR) using predicted maximal heart rate ($HR_{max}$) and the heart rate reserve (HRR) method (Karvonen formula) with recommended intensity percentages based on client fitness level, medical considerations, and goals | • $HR_{max}$: 220 − age<br>• THR = 220 − age × 0.64 (low)<br>• THR = 220 − age × 0.94 (high)<br>• Intensity: 64/70% − 94%<br>• HRR: $HR_{max}$ − resting HR ($HR_{rest}$)<br>• THR = [(0.4) × HRR] + $HR_{rest}$<br>• THR = [(0.85) × HRR] + $HR_{rest}$<br>• Intensity: 40%/50% − 85% | *ACSM's Resources for the Personal Trainer*, 4th edition (10)<br>• Chapter 15<br>*ACSM's Guidelines for Exercise Testing and Prescription* (GETP), 9th edition (15)<br>• Chapter 7 |
| **Knowledge** of periodization for CV, resistance training, and conditioning program design and progression of exercises when necessary to avoid training plateaus or injury. | • Systematic variations in the prescribed volume and intensity during different phases of training program<br>• Recognize signs of overtraining.<br>• Make appropriate modifications for injuries and plateaus. | *ACSM's Resources for the Personal Trainer*, 4th edition (10)<br>• Chapters 13, 14, and 15<br>• Tables 13.5 and 16.1–16.3, |
| **Knowledge** of repetitions (reps) sets, load, and rest periods necessary for desired outcome goals. | • Intensity and reps are inversely related.<br>• Reps and rest time are inversely related.<br>• Muscle strength = 8 − 12 reps (60%–80% one repitition maximum [1-RM])<br>• Muscle endurance = 15–25 reps (no more than 50% of 1-RM) | *ACSM's Resources for the Personal Trainer*, 4th edition (10)<br>• Chapter 14<br>*ACSM's Guidelines for Exercise Testing and Prescription* (GETP), 9th edition (15)<br>• Chapter 7 |
| **Knowledge** of using rep maximum test results procedure to determine resistance training loads | • Use a percentage of 1-RM (70%–85%)<br>• RM: maximum load that can be lifted for a specific number of reps<br>• Absolute resistance: only a specific number of reps | *ACSM's Resources for the Personal Trainer*, 4th edition (10)<br>• Chapter 14 |

CPT

## D. Review proposed program with client; demonstrate and instruct the client to perform exercises safely and effectively.

| Knowledge or Skill Statement | Explanation/Examples | Resources |
|---|---|---|
| **Knowledge** of and ability to describe the unique adaptations to exercise training regarding strength, functional capacity (FC), and motor skills. | • FC relates to physiological adaptations to aerobic exercise<br>• Strength adaptations related to physiological adaptations of resistance training<br>• Motor skills adaptations occur through<br>• Cardiovascular (CV) training (intervals); resistance and plyometric training; and flexibility, balance, and agility training | *ACSM's Resource Manual for Guidelines for Exercise Testing and Prescription*, 7th edition (15)<br>• Chapters 31 and 33<br>*ACSM's Resources for the Personal Trainer*, 4th edition (10)<br>• Chapters 13–16<br>"ACSM Position Stand: Progressive Models in Resistance Training" (16) |
| **Knowledge** of and the ability to safely demonstrate exercises designed to enhance CV endurance, muscular strength and endurance, balance, and range of motion | • Each exercise requires understanding of joint range of motion and surrounding muscle anatomy; different modes and techniques, biomechanics, precautions for individuals with health concerns, specifics concerning the movement, key points, details, and safety considerations.<br>• Demonstration involves modeling the exercise accurately, precisely, and correctly — at normal speed and at slower speed/in phases. | *ACSM's Resources for the Personal Trainer*, 4th edition (10)<br>• Chapters 3, 5, and 13–16 |
| **Knowledge** of appropriate teaching techniques and the ability to demonstrate exercises for improving range of motion of all major joints | • Understanding of joint range of motion and surrounding muscle origins and insertions<br>• Communicate clearly and accurately the guidelines or how to perform and check for understanding.<br>• Model proper technique including alignment, position, breathing, and specifics concerning the technique used.<br>• Engage client in exercise — practice.<br>• Evaluate client performance.<br>• Provide feedback to client.<br>• Have client perform exercise again while cuing for corrections. | *ACSM's Resources for the Personal Trainer*, 4th edition (10)<br>• Chapter 16<br>• Table 16.1<br>• Figure 16.2; all figures in chapter are useful<br>*ACSM's Guidelines for Exercise Testing and Prescription* (GETP), 9th edition (15)<br>• Chapter 7 |
| **Knowledge** of and the ability to safely demonstrate a wide range of resistance training modalities and activities including variable resistance devices, dynamic constant external resistance devices, kettlebells, static resistance devices, and other resistance devices | • Each exercise requires understanding of joint range of motion and surrounding muscle anatomy; different modes and techniques, biomechanics, precautions for individuals with health concerns, specifics concerning the movement, key points, details, and safety considerations.<br>• Demonstration involves modeling the exercise accurately, precisely, and correctly — at normal speed and at slower speed/in phases.<br>• Communicate clearly and accurately how to perform and check for understanding.<br>• Model proper technique including alignment, position, breathing, and specifics concerning the technique used.<br>• Choice of modality based on availability, needs, goals, experience, and limitations of the client | *ACSM's Resources for the Personal Trainer*, 4th edition (10)<br>• Chapters 13, 14, and 18<br>*ACSM's Resource Manual for Guidelines for Exercise Testing and Prescription*, 7th edition (18)<br>• Chapters 33 and 34<br>KettleBell Concepts (26) |

## D. Review proposed program with client; demonstrate and instruct the client to perform exercises safely and effectively. (cont.)

| Knowledge or Skill Statement | Explanation/Examples | Resources |
|---|---|---|
| **Knowledge** of and ability to safely demonstrate a wide variety of functional training exercises involving nontraditional equipment such as stability balls, balance boards, resistance bands, medicine balls, and foam rollers | • Each exercise requires understanding of joint range of motion and surrounding muscle anatomy; different modes and techniques, biomechanics, precautions for individuals with health concerns, specifics concerning the movement, key points, details, and safety considerations.<br>• Demonstration involves modeling the exercise accurately, precisely, and correctly — at normal speed and at slower speed/in phases.<br>• Communicate clearly and accurately how to perform and check for understanding.<br>• Model proper technique including alignment, position, breathing, and specifics concerning the technique used.<br>• Choice of modality based on availability, needs, goals, experience, and limitations of the client | *ACSM's Resource Manual for Guidelines for Exercise Testing and Prescription*, 7th edition (18)<br>• Chapters 31, 33, and 34<br>*ACSM's Resources for the Personal Trainer*, 4th edition<br>• Chapters 13 and 18<br>ACSM Brochures (1)<br>Perform Better (33)<br>Thera-Band Academy (37) |
| **Knowledge** of the physiological effects of the Valsalva maneuver and the associated risks | • Forced exhalation against a closed glottis that results in increases in intrathoracic pressure<br>• Increased blood pressure (BP) response; changes in cardiac physiology | *ACSM's Resource Manual for Guidelines for Exercise Testing and Prescription*, 7th edition (18)<br>• Chapter 31 |
| **Knowledge** of the biomechanical principles for the performance of common physical activities (*e.g.*, walking, running, swimming, cycling, resistance training, yoga, Pilates, functional training) | • Understanding biomechanical laws and principles as it influences gait, ground force reaction, inertia, joint angles, body position, lifting and carrying, and external resistive forces (*e.g.*, water, wind) | *ACSM's Resources for the Personal Trainer*, 4th edition (10)<br>• Chapter 4<br>*ACSM's Resource Manual for Guidelines for Exercise Testing and Prescription*, 7th edition (18)<br>• Chapter 30 |
| **Knowledge** of the concept of detraining or reversibility of conditioning and effects on fitness and functional performance | • When physical training is stopped or reduced, systems readjust in accordance with diminished physiologic stimuli and adaptations to exercise are gradually reduced or lost. | *ACSM's Resource Manual for Guidelines for Exercise Testing and Prescription*, 7th edition (18)<br>• Chapter 5 |
| **Knowledge** of signs and symptoms of overreaching/overtraining and recommendations to prevent and/or reverse the detrimental effects | • Signs and symptoms — physical, metabolic, and physiological indicators<br>• Proper program design, periodization (planned volume and variation of work), nutrition, and sufficient recovery time<br>• Rest and/or decrease in volume can reverse effects | *ACSM's Resource Manual for Guidelines for Exercise Testing and Prescription*, 7th edition (18)<br>• Chapters 33 and 37 |

**CPT**

## D.  Review proposed program with client; demonstrate and instruct the client to perform exercises safely and effectively. (cont.)

| Knowledge or Skill Statement | Explanation/Examples | Resources |
|---|---|---|
| **Knowledge** of improper exercise form and/or techniques to modify/prevent musculoskeletal injury | • Intrinsic and extrinsic risk factors<br>• Improper biomechanics, improper training techniques, excessive training, misuse of weight-training equipment, fatigue, high intensity, speed of movement, common lifting and movement errors<br>• Teach proper alignment or technique and monitor rehearsal of movements. | *ACSM's Resource Manual for Guidelines for Exercise Testing and Prescription*, 7th edition (18)<br>• Chapters 33 and 37 |
| **Knowledge** of appropriate exercise attire (*e.g.*, footwear, layering for cold, light colored in heat) for specific activities, environments, and conditions | • Clothing should be comfortable, breathable, and allows movement. Footwear should fit properly, not show excessive wear and be suitable for particular exercise and surfaces.<br>• Clothing can restrict the maximum rate of evaporative cooling in the heat. Covered area, fabric weave, weight, color, air spaces, and *proper fit* are important.<br>• Proper clothing is a primary mechanism for achieving thermal balance during *heat* and cold stress. Adequate layers of insulation, wind protection, and area covered are important. | *ACSM's Resource Manual for Guidelines for Exercise Testing and Prescription*, 7th edition (18)<br>• Chapters 3 and 32 |
| **Knowledge** of communication techniques for effective teaching and client retention with awareness of visual, auditory, and kinesthetic learning styles | • Visual: learn through seeing; demonstration; images and diagrams, watching a video, use of imagery, visual cues for proper body alignment, use mirrors for feedback<br>• Auditory: learn through hearing; verbal instruction and cuing, clear verbal presentation<br>• Kinesthetic: learn by direct involvement after short and concise explanation; palpate muscle used, guide clients physically through movement, practice without resistance to review movement pattern | *ACSM's Resources for the Personal Trainer*, 4th edition (10)<br>• Chapter 9 |
| **Knowledge** of proper spotting positions and techniques for injury prevention and exercise assistance | • Goal of spotting is to prevent injury.<br>• Be in a position to assist client with lift if unable to perform correctly, break form, or possible loss of balance.<br>• Good communication<br>• Know proper hand grip positions.<br>• Know proper exercise technique.<br>• Know number of reps lifter intends to do.<br>• Know plan of action if serious injury occurs. | *ACSM's Resource Manual for Guidelines for Exercise Testing and Prescription*, 7th edition (18)<br>• Chapters 31 and 33<br>*ACSM's Resources for the Personal Trainer*, 4th edition (10)<br>• Chapters 14 and 17 |

## E. Monitor client technique and response to exercise modifying as necessary.

| Knowledge or Skill Statement | Explanation/Examples | Resources |
|---|---|---|
| **Knowledge** of normal and abnormal responses to exercise and criteria for termination of exercise (*e.g.*, shortness of breath (SOB), unusual joint pain, dizziness, abnormal heart rate response) | • Normal response — heart rate (HR), systolic blood pressure (SBP), and respiratory rate increase as work increases<br>• Termination: abnormal response in HR, blood pressure (BP), chest pain, or change in heart rhythm; poor perfusion; physical or verbal manifestations of severe fatigue, SOB, wheezing, leg cramps, etc. | *ACSM's Resources for the Personal Trainer*, 4th edition (10)<br>• Chapters 5 and 15<br>*ACSM's Guidelines for Exercise Testing and Prescription* (GETP), 9th edition (15)<br>• Chapter 4<br>• Box 4.5 |
| **Knowledge** of proper and improper form and technique while using cardiovascular conditioning equipment (*e.g.*, stair-climbers, stationary cycles, treadmills, and elliptical trainers) | • Provide cues for proper alignment and posture based on biomechanics.<br>• Review manufacturer's instructions and warranty information.<br>• Provide safety instructions for mounting and dismounting equipment. | *ACSM's Resources for the Personal Trainer*, 4th edition (10)<br>• Chapter 15 |
| **Knowledge** of proper and improper form and technique while performing resistance exercises (*e.g.*, resistance machines, stability balls, free weights, resistance bands, calisthenics/body weight) | • Proper posture, body alignment, and breathing<br>• Line up joint with axis of rotation.<br>• Exercises use full range of motion conducted in a deliberate, controlled manner and involve concentric and eccentric muscle actions.<br>• Provide safety instructions.<br>• Instruct, demonstrate, and provide feedback. | *ACSM's Resources for the Personal Trainer*, 4th edition (10)<br>• Chapter 14<br>*ACSM's Guidelines for Exercise Testing and Prescription* (GETP), 9th edition (15)<br>• Chapter 7 |
| **Knowledge** of proper and improper form and technique for flexibility exercises (*e.g.*, static stretching, dynamic, partner stretching) | • Proper posture and alignment<br>• Emphasize proper breathing.<br>• Hold endpoints.<br>• Exhale when you feel the muscle being stretched, relaxed, and softened.<br>• Slowly reposition and allow muscle to recover.<br>• Do not bounce or force a stretch while holding breath.<br>• Do not stretch beyond limits. | *ACSM's Resources for the Personal Trainer*, 4th edition (10)<br>• Chapters 13 and 16 |
| **Skill** in interpreting client understanding/comprehension and body language during exercise | • Use established rapport.<br>• Knowledge of common body language cues<br>• Observe; confirm observations verbally with client. | *ACSM's Resources for the Personal Trainer*, 4th edition (10)<br>• Chapters 9, 10, and 17 |
| **Skill** in effective communication, including active listening, cuing, and providing constructive feedback during and after exercise | • Customer service skills on body language, communication, greeting<br>• Feedback should be immediate, specific, and based on performance standards. It should also be objective, nonthreatening, clarifying, and supportive.<br>• Cues can be verbal, visual, and/or physical. | *ACSM's Resources for the Personal Trainer*, 4th edition (10)<br>• Chapters 9 and 17 |

## F.    Modify FITT to improve or maintain the client's physical fitness level.

| Knowledge or Skill Statement | Explanation/Examples | Resources |
|---|---|---|
| **Knowledge** of specific exercises and program modifications for healthy adults, seniors, children and adolescents, and pregnant women | • Once competency of basic exercises is established, add advanced exercises and progress by increasing intensity or duration.<br>• Modifications for specific population based on structural, physiological effects of maturation and/or condition | *ACSM's Resources for the Personal Trainer*, 4th edition (10)<br>• Chapters 12, 13, and 19<br>*ACSM's Guidelines for Exercise Testing and Prescription* (GETP), 9th edition (15)<br>• Chapter 8 |
| **Knowledge** of specific exercises and program modifications for individuals with chronic disease who are medically cleared to exercise — stable coronary artery disease, other cardiovascular (CV) diseases, diabetes mellitus, obesity, metabolic syndrome, hypertension, arthritis, chronic back pain, osteoporosis, chronic pulmonary disease, and chronic pain | • Once competency of basic exercises is established, add advanced exercises and progress by increase intensity or duration.<br>• Modifications for specific population based on structural, physiological effects of maturation and/or condition | *ACSM's Resources for the Personal Trainer*, 4th edition (10)<br>• Chapters 12, 13, and 19<br>*ACSM's Guidelines for Exercise Testing and Prescription* (GETP), 9th edition (15)<br>• Chapters 8–10<br>*ACSM's Resource Manual for Guidelines for Exercise Testing and Prescription*, 7th edition (18)<br>• Chapters 30 and 32 |
| **Knowledge** of principles of progressive overload, specificity, and program progression to avoid training plateaus and promote continued improvement and goal achievement | • Progressive overload: as the body adapts to a given stimulus, an increase in stimulus is required for further adaptation and improvement (increase load or volume).<br>• Specificity: only muscles that are trained will adapt and change (training two to three times per week for each body part).<br>• Progression: modify volume and add advanced exercises once competency is achieved.<br>• Be wary of signs and symptoms of overtraining. | *ACSM's Resources for the Personal Trainer*, 4th edition (10)<br>• Chapters 13 and 14<br>*ACSM's Resource Manual for Guidelines for Exercise Testing and Prescription*, 7th edition (18)<br>• Chapters 31 and 33 |
| **Knowledge** of appropriate methods to teach progression of exercises for all major muscle groups (*e.g.*, progression of standing lunge to walking lunge to walking lunge with resistance) | • Progressions: move from wide to smaller base of support, supported to unsupported movement, bilateral to unilateral, short to long lever, simple to complex, single joint to compound exercises | *ACSM's Resources for the Personal Trainer*, 4th edition (10)<br>• Chapters 13 and 14 |
| **Knowledge** of modifications to periodized conditioning programs to increase or maintain muscular strength and/or endurance, hypertrophy, power, CV endurance, balance, and range of motion/flexibility | • Hypertrophy: high volume — short rest periods<br>• Strength/power: reduced volume, increased load and rest periods<br>• CV endurance: once frequency and baseline conditioning is established, increase intensity and vary modes (interval training).<br>• Balance: vary base of support, use unstable surfaces, change perturbations<br>• Flexibility: use different modes and techniques; increase frequency. | *ACSM's Resources for the Personal Trainer*, 4th edition (10)<br>• Chapters 14–16 |

## G.  Seek client feedback to ensure satisfaction and enjoyment of the program.

| Knowledge or Skill Statement | Explanation/Examples | Resources |
|---|---|---|
| **Knowledge** of effective techniques for program evaluation and client satisfaction (*e.g.*, survey, written follow-up, verbal feedback) | • Use of assessments<br>• Feedback vehicles both written and verbal<br>• Track response rate.<br>• Establish best practices.<br>• Track programs year over year (client database).<br>• Timely follow-up and feedback<br>• Positive reinforcement | *ACSM's Resources for the Personal Trainer*, 4th edition (10)<br>• Chapters 8 and 13<br>*ACSM's Resource Manual for Guidelines for Exercise Testing and Prescription*, 7th edition (18)<br>• Chapter 48 |
| **Knowledge** of client goals and appropriate review and modification | • Use of assessments on a periodic basis (4 wk to 3 mo) as a measure of success for achieving goals and motivation<br>• Consistency of workouts; check motivation levels, self-efficacy. | *ACSM's Resources for the Personal Trainer*, 4th edition (10)<br>• Chapters 12, 13, and 17<br>*ACSM's Resource Manual for Guidelines for Exercise Testing and Prescription*, 7th edition (18)<br>• Chapters 45 and 48 |

# DOMAIN III: LEADERSHIP AND EDUCATION IMPLEMENTATION

## A.  Create a positive exercise experience in order to optimize participant adherence by applying effective communication techniques, motivation techniques, and behavioral strategies.

| Knowledge or Skill Statement | Explanation/Examples | Resources |
|---|---|---|
| **Knowledge** of effective and timely uses of a wide variety of communication modes (*i.e.*, e-mail, telephone, Web site, newsletters) | • Analyze effectiveness, timeliness, cost, return on investment, number of people reached, audience, and number of responses.<br>• Monitor consistency, reliability, and credibility of message delivery. | *ACSM's Resource Manual for Guidelines for Exercise Testing and Prescription*, 7th edition (18)<br>• Chapter 45 |
| **Knowledge** of verbal and nonverbal behaviors that communicate positive reinforcement and encouragement (*i.e.*, eye contact, targeted praise, empathy) | • Positive body language, facial expressions, head movements, positive client-centered approach, eye contact<br>• Accept clients. | *ACSM's Resources for the Personal Trainer*, 4th edition (10)<br>• Chapters 9 and 10 |
| **Knowledge** of and skill in engaging active listening techniques | • Use of reflective statements to clarify and summarize client issues<br>• Nonjudgmental<br>• Undivided attention<br>• Eye contact<br>• Empathy | *ACSM's Resources for the Personal Trainer*, 4th edition (10)<br>• Chapters 9 and 10 |
| **Knowledge** of different types of learners (auditory, visual, kinesthetic) and how to apply teaching and training techniques to optimize a client's training session | • Visual: learn through seeing; demonstration; alignment cuing<br>• Auditory: learn through hearing; verbal instruction<br>• Kinesthetic: learn by direct involvement; moving, experiencing | *ACSM's Resources for the Personal Trainer*, 4th edition (10)<br>• Chapters 7, 8, 9, and 17 |

**A. Create a positive exercise experience in order to optimize participant adherence by applying effective communication techniques, motivation techniques, and behavioral strategies. (cont.)**

| Knowledge or Skill Statement | Explanation/Examples | Resources |
|---|---|---|
| **Knowledge** of different types of feedback (*i.e.*, evaluative, supportive, descriptive) and the ability to use feedback to optimize a client's training session | • Corrective feedback should be immediate <br> • All feedback should be nonthreatening, objective, clarifying, reflective, and supportive. | *ACSM's Resources for the Personal Trainer*, 4th edition (10) <br> • Chapter 9 |
| **Knowledge** of and the application of health behavior change models (socioecological model, readiness to change model, social cognitive theory, and theory of planned behavior, etc.) and effective strategies that support and facilitate exercise adherence | • Behavior change pyramid moves clients through stages to their goal. <br> • Action-oriented process of making a commitment, identifying and eliminating cues that produce problem behavior; provide healthy substitutions; elicit social support and provide reinforcement | *ACSM's Resources for the Personal Trainer*, 4th edition (10) <br> • Chapters 7 and 8 <br> *ACSM's Resource Manual for Guidelines for Exercise Testing and Prescription*, 7th edition (18) <br> • Chapters 44, 45, and 46 <br> *ACSM's Guidelines for Exercise Testing and Prescription* (GETP), 9th edition (15) <br> • Chapter 11 |
| **Knowledge** of barriers to exercise adherence and compliance (*e.g.*, time management, injury, fear, lack of knowledge, weather) | • Identify solutions to common barriers: personal, behavioral, environmental, social, and programmatic. <br> • Discuss and brainstorm solutions such as scheduling workouts, alternative training environments, progressive plans, educating clients, home exercise recommendations, and incentives. | *ACSM's Resources for the Personal Trainer*, 4th edition (10) <br> • Chapter 8 <br> *ACSM's Resource Manual for Guidelines for Exercise Testing and Prescription*, 7th edition (18) <br> • Chapter 45 <br> *ACSM's Guidelines for Exercise Testing and Prescription* (GETP), 9th edition (15) <br> • Chapter 11 <br> • Table 11.1 |
| **Knowledge** of triggers to relapse and prevention strategies | • Plan for common lapses in healthy behavior such as work pressures, travel, and boredom. <br> • Prevention strategies: stress management skills, goal setting, variety of activities, places to exercise, and competitive events | *ACSM's Resources for the Personal Trainer*, 4th edition (10) <br> • Chapters 8 and 9 <br> *ACSM's Resource Manual for Guidelines for Exercise Testing and Prescription*, 7th edition (18) <br> • Chapters 44–46 |
| **Knowledge** of specific techniques to facilitate motivation (*e.g.*, goal setting, incentive programs, achievement recognition, social support) | • Use goal setting to establish level of concern. <br> • Pleasant training environment <br> • Tracking progress and knowledge of results to establish success; rewarding achievement | *ACSM's Resources for the Personal Trainer*, 4th edition (10) <br> • Chapters 8 and 9 <br> *ACSM's Resource Manual for Guidelines for Exercise Testing and Prescription*, 7th edition (18) <br> • Chapter 45 |
| **Knowledge** of extrinsic and intrinsic reinforcement strategies (*e.g.*, T-shirt, improved self-esteem) | • Extrinsic: identify outside factors that support a desire to attain a goal. <br> • Intrinsic: remain important long after goal is achieved. <br> • Strategies: motivational interviewing, disadvantages of current behavior, and advantage to change | *ACSM's Resources for the Personal Trainer*, 4th edition (10) <br> • Chapters 8 and 9 |

## A. Create a positive exercise experience in order to optimize participant adherence by applying effective communication techniques, motivation techniques, and behavioral strategies. (cont.)

| Knowledge or Skill Statement | Explanation/Examples | Resources |
|---|---|---|
| **Knowledge** of strategies to increase nonstructured physical activity levels (*e.g.*, stair walking, parking farther away, bike to work) | • Walking or biking short distances when one would normally drive a car.<br>• Take the stairs instead of elevator or escalator.<br>• Park at far end of parking lot when shopping.<br>• Take a walk for half of your lunch hour.<br>• Get off one stop before destination and walk the rest of the way.<br>• Pace while talking on the phone.<br>• Walk to the next office instead of sending an e-mail or phoning.<br>• Get up and walk around for 10 min out of every hour while at work.<br>• Use a pedometer to track the number of steps taken per day.<br>• Physical activity can be part of the routine activities of day-to-day living, such as farming, gardening, walking or cycling to work, walking to catch a bus, house cleaning, or doing household chores. | "Physical Activity and Public Health: Updated Recommendation for Adults from the American College of Sports Medicine and the American Heart Association" (13) |
| **Knowledge** of health coaching principles and lifestyle management techniques related to behavior change | • Goal setting; connecting goals to deeper motivation; adopt a being curious attitude; ask clients what they are willing to do; create manageable weekly goals between sessions; focus on what's working. | *ACSM's Resources for the Personal Trainer*, 4th edition (10)<br>• Chapters 7 and 8 |
| **Knowledge** of specific, age-appropriate leadership techniques, and educational methods to increase client engagement | • Social support and participation of similar niches<br>• Community-based programs<br>• Appropriate music and intensity level<br>• Fun | *ACSM's Resource Manual for Guidelines for Exercise Testing and Prescription*, 7th edition (18)<br>• Chapter 45 |

## B. Educate clients using scientifically sound health and fitness information and resources to enhance client's knowledge base, program enjoyment, adherence, and overall awareness of health- and fitness-related information.

| Knowledge or Skill Statement | Explanation/Examples | Resources |
|---|---|---|
| **Knowledge** of the influence of lifestyle factors, including nutrition and physical activity habits, on lipid and lipoprotein profiles | • Chronic adaptations to cardiovascular exercise<br>• Fundamentals of nutrition and fat metabolism<br>• Good sources of fats | *ACSM's Resources for the Personal Trainer*, 4th edition (10)<br>• Chapters 5 and 6<br>• Table 5.2 |

**B.  Educate clients using scientifically sound health and fitness information and resources to enhance client's knowledge base, program enjoyment, adherence, and overall awareness of health- and fitness-related information. (cont.)**

| Knowledge or Skill Statement | Explanation/Examples | Resources |
|---|---|---|
| **Knowledge** of the value of carbohydrates, fats, and proteins as fuels for exercise and physical activity | • Explain the functions of carbohydrates as preferred fuel, quick energy source, protein sparing, oxidation of fat, and storage forms.<br>• Explain the functions of fats as an insulation from extreme temperatures, cushion for concussion forces, satiety, and carrier of essential nutrients.<br>• Explain the functions of protein in hormone production, acid–base balance, growth and tissue maintenance, transport of nutrients, fluid balance enzyme synthesis. | *ACSM's Resources for the Personal Trainer*, 4th edition (10)<br>• Chapter 6 |
| **Knowledge** of the following terms: body composition, body mass index (BMI), lean body mass, anorexia nervosa, bulimia nervosa, and body fat distribution | • Body composition: explain the relative proportion of fat and fat-free mass.<br>• BMI: technique of using weight relative to height<br>• Lean body mass: term used to describe a collection of tissues (muscle, bone, etc.) other than fat, which make up total body weight.<br>• Anorexia nervosa: eating disorder characterized by restrictive eating due to being afraid of gaining weight, even though at least 15% below expected weight for age and height.<br>• Bulimia nervosa: eating disorder of usually normal weight individuals characterized by cycles of overeating and purging or other compensatory behaviors. | *ACSM's Resources for the Personal Trainer*, 4th edition (10)<br>• Chapter 12<br>"ACSM Position Stand: The Female Athlete Triad" (14) |
| **Knowledge** of the relationship between body composition and health | • Explanation of the strong correlation between obesity and the increased risk of chronic diseases | *ACSM's Resources for the Personal Trainer*, 4th edition (10)<br>• Chapter 12 |
| **Knowledge** of the effectiveness of diet, exercise, and behavior modification as a method for modifying body composition | • Explain the effectiveness a healthy and balanced diet, consisting of portion control, healthy food choices and food preparation, caloric intake on weight, and body composition.<br>• Explain the relationship between type, intensity, frequency, and duration of exercise and caloric expenditure<br>• Explain the common behavioral strategies such as nonsupervised and supervised exercise, occupational and leisure time activities as mean to increase physical activity. | "ACSM Position Stand: Appropriate Physical Activity Intervention strategies for Weight Loss and Prevention of Weight Regain for Adults" (11) |

## B. Educate clients using scientifically sound health and fitness information and resources to enhance client's knowledge base, program enjoyment, adherence, and overall awareness of health- and fitness-related information. (cont.)

| Knowledge or Skill Statement | Explanation/Examples | Resources |
|---|---|---|
| **Knowledge** of the importance of maintaining hydration before, during, and after exercise | • Explain the goal of prehydration is to start activity hydrated and with normal plasma electrolyte levels.<br>• Explain the goal of drinking during physical activity is to prevent dehydration.<br>• Explain the goal of hydration after exercise is to replace any electrolyte fluid deficit.<br>• Explain individual fluid replacement rate is based on individual sweat rates, choice of beverages, length and intensity of activity, and environmental conditions. | "ACSM Position Stand: Exercise and Fluid Replacement" (17)<br>*ACSM's Resources for the Personal Trainer*, 4th edition (10)<br>• Chapter 6 |
| **Knowledge** of the U.S. Department of Agriculture (USDA) Food Guide Pyramid and American College of Sports Medicine (ACSM)–endorsed Dietary Guidelines (American Dietetic Association) | • Guidelines explaining the different food groups, sources, and portions of a balanced and healthy eating plan<br>• USDA Dietary Guidelines 2010 is the federal government's evidence-based nutritional guidance to promote health, reduce the risk of chronic diseases, and reduce the prevalence of overweight and obesity through improved nutrition and physical activity.<br>• American Dietetic Association is the world's largest organization of food and nutrition professionals. | ChooseMyPlate, formerly known as USDA Food Guide Pyramid (39)<br>"USDA Dietary Guidelines for Americans" (40)<br>Academy of Nutrition and Dietetics formerly known as American Dietetic Association (20) |
| **Knowledge** of the Female Athlete Triad | • Explain the interrelationships between energy availability, menstrual cycle, and bone mineral density of women and girls who participate in athletics on the clinical manifestations of eating disorders, amenorrhea, and osteoporosis and possible interventions and/or educational measures used to prevent or mitigate the effects. | "ACSM Position Stand: The Female Athlete Triad" (14) |
| **Knowledge** of the myths and consequences associated with inappropriate weight loss methods (*e.g.*, fad diets, dietary supplements, overexercising, starvation diets) | • Explain scientifically based safe methods of weight loss using the proper eating habits and appropriate physical activity guidelines and issues associated with diets based on extreme or exclusive principles. | *ACSM's Resources for the Personal Trainer*, 4th edition (10)<br>• Chapter 6<br>*ACSM's Resource Manual for Guidelines for Exercise Testing and Prescription*, 7th edition (18)<br>• Chapter 35 |
| **Knowledge** of the number of kilocalories in 1 g of carbohydrate, fat, protein, and alcohol | • Carbohydrate = 4 kcal $\cdot$ g$^{-1}$<br>• Fat = 9 kcal $\cdot$ g$^{-1}$<br>• Protein = 4 kcal $\cdot$ g$^{-1}$<br>• Alcohol = 7 kcal $\cdot$ g$^{-1}$ | *ACSM's Resources for the Personal Trainer*, 4th edition (10)<br>• Chapter 6 |

| B. Educate clients using scientifically sound health and fitness information and resources to enhance client's knowledge base, program enjoyment, adherence, and overall awareness of health- and fitness-related information. (cont.) | | |
|---|---|---|
| **Knowledge or Skill Statement** | **Explanation/Examples** | **Resources** |
| **Knowledge** of the ACSM's guidelines for caloric intake for individuals desiring to lose or gain weight | • Weight loss = calories out > calories in <br> • Weight gain = calories in > calories out <br> • Explain the physical activity expenditure recommendations for weight loss and weight maintenance in minutes and the associated caloric equivalent. | "ACSM Position Stand: Appropriate Physical Activity Intervention Strategies for Weight Loss and Prevention of Weight Regain for Adults" (11) <br> *ACSM's Resources for the Personal Trainer*, 4th edition (10) <br> • Chapter 6 <br> *ACSM's Resource Manual for Guidelines for Exercise Testing and Prescription*, 7th edition (18) <br> • Chapter 35 |
| **Knowledge** of accessing and dissemination of scientifically based, relevant health, exercise, and wellness-related resources and information | • Identify competent and reputable sources of current information such as ACSM Web site, National Institute of Health (NIH) Web site, peer-reviewed journals, and others. | ACSM's Web site and resources (1,2,3) <br> National Institute of Health (30,31) <br> "WebMD Healthy Living" (44) <br> "Mayo Clinic Health Information" (27) |
| **Knowledge** of community-based exercise programs that provide social support and structured activities (*e.g.*, walking clubs, intramural sports, golf leagues, cycling clubs) | • Identify national and local programs targeted toward specific conditions, age, sponsoring organizations, sport categories, and level of fitness. <br> • Contact chamber of commerce, rotary club, or civic organizations. | "National Blueprint: Increasing Physical Activity among Adults" (29) <br> President's Council on Fitness, Sports, and Nutrition (34) <br> "Exercise is Medicine" (24) <br> National Physical Activity Plan (32) <br> "The Community Guide to Promoting Physical Activity" (25) |
| **Knowledge** of stress management and relaxation techniques (*e.g.*, progressive relaxation, guided imagery, massage therapy) | • Explain the differences between common relaxation and stress management techniques. <br> • Knowledge of proper breathing techniques | "WebMD Stress Management Health Center" (45) <br> "Stress Management Techniques" (36) <br> "Relaxation Technique for Stress Relief" (35) |

# DOMAIN IV: LEGAL, PROFESSIONAL, BUSINESS, AND MARKETING

| A. Obtain medical clearance for all clients prior to starting an exercise program. | | |
|---|---|---|
| **Knowledge or Skill Statement** | **Explanation/Examples** | **Resources** |
| **Knowledge** of risk stratification and medical clearance procedures in order to decrease client injury and/or medical complications thereby minimizing Certified Personal Trainer negligence and risk of liability | • Properly identify those who pose an increased risk of experiencing exercise-related cardiovascular incident. | *ACSM's Resources for the Personal Trainer*, 4th edition (10) <br> • Chapters 11, 19, and 21 <br> *ACSM's Health/Fitness Facility Standards and Guidelines*, 3rd edition (19) <br> • Chapter 2 <br> • Table 2.1 |

## A.  Obtain medical clearance for all clients prior to starting an exercise program. (cont.)

| Knowledge or Skill Statement | Explanation/Examples | Resources |
|---|---|---|
| **Knowledge** of the application of the ACSM risk stratification process | • High risk clients are those who are symptomatic or with known cardiac, pulmonary, or metabolic disease.<br>• Moderate-risk clients are asymptomatic and have two or more risk factors. | *ACSM's Resources for the Personal Trainer*, 4th edition (10)<br>• Chapter 11<br>• Figures 11.5 and 11.6<br>• Tables 11.1 and 11.2 |
| **Knowledge** of medical clearance requirements prior to exercise testing and program participation | • High-risk clients: recommended medical exam and graded exercise test (GXT) prior to exercise program for moderate and vigorous exercise; medical doctor (MD) supervision of exercise test recommended<br>• Moderate-risk clients: recommended medical exam and GXT with medical supervision prior to exercise program for vigorous exercise.<br>• Medical examination and GXT not necessary for moderate exercise for moderate-risk clients | *ACSM's Resources for the Personal Trainer*, 4th edition (10)<br>• Chapter 11<br>• Figures 11.5 and 11.6<br>• Tables 11.1 and 11.2 |
| **Knowledge** of the appropriate level of supervision and monitoring recommended for individuals with known disease based on disease-specific risk stratification guidelines and current health status | • May need to use a facility with medically qualified staff | *ACSM's Resources for the Personal Trainer*, 4th edition (10)<br>• Chapter 11<br>• Figure 11.2 |

## B.  Collaborate with various health care professionals and organizations in order to provide clients with a network of providers that minimizes liability and maximizes program effectiveness.

| Knowledge or Skill Statement | Explanation/Examples | Resources |
|---|---|---|
| **Knowledge** of reputable professional resources and referral sources to ensure client safety and program effectiveness | • Establish a local network of health care professionals.<br>• Establish policies, procedures, and forms for matching clients with appropriate professionals, services, appraisals, programs, and referrals. | *ACSM's Resources for the Personal Trainer*, 4th edition (10)<br>• Chapter 11 |
| **Knowledge** of the scope of practice for the Certified Personal Trainer and the need to practice within this scope | • Scope: fitness professional who develops and implements safe and sound programs through an individualized approach to exercise leadership in healthy populations and/or those individuals with medical clearance to exercise.<br>• Minimize risk of exposure to liability. | ACSM Web site (7)<br>*ACSM's Resources for the Personal Trainer*, 4th edition (10)<br>• Chapters 1 and 21 |

## B. Collaborate with various health care professionals and organizations in order to provide clients with a network of providers that minimizes liability and maximizes program effectiveness. (cont.)

| Knowledge or Skill Statement | Explanation/Examples | Resources |
|---|---|---|
| **Knowledge** of effective and professional communication with allied health and fitness professionals | • Proper spelling and grammar used<br>• Confidential cover sheet<br>• Contact prior to sending fax.<br>• Secure network if using e-mail.<br>• Up-to-date self-credentials and contact information. | *ACSM's Resources for the Personal Trainer*, 4th edition (10)<br>• Chapter 9<br>U.S. Department of Health and Human Services, Health Information Privacy (42,43) |
| **Knowledge** of identifying individuals requiring referral to a physician or allied health services such as physical therapy, dietary counseling, stress management, weight management, and psychological and social services | • Knowledge of conditions, signs, or indicators that fall outside of scope of practice<br>• Establish local network of health care professionals.<br>• Establish policies, procedures, and forms for matching clients with appropriate services, appraisals, programs, and referrals. | *ACSM's Resources for the Personal Trainer*, 4th edition (10)<br>• Chapter 11 |

## C. Develop a comprehensive risk management program (including emergency action plan and injury prevention program) to enhance the standard of care and reflect a client-focused mission.

| Knowledge or Skill Statement | Explanation/Examples | Resources |
|---|---|---|
| **Knowledge** of and skill in obtaining basic life support, automated external defibrillator (AED), and cardiopulmonary resuscitation (CPR) certification | • Current certification that includes demonstration of practical skills | *American Red Cross First Aid/CPR/ AED Participant Manual* (21)<br>American Heart Association Basic Life Support (BLS) or Lifesaver Certification (23) |
| **Knowledge** of appropriate emergency procedures (*i.e.*, telephone procedures, written emergency procedures, personnel responsibilities) in a health and fitness setting | • Written plan that addresses major emergency situations<br>• Explicit steps and instructions on how each emergency situation is handled and the roles of responders<br>• Emergency medical services (EMS) contact information, emergency equipment location<br>• Rehearsal of plan four times a year<br>• Proper follow-up and documentation | *ACSM's Resources for the Personal Trainer*, 4th edition (10)<br>• Chapter 21<br>• Box 21.3<br>*ACSM's Health/Fitness Facility Standards and Guidelines*, 3rd edition (10)<br>• Chapter 4<br>• Appendix D and Form 26 |
| **Knowledge** of basic first aid procedures for exercise-related injuries, such as bleeding, strains/sprains, fractures, and exercise intolerance (dizziness, syncope, heat injury) | • Rest, ice, compression, and elevation (RICE) for strains/sprains<br>• Direct pressure for bleeding<br>• Let professionals treat fractures and serious injuries out of scope of training.<br>• Supine with legs elevated for fainting | *American Red Cross First Aid/CPR/ AED Participant Manual* (21)<br>• Chapters 5–8<br>*ACSM's Resource Manual for Guidelines for Exercise Testing and Prescription*, 7th edition (18)<br>• Chapter 37 |

## C. Develop a comprehensive risk management program (including emergency action plan and injury prevention program) to enhance the standard of care and reflect a client-focused mission. (cont.)

| Knowledge or Skill Statement | Explanation/Examples | Resources |
|---|---|---|
| **Knowledge** of precautions taken in an exercise setting to ensure participant safety (*e.g.*, equipment placement, facility cleanliness, floor surface) | • Signage for potential risk; conform to relevant laws, regulations, and published standards<br>• ADA requirements for passageway width, signage, and clear floor space<br>• Circulation areas adjacent to physical activity areas<br>• Proper signage on any equipment or areas of facility that are out of order or unusable | *ACSM's Resources for the Personal Trainer*, 4th edition (10)<br>• Chapter 21<br>*ACSM's Health/Fitness Facility Standards and Guidelines*, 3rd edition (19)<br>• Chapters 6 and 7<br>*Risk Management for Health/Fitness Professionals* (9)<br>• Chapter 10 |
| **Knowledge** of the following terms related to musculoskeletal injuries (*e.g.*, shin splints, sprain, strain, bursitis, fractures, tendonitis, patellofemoral pain syndrome, low back pain, plantar fasciitis) | • Sprain: injury to a ligament<br>• Strain: injury to a muscle<br>• Bursitis: inflammation of bursa<br>• Tendonitis: inflammation of tendon<br>• Fracture: broken bone<br>• Plantar fasciitis: chronic inflammatory condition that results in pain at the calcaneal insertion<br>• Patellofemoral pain syndrome: common disorder in young athletes that produces anterior knee pain | *ACSM's Resources for the Personal Trainer*, 4th edition (10)<br>• Chapter 3 |
| **Knowledge** of contraindicated exercises/postures and potential risks associated with certain exercises (*e.g.*, straight-leg sit-ups, double-leg raises, full squats, hurdler's stretch, cervical and lumbar hyperextension, and standing bent-over-toe touch) | • Potential risks: correct body alignment and joint position are critical for maximum results and minimal risk of injury.<br>• Potentially harmful postures/exercises should be modified to safer joint positions.<br>• Any exercises, which are contraindicated by physician should be avoided. | *ACSM's Resources for the Personal Trainer*, 4th edition (10)<br>• Chapter 16 |
| **Knowledge** of the responsibilities, limitations, and the legal implications for the Certified Personal Trainer of carrying out emergency procedures | • Duty of care<br>• Current certifications, including CPR/AED; familiarity of facility emergency plan; documentation of incident; professional liability insurance | *ACSM's Resources for the Personal Trainer*, 4th edition (10)<br>• Chapter 21<br>*Risk Management for Health/Fitness Professionals* (9)<br>• Chapter 11 |
| **Knowledge** of potential musculoskeletal injuries (*e.g.*, knowledge of contusions, sprains, strains, fractures), cardiovascular/pulmonary complications (*e.g.*, chest pain, palpitations/arrhythmias, tachycardia, bradycardia, hypotension/hypertension, hyperventilation), and metabolic abnormalities (*e.g.*, fainting/syncope, hypoglycemia/hyperglycemia, hypothermia/hyperthermia) | • Cardiovascular/pulmonary complications: identification — Table 37.5; basic first aid guidelines — Table 37.6<br>• Potential musculoskeletal injuries — Table 37.2<br>• Metabolic abnormalities: basic first aid guidelines — Table 37.6<br>• Environmental conditions: basic first aid — Table 37.8; Box 37.11 | *ACSM's Resources for the Personal Trainer*, 4th edition (10)<br>• Chapter 3<br>*American Red Cross First Aid/CPR/AED Participant Manual* (21)<br>*ACSM's Resource Manual for Guidelines for Exercise Testing and Prescription*, 7th edition (18)<br>• Chapter 37 |

**CPT**

| C. Develop a comprehensive risk management program (including emergency action plan and injury prevention program) to enhance the standard of care and reflect a client-focused mission. (cont.) | | |
|---|---|---|
| **Knowledge or Skill Statement** | **Explanation/Examples** | **Resources** |
| **Knowledge** of the initial management and first aid techniques associated with open wounds, musculoskeletal injuries, cardiovascular/pulmonary complications, and metabolic disorders | • Open wounds — Chapter 7<br>• Musculoskeletal injuries — Chapter 8<br>• Breathing and cardiac emergencies — Chapters 2–4<br>• Sudden illness — Chapter 5 | *American Red Cross First Aid/CPR/AED Participant Manual* (21)<br>• Chapters 2–5, 7, and 8<br>*ACSM's Guidelines for Exercise Testing and Prescription* (GETP), 9th edition (15)<br>• Chapter 7<br>*ACSM's Resource Manual for Guidelines for Exercise Testing and Prescription*, 7th edition (18)<br>• Chapter 37 |
| **Knowledge** of the need for and components of an equipment service plan/agreement and how it may be used to evaluate the condition of exercise equipment to reduce the potential risk of injury | • Daily, weekly, and monthly care for all equipment<br>• Regular inspection and preventative maintenance of equipment and documentation of inspection and repairs<br>• Knowledge of equipment warranty and repair information<br>• Follow manufacturer's recommendations. | *ACSM's Health/Fitness Facility Standards and Guidelines*, 3rd edition (19)<br>• Chapter 7<br>• Tables 7.3 and 7.4<br>• Appendix A<br>• Supplements 3 and 4<br>*Risk Management for Health/Fitness Professionals* (9)<br>• Chapter 9 |
| **Knowledge** of the need for and use of safety policies and procedures (*e.g.*, incident/accident reports, emergency procedure training) and legal necessity thereof | • Duty to public to provide safe facility and programs<br>• Emergency response system critical to providing safe environment<br>• Address major emergency situation.<br>• Elicit instructions and roles of how to respond.<br>• Document system (training, instructions)<br>• Rehearsal 4 times a year<br>• Available first aid and emergency equipment<br>• Coordination with local EMS | *ACSM's Resources for the Personal Trainer*, 4th edition (10)<br>• Chapter 21<br>*ACSM's Health/Fitness Facility Standards and Guidelines*, 3rd edition (19)<br>• Chapter 4<br>*Risk Management for Health/Fitness Professionals* (9)<br>• Chapter 11 |
| **Knowledge** of the need for and components of an emergency action plan. | • Written emergency action plan with explicit steps and instructions on how each emergency situation is handled and the roles of responders<br>• EMS contact information, emergency equipment location<br>• Rehearsal<br>• Knowledge of fire safety and facility evacuation procedures<br>• Proper follow-up and documentation | *ACSM's Resources for the Personal Trainer*, 4th edition (10)<br>• Chapter 21<br>*ACSM's Health/Fitness Facility Standards and Guidelines*, 3rd edition (19)<br>• Chapter 4<br>*ACSM's Guidelines for Exercise Testing and Prescription* (GETP), 9th edition (15)<br>• Appendix B<br>*Risk Management for Health/Fitness Professionals* (9)<br>• Chapter 11 |

## C. Develop a comprehensive risk management program (including emergency action plan and injury prevention program) to enhance the standard of care and reflect a client-focused mission. (cont.)

| Knowledge or Skill Statement | Explanation/Examples | Resources |
|---|---|---|
| **Knowledge** of effective communication skills and the ability to inform staff and clients of emergency policies and procedures for the facility or program | • Establish who is responsible for communication to EMS and within facility as part of the emergency action plan.<br>• Telephone number for emergency assistance should be clearly posted near all phones. Emergency communication devices must be readily available and working properly.<br>• Plans should include medical, fire, evacuations, and other emergencies.<br>• Rehearse plan, including communication portion every 3 mo.<br>• Unsupervised facility: signage of what steps members should take in the event of a witnessed emergency situation. | *ACSM's Resource Manual for Guidelines for Exercise Testing and Prescription*, 7th edition (18)<br>• Chapter 37<br>*Risk Management for Health/Fitness Professionals* (9)<br>• Chapter 11<br>*ACSM's Health/Fitness Facility Standards and Guidelines*, 3rd edition (19)<br>• Chapter 8<br>*ACSM's Guidelines for Exercise Testing and Prescription* (GETP), 9th edition (15)<br>• Appendix B |
| **Skill** in demonstrating and carrying out emergency procedures during exercise testing and/or training | • Emergency drills convened four times a year<br>• Follow-up evaluation of personnel and response and documentation of drills | *ACSM's Health/Fitness Facility Standards and Guidelines*, 3rd edition (19)<br>• Chapter 4<br>*ACSM's Guidelines for Exercise Testing and Prescription* (GETP), 9th edition (15)<br>• Appendix B |
| **Skill** in assisting, spotting, and monitoring a client safely and effectively during exercise testing and/or training | • Knowledge of exercise being performed, possible adverse effects, common errors in performing, proper positioning to assist lift, being alert, good communication | *ACSM's Resources for the Personal Trainer*, 4th edition (10)<br>• Chapters 14 and 17<br>*ACSM's Resource Manual for Guidelines for Exercise Testing and Prescription*, 7th edition (18)<br>• Chapters 31 and 33 |

## D. Participate in approved continuing education programs on a regular basis to maximize effectiveness, increase professionalism, and enhance knowledge and skills in the field of health and fitness.

| Knowledge or Skill Statement | Explanation/Examples | Resources |
|---|---|---|
| **Knowledge** of the role of continuing education, professional resources, and requirements for certification and recertification | • Obligation to public and clients to keep current with science and practice-related research<br>• Certification requirements: 18 yr old; high school diploma (general education development [GED]); adult cardiopulmonary resuscitation (CPR) certification<br>• American College of Sports Medicine (ACSM) Certification is valid for 3 yr.<br>• Recertification: 45 credits | ACSM Web site (5,6)<br>*ACSM's Resources for the Personal Trainer*, 4th edition (10)<br>• Chapters 1 and 2 |

CPT

## D.  Participate in approved continuing education programs on a regular basis to maximize effectiveness, increase professionalism, and enhance knowledge and skills in the field of health and fitness. (cont.)

| Knowledge or Skill Statement | Explanation/Examples | Resources |
|---|---|---|
| **Knowledge** of the requirements for obtaining and maintaining continuing education credits (CEC) and where one can obtain ACSM-approved CEC<br>**Knowledge** of the continually evolving field of health and fitness and the need for Certified Personal Trainers to keep abreast of new research and applications in the field of exercise science | • Identify ACSM-approved providers for CEC.<br>• Identify credible health/fitness resources to obtain CEC in person (workshops) and via Internet. | ACSM Web site (5,6)<br>*ACSM's Resources for the Personal Trainer*, 4th edition (10)<br>• Chapters 1 and 2<br>ACSM Journals (4) |

## E.  Adhere to American College of Sports Medicine's (ACSM's) Code of Ethics by practicing in a professional manner within the scope of practice of a Certified Personal Trainer.

| Knowledge or Skill Statement | Explanation/Examples | Resources |
|---|---|---|
| **Knowledge** of the components of both the ACSM's Code of Ethics as well as the ACSM Certified Personal Trainer scope of practice | • Code of Ethics: improve knowledge and skill, maintain high professional and scientific standards, safeguard the public, and improving both the health and well-being of the individual and the community.<br>• Scope: fitness professional who develops and implements an individualized approach to exercise leadership in healthy populations and/or those individuals with medical clearance to exercise | ACSM Web site (8)<br>*ACSM's Resources for the Personal Trainer*, 3rd edition (10)<br>• Chapters 1 and 2 |
| **Knowledge** of appropriate work attire and professional behavior | • Work attire may be dictated by professional work environments.<br>• Professional behavior established via code of ethics and scope of practice; good communication skills, ability to build relationships | *ACSM's Resources for the Personal Trainer*, 4th edition (10)<br>• Chapters 1 and 2 |
| **Skill** in conducting all professional activities within the scope of practice of the ACSM Certified Personal Trainer | • Leading and demonstrating safe and effective methods of exercise by applying the fundamental principles of exercise science.<br>• Writing appropriate exercise recommendations.<br>• Motivating individuals to begin and to continue with their healthy behaviors. | ACSM Web site (1,4)<br>*ACSM's Resources for the Personal Trainer*, 4th edition (10)<br>• Chapters 1 and 2 |

## F. Develop a business plan to establish mission, business, budgetary, and sales objectives.

| Knowledge or Skill Statement | Explanation/Examples | Resources |
|---|---|---|
| **Knowledge** of implementation methods for effective, ethical, and professional business practices | • Create vision, mission statement, core business values, services, and operational policies.<br>• Collect and review the most recent publications of standards and guidelines by national organizations. | *ACSM's Resources for the Personal Trainer*, 4th edition (10)<br>• Chapter 20<br>*ACSM's Resource Manual for Guidelines for Exercise Testing and Prescription*, 7th edition (18)<br>• Chapters 10 and 19 |
| **Knowledge** of various business models (*i.e.*, sole proprietorship, independent contractor, partnership, corporation, S corporation) | • Sole: one person owned business<br>• Individual contractor: provides services for an individual or business<br>• Partner: two or more people with a contract filed with local or state gov't<br>• Corporation: formal business entity subject to laws, regulations, and demands of stockholders<br>• Limited liability corporation (LLC): similar to a corporation, owners have limited personal liability for the debts and actions of the LLC. Other features of LLCs are more like a partnership, providing management flexibility, and the benefit of pass-through taxation. (from Internal Revenue Service [IRS] Web site: http://www.irs.gov/businesses/small/article/0,,id=98277,00.html)<br>• S corporation: alternative for small business that combines advantages of the other business models. | *ACSM's Resources for the Personal Trainer*, 4th edition (10)<br>• Chapter 20 |
| **Skill** in the development of a basic business plan, which includes establishing a budget (*i.e.*, billing, cancellation policy, late arrival policy, payment methods/plans) | • Demographic and competitive analysis<br>• Establish a budget.<br>• Revenue and expense management<br>• Develop management policies, marketing, sales and pricing. | *ACSM's Resources for the Personal Trainer*, 4th edition (10)<br>• Chapter 20<br>*ACSM's Resource Manual for Guidelines for Exercise Testing and Prescription*, 7th edition (18)<br>• Chapter 19 |
| **Skill** in the development of business objectives (*i.e.*, clearly define business mission statement, business, goals, benchmarks, membership/financial goals, program evaluation) | • Define philosophy and purpose of program or center.<br>• Use mock business plans as a template.<br>• Knowledge of industry standards for goals and benchmarks<br>• Results outcomes expected/projected for all categories<br>• Measure key performance indicators. | *ACSM's Resources for the Personal Trainer*, 4th edition (10)<br>• Chapter 20<br>*ACSM's Resource Manual for Guidelines for Exercise Testing and Prescription*, 7th edition (18)<br>• Chapter 19 |
| **Skill** in market niches and the components of a mission statement (*i.e.*, vision, values, service description) | • Using demographics to identify niches based on client type, training needs, or location | *ACSM's Resources for the Personal Trainer*, 4th edition (10)<br>• Chapter 20 |
| **Skill** in using spreadsheet software to develop and manage budget | • Use QuickBooks or Mind Your Own Business (MYOB) software programs | Microsoft Excel (28) |

## F. Develop a business plan to establish mission, business, budgetary, and sales objectives. (cont.)

| Knowledge or Skill Statement | Explanation/Examples | Resources |
|---|---|---|
| **Skill** in career development practices (*i.e.,* hiring, setting training standards) | • Steps to hiring personal trainers<br>• Establish training standards.<br>• Train and empower staff.<br>• Manage staff and business.<br>• Provide education to staff. | *ACSM's Resources for the Personal Trainer*, 4th edition (10)<br>• Chapters 2 and 20<br>*ACSM's Resource Manual for Guidelines for Exercise Testing and Prescription*, 7th edition (18)<br>• Chapters 10 and 19 |

## G. Develop marketing materials and engage in networking/business exchanges to build client base, promote services, and increase resources.

| Knowledge or Skill Statement | Explanation/Examples | Resources |
|---|---|---|
| **Knowledge** of management policies, marketing, sales, and pricing | • Operational policies such as billing, cancellation, payment methods<br>• Marketing: lead boxes, referrals, advertising, direct mail, and multimedia<br>• Sales: eight-step sales generation process and sales checklist<br>• Pricing based on education, experience, environment/location, and expenses | *ACSM's Resources for the Personal Trainer*, 4th edition (10)<br>• Chapter 20<br>*ACSM's Resource Manual for Guidelines for Exercise Testing and Prescription*, 7th edition (18)<br>• Chapter 48 |
| **Knowledge** of marketing materials to promote the business (*i.e.,* brochures, business cards, web pages, blogs, video clips, e-marketing) | • Converts leads to prospects and prospects to members.<br>• Create positive image.<br>• Web sites, print/video brochures | *ACSM's Resources for the Personal Trainer*, 4th edition (10)<br>• Chapter 20 |
| **Knowledge** of various methods for distribution and promotion of the personal training business (*i.e.,* social networking, press releases, feature newspaper articles) | • External signage, Web sites, radio, TV, billboards, community involvement<br>• Create a positive image and educate consumers. | *ACSM's Resources for the Personal Trainer*, 4th edition (10)<br>• Chapter 20 |
| **Skill** in the development of various marketing materials via computer applications (*i.e.,* Microsoft Word, Microsoft Power Point, PDF, Publisher) | • Use online assistance for each application.<br>• Marketing should not be too busy, eye-catching, colorful, and targeted. | *ACSM's Resources for the Personal Trainer*, 4th edition (10)<br>• Chapter 20 |

## H. Obtain appropriate personal training and liability insurance and follow industry-accepted professional, ethical, and business standards in order to optimize safety and to reduce liability.

| Knowledge or Skill Statement | Explanation/Examples | Resources |
|---|---|---|
| **Knowledge** of professional liability and common types of negligence seen in training environments | • Negligence is failing to do something that a reasonable, prudent person would have done under same or similar circumstances or doing something that a reasonable, prudent person would not have done.<br>• Types: gross, contributory, comparative, omission<br>• Duty of care, breach of duty, causation, damages<br>• Level of responsibility to protect from harm<br>• Safe premises, equipment usage, scope of practice, qualifications, emergency preparedness | *ACSM's Resources for the Personal Trainer*, 4th edition (10)<br>• Chapter 21<br>*ACSM's Resource Manual for Guidelines for Exercise Testing and Prescription*, 7th edition (18)<br>• Chapter 10<br>*Risk Management for Health/Fitness Professionals* (9)<br>• Chapter 2 |
| **Knowledge** of legal issues pertinent to health care delivery by licensed and nonlicensed health care professionals providing rehabilitative services and exercise testing and legal risk management techniques | • Higher standard level of care expected at medical facilities<br>• Refer to appropriate health care professional if not within scope of practice.<br>• Establish strategic alliances. | *ACSM's Resources for the Personal Trainer*, 4th edition (10)<br>• Chapter 21<br>*ACSM's Resource Manual for Guidelines for Exercise Testing and Prescription*, 7th edition (18)<br>• Chapter 48 |
| **Knowledge** of equipment maintenance such to decrease risk of injury and liability (*i.e.*, maintenance plan, service schedule, safety considerations for each piece) | • Follow manufacturer's recommendations.<br>• Regular inspection and preventative cleaning and maintenance<br>• Documentation of maintenance for each piece of equipment<br>• Out of order sign if not in proper working condition<br>• Signage for proper usage of equipment with varying degrees (danger, warning, caution) | *ACSM's Resources for the Personal Trainer*, 4th edition (10)<br>• Chapter 21<br>*ACSM's Health/Fitness Facility Standards and Guidelines*, 3rd edition (19)<br>• Chapter 7<br>• Tables 7.3 and 7.4<br>*Risk Management for Health/Fitness Professionals* (9)<br>• Chapter 9 |

## I. Engage in healthy lifestyle practices in order to be a positive role model for all clients.

| Knowledge or Skill Statement | Explanation/Examples | Resources |
|---|---|---|
| **Knowledge** of appropriate professional behavior (*i.e.*, not smoking, substance-free, nonoffensive dress, courtesy, politeness, active listening skills) | • Model healthy lifestyle.<br>• Be prompt and prepared.<br>• Customer service skills<br>• Educated<br>• Current certifications | *ACSM's Resources for the Personal Trainer*, 4th edition (10)<br>• Chapters 1, 2, and 9 |
| **Knowledge** of environmental influences that may negatively impact client satisfaction/compliance (*i.e.*, music choice/volume level, personal hygiene, scent sensitivity) | • Use facility standards and guidelines to ensure proper range of environmental factors.<br>• Ask for feedback through surveys, comment cards, feedback books, etc.<br>• Create facility policies to ensure comfortable, safe atmosphere for all. | *ACSM's Resources for the Personal Trainer*, 4th edition (10)<br>• Chapters 8 and 17<br>*ACSM's Health/Fitness Facility Standards and Guidelines*, 3rd edition (19) |

## I. Engage in healthy lifestyle practices in order to be a positive role model for all clients.

| Knowledge or Skill Statement | Explanation/Examples | Resources |
|---|---|---|
| **Knowledge** of the need to avoid distractions during a training session (*i.e.*, texting, cell phone calls, in-person conversation with others) | • Client deserves and pays for your full attention.<br>• Manage your energy level through proper sleep, eating well, regular exercise, and good self-care.<br>• Administrative time used for correspondence<br>• If unavoidable, temporarily excuse yourself, keep it brief, and refer to other floor staff. | *ACSM's Resources for the Personal Trainer*, 4th edition (10)<br>• Chapters 1, 9, and 17 |

## J. Respect copyrights to protect original and creative work, media, etc. by legally securing copyright material and other intellectual property based on national and international copyright laws.

| Knowledge or Skill Statement | Explanation/Examples | Resources |
|---|---|---|
| **Knowledge** of and application of national and international copyright laws | • Copyright, a form of intellectual property law, protects original works of authorship including literary, dramatic, musical, and artistic works, such as poetry, novels, movies, songs, computer software, and architecture. Copyright does not protect facts, ideas, systems, or methods of operation, although it may protect the way these things are expressed. | *ACSM's Resources for the Personal Trainer*, 4th edition (10)<br>• Chapter 1<br>United States Copyright Office (38) |
| **Knowledge** of documentation of nonoriginal work | • Part of code of ethics: Credentialed professionals take credit, including authorship, only for work they have actually performed and give credit to the contributions of others if warranted.<br>• All nonoriginal ideas must be cited. Parenthetically, most common: authors last name and year of publication. On the reference page, list all authors for works with three, four, or five authors. | *ACSM's Resources for the Personal Trainer*, 4th edition<br>• Chapter 1<br>"Bates College: How to Cite Sources" (22) |
| **Skill** in developing original educational material | • Research a variety of sources.<br>• Discuss in laymen's terms.<br>• Highlight important points.<br>• Length of material will vary based on space and audience.<br>• Create an eye-appealing format and a catchy title.<br>• Use templates as a starting point. | ACSM Web site (1,2,3) |

## K.  Safeguard client confidentiality and privacy rights unless formally waived or in emergency situations.

| Knowledge or Skill Statement | Explanation/Examples | Resources |
| --- | --- | --- |
| **Knowledge** of practices/systems for maintaining client confidentiality with electronic and hard copy files | • American College of Sports Medicine (ACSM) guideline: A facility should ensure that fitness testing, health promotion, and wellness have a system that provides for and protects the complete confidentiality of all user records and meetings. <br>• Permitting only certain authorized individuals access to information, with the understanding that they will disclose it only to authorized individuals. <br>• User records should only be released with an individual's signed authorization. | *ACSM's Resources for the Personal Trainer*, 4th edition (10) <br>• Chapters 10 and 21 <br>*Risk Management for Health/Fitness Professionals* (9) <br>• Chapter 6 |
| **Knowledge** of the importance of client privacy (*i.e.*, client personal safety, legal liability, client credit protection, client medical disclosure) | • Protection against theft or injury, prevention of potential harm to a client's reputation, maintain trust and provide a safe environment, prevent litigation | *ACSM's Resources for the Personal Trainer*, 4th edition (10) <br>• Chapters 10 and 21 |
| **Knowledge** of the Family Educational Rights and Privacy Act (FERPA) and Health Insurance Portability and Accountability Act (HIPAA) laws depending on setting and state that the personal training business resides in | • HIPAA: strict policies regarding safety and security of private records <br>• FERPA: policy for the stewards of education data to ensure students' personal information is properly safeguarded and is used only for legitimate purposes and only when absolutely necessary | *ACSM's Resources for the Personal Trainer*, 4th edition (10) <br>• Chapter 21 <br>U.S. Department of Health and Human Services, Health Insurance Portability and Accountability Act (42,43) <br>U.S. Department of Education, Family Educational Rights and Privacy Act (41) <br>*Risk Management for Health/Fitness Professionals* (9) <br>• Chapter 6 |
| **Skill** in obtaining and maintaining rapid access to client health history and emergency contact information | • Create a secure, accurate, current, and alphabetized filing system for active client files. | *ACSM's Resources for the Personal Trainer*, 4th edition (10) <br>• Chapter 21 |

CPT

# REFERENCES

## ACSM REFERENCES:

1. American College of Sports Medicine. ACSM brochures. *American College of Sports Medicine* [Internet]. [cited 2011 Sep 22]. Available from: http://www.acsm.org/access-public-information/brochures-fact-sheets/brochures

2. American College of Sports Medicine. ACSM current comment fact sheet. *American College of Sports Medicine* [Internet]. [cited 2011 Sep 22]. Available from: http://www.acsm.org/access-public-information/brochures-fact-sheets/fact-sheets

3. American College of Sports Medicine. ACSM fit society page. *American College of Sports Medicine* [Internet]. [cited 2011 Sep 22]. Available from: http://www.acsm.org/access-public-information/newsletters/fit-society-page

4. American College of Sports Medicine. ACSM journals. *American College of Sports Medicine* [Internet]. [cited 2012 Mar 4]. Available from http://www.acsm.org/access-public-information/acsm-journals

5. American College of Sports Medicine. Certified personal trainer ACSM certification/renewal form. *American College of Sports Medicine* [Internet]. [cited 2011 Sep 22]. Available from: http://forms.acsm.org/_frm/crt/New/certification_renewal_form.asp

6. American College of Sports Medicine. Certified personal trainer renewing your ACSM certification. *American College of Sports Medicine* [Internet]. [cited 2011 Sep 22]. Available from: http://certification.acsm.org/renew-your-certification

7. American College of Sports Medicine. Certified personal trainer scope of practice. *American College of Sports Medicine* [Internet]. [cited 2011 Sep 22]. Available from: http://certification.acsm.org/acsm-certified-personal-trainer

8. American College of Sports Medicine. Code of ethics of American College of Sports Medicine. *American College of Sports Medicine* [Internet]. [cited 2011 Sep 22]. Available from: http://www.acsm.org/Content/NavigationMenu/MemberServices/MemberResources/CodeofEthics/Code_of_Ethics.htm

9. Bickhoff-Schemek J, Herbert DL, Connaughton DP. *ACSM Risk Management for Health/Fitness Professionals: Legal Issues and Strategies.* Philadelphia (PA): Lippincott Williams & Wilkins; 2009. 407 p.

10. Bushman BA, senior editor. *ACSM's Resources for the Personal Trainer.* 4th ed. Baltimore (MD): Lippincott Williams & Wilkins; 2014.

11. Donnelly JE, Blair SN, Jakicic JM, et al. American College of Sports Medicine position stand. Appropriate physical activity intervention strategies for weight loss and prevention of weight regain for adults. *Med Sci in Sports Exerc.* 2009;41(2):459–71.

12. Garber CE, Blissmer B, Deschenes MR, et al. American College of Sports Medicine position stand. Quantity and quality of exercise for developing and maintaining cardiorespiratory, musculoskeletal, and neuromotor fitness in apparently healthy adults: guidance for prescribing exercise. *Med Sci Sports Exerc.* 2011;43(7):1334–59.

13. Haskell WL, Lee IM, Pate RR, et al. Physical activity and public health: updated recommendation for adults from the American College of Sports Medicine and the American Heart Association. *Med Sci Sports Exerc.* 2007;39(8):1423–34.

14. Nattiv A, Loucks AB, Manore MM, et al. American College of Sports Medicine position stand. The female athlete triad. *Med Sci Sports Exerc.* 2007;39(10):1867–82.

15. Pescatello LS, editor. *ACSM's Guidelines for Exercise Testing and Prescription.* 9th ed. Philadelphia (PA): Lippincott Williams & Wilkins; 2014.

16. Ratamess NA, Alvar BA, Evetock TK, et al. American College of Sports Medicine position stand. Progressive models in resistance training. *Med Sci Sports Exercise.* 2009;41(3):687–708.

17. Sawka MN, Burke LM, Eichner ER, et al. American College of Sports Medicine position stand. Exercise and fluid replacement. *Med Sci Sports Exerc.* 2007;39(2):377–90.

18. Swain DP, senior editor. *ACSM's Resource Manual for Guidelines for Exercise Testing and Prescription.* 7th ed. Baltimore (MD): Lippincott Williams & Wilkins; 2014.

19. Tharrett SJ, McInnis KJ, Peterson JA. *ACSM's Health/Fitness Facility Standards and Guidelines.* 3rd ed. Champaign (IL): Human Kinetics; 2007. 203 p.

## NON-ACSM REFERENCES:

20. Academy of Nutrition and Dietetics Web site [Internet]. Chicago (IL): Academy of Nutrition and Dietetics. [cited 2012 Mar 4]. Available from: www.eatright.org

21. American Red Cross. *American Red Cross First Aid/CPR/AED Participant Manual.* Yardley (PA): Staywell; 2011. 181 p.

22. Purdue Online Writing Lab. MLA In-Text Citations: the basics. *Purdue University* [Internet]. [cited 2012 Sep 8]. Available from: http://owl.english.purdue.edu/owl/resource/747/02/

23. Bureau of Labor Statistics. Occupational outlook handbook, 2010–2011 edition, fitness workers. *Bureau of Labor Statistics* [Internet]. [cited 2011 Sep 22]. Available from: http://www.bls.gov/oco/ocos296.htm

24. Exercise is Medicine. Additional resources. *Exercise is Medicine* [Internet]. [cited 2011 Sep 22]. Available from: http://exerciseismedicine.org/resources.htm

25. The Guide to Community Preventive Services. Community guide topics. Promoting physical activity. *The Guide to Community Preventive Services* [Internet]. [cited 2012 Mar 4]. Available from: http://www.thecommunityguide.org/pa/index.html

26. KettleBell Concepts Web site [Internet]. New York (NY): KettleBell Concepts; [cited 2012 Mar 4]. Available from: http://www.kettlebellconcepts.com/index.php

27. Mayo Clinic. Health information. Diseases and conditions. *Mayo Clinic* [Internet]. [cited 2012 Mar 4]. Available from: http://www.mayoclinic.com/health-information/

28. Microsoft Excel. Manage your personal budget with Excel. *Microsoft Office* [Internet]. [cited 2012 Mar 4]. Available from: http://office.microsoft.com/en-us/excel-help/manage-your-personal-budget-with-excel-HA001045087.aspx

29. National blueprint: increasing physical activity among adults aged 50 and older. Active aging partnerships. *Blueprint Partners* [Internet]. [cited 2012 Mar 4]. Available from: http://www.agingblueprint.org/partnership.cfm

30. National Institute of Health. Health information, health topics. *National Institute of Health* [Internet]. [cited 2012 Mar 4]. Available from: http://health.nih.gov/see_all_topics.aspx

31. National Institute of Health. Research and training. Science education. *National Institute of Health* [Internet]. [cited 2012 Mar 4]. Available from: http://www.nih.gov/science/education.htm

32. National Physical Activity Plan Web site [Internet]. Columbia (SC): National Physical Activity Plan [cited 2012 Mar 4]. Available from: http://www.physicalactivityplan.org

33. Perform Better. Balance and stabilization training exercises. *Perform Better* [Internet]. [cited 2012 Mar 4]. Available from: www.performbetter.com

34. President's Council on Fitness, Sports & Nutrition. Resources. *President's Council on Fitness, Sports & Nutrition* [Internet]. [cited 2012 Mar 4]. Available from: http://www.fitness.gov/resources-and-grants/resources/

35. Robinson L, Segal R, Segal J, et al. Relaxation technique for stress relief. *Helpguide* [Internet]. [cited 2012 Mar 4]. Available

from: http://helpguide.org/mental/stress_relief_meditation_yoga_relaxation.htm

36.  Stoppler MC, Sheil WC, editor. Stress management techniques. *MedicineNet* [Internet]. [cited 2012 Mar 4]. Available from: http://www.medicinenet.com/stress_management_techniques/page3.htm

37.  Thera-Band Academy. Theraband exercises. *Thera-Band Academy* [Internet]. [cited 2012 Mar 4].Available from: http://www.thera-bandacademy.com/

38.  U.S. Copyright Office Web site [Internet]. Washington (DC): U.S. Copyright Office; [cited 2012 Mar 4]. Available from: http://www.copyright.gov/

39.  U.S. Department of Agriculture. USDA center for nutrition policy and promotion. *United States Department of Agriculture* [Internet]. [cited 2011 Sep 26]. Available from: http://www.choosemyplate.gov/index.html

40.  U.S. Department of Agriculture. USDA dietary guidelines for Americans. *United States Department of Agriculture* [Internet]. [cited 2011 Sep 26]. Available from: http://www.cnpp.usda.gov/DietaryGuidelines.htm

41.  U.S. Department of Education. Family educational rights and privacy act. *U.S. Department of Education* [Internet]. [cited 2012 Mar 4]. Available from: www2.ed.gov/offices/OM/fpco/ferpa/index.html

42.  U.S. Department of Health & Human Services. Health information privacy. *U.S. Department of Health & Human Services* [Internet]. [cited 2012 Mar 4]. Available from: http://www.hhs.gov/ocr/privacy/

43.  U.S. Department of Health & Human Services. Summary of the HIPPA privacy rule. *U.S. Department of Health & Human Services* [Internet]. [cited 2011 Sep 22]. Available from: http://www.hhs.gov/ocr/privacy/hipaa/understanding/summary/privacysummary.pdf

44.  WebMD. Healthy living A–Z. *WebMD* [Internet]. [cited 2012 Mar 4]. Available from: http://www.webmd.com/a-to-z-guides/healthy-living/default.htm

45.  WebMD. Stress management health center. *WebMD* [Internet]. [cited 2012 Mar 4]. Available from: http://www.webmd.com/balance/stress-management/stress-management-relieving-stress

DIRECTIONS: Each of the numbered items or incomplete statements in this section is followed by answers or by completions of the statement. Select the ONE lettered answer or completion that is BEST in each case.

1. Which of the following exercise modes allows buoyancy to reduce the potential for musculoskeletal injury?
   A) Cycling
   B) Walking
   C) Skiing
   D) Water exercise

2. In which stage of motivational readiness is a person who is an irregular exerciser?
   A) Precontemplation
   B) Contemplation
   C) Preparation
   D) Action

3. Which of the following medications is designed to modify blood cholesterol levels?
   A) Nitrates
   B) β-blockers
   C) Antihyperlipidemics
   D) Aspirin

4. Which of the following represents more than 90% of the fat stored in the body and is composed of a glycerol molecule connected to three fatty acids?
   A) Phospholipids
   B) Cholesterol
   C) Triglycerides (TG)
   D) Free fatty acids

5. Limited flexibility of which of the following muscle groups increases the risk of low back pain?
   A) Quadriceps
   B) Hamstrings
   C) Hip flexors
   D) Gluteus maximus

6. Calcium, phosphorus, magnesium, potassium, sulfur, sodium, and chloride are examples of _____.
   A) Macrominerals
   B) Microminerals
   C) Proteins
   D) Vitamins

7. Which of the following terms represents an imaginary horizontal plane passing through the midsection of the body and dividing it into upper and lower portions?
   A) Sagittal
   B) Frontal
   C) Transverse
   D) Superior

8. A personal trainer fails to spot a client performing heavy incline dumbbell presses and the client injures himself when the dumbbell is dropped on his face. Which of the following identify the appropriate type of negligence displayed in this scenario?
   A) Admission
   B) Commission
   C) Omission
   D) Legal

9. Which of the following blood pressure (BP) readings would characterize hypertension in the adult?
   A) 100/60 mm Hg
   B) 110/70 mm Hg
   C) 120/80 mm Hg
   D) 140/90 mm Hg

10. Which of the following stages define people having the greatest risk of relapse?
    A) Precontemplation
    B) Contemplation
    C) Preparation
    D) Action

11. Uncoordinated gait, headache, dizziness, vomiting, and elevated body temperature are signs and symptoms of _____.
    A) Acute exposure to the cold
    B) Hypothermia
    C) Heat exhaustion and heat stroke
    D) Acute altitude sickness

12. Moving the hand from palm up to palm down with the elbow flexed at 90 degrees _____.
    A) Adducts the ulna
    B) Internally rotates the radius
    C) Internally rotates the humerus
    D) Flexes the ulna

13. What is a subject's work rate in watts if he pedals on a Monark cycle ergometer at 50 revolutions per minute (RPM) at a resistance of 2.0 kp? Assume that one revolution of the cycle ergometer flywheel is 6 m long.
    A) 10 W
    B) 50 W
    C) 100 W
    D) 200 W

14. Relative proportions of fat and fat-free (lean) tissue can be reported as _____.
    A) Percentage body fat
    B) Body composition
    C) Body mass index (BMI)
    D) Weight-to-waist circumference ratio

15. How many calories are contained in a food bar that contains 5 g of fat, 30 g of carbohydrates including 4 g of fiber, and 3 g of protein?
    A) 161 kcal
    B) 168 kcal
    C) 177 kcal
    D) 193 kcal

16. Verbal encouragement, material incentives, self-praise, and use of specific contingency contracts are examples of _____.
    A) Shaping
    B) Reinforcement
    C) Antecedent control
    D) Setting goals

17. Which physiologic response(s) would be expected to occur under conditions of high ambient temperature?
    A) Decreased maximal oxygen uptake
    B) Decreased heart rate at rest
    C) Increased heart rate at submaximal workload
    D) Decreased maximal heart rate

18. Regular exercise will result in what chronic adaptation in cardiac output (CO) during exercise at the same workload?
    A) Increase
    B) Decrease
    C) No change
    D) Increase during dynamic exercise only

19. Which of the following conditions is characterized by a decrease in bone mass and density, producing bone porosity and fragility?
    A) Osteoarthritis
    B) Osteomyelitis
    C) Epiphyseal osteomyelitis
    D) Osteoporosis

20. Studies designed to measure the success of a program based on some quantifiable data that can be analyzed examine _____.
    A) Incomes
    B) Outcomes
    C) Client progress notes
    D) Attendance records

21. When using the original Borg scale (6–20) for the general public, exercise intensity should be maintained between _____.
    A) 7 and 10
    B) 12 and 16
    C) 17 and 18
    D) 19 and 20

22. Rotation of the anterior surface of a bone toward the midline of the body is called _____.
    A) Medial rotation
    B) Lateral rotation
    C) Supination
    D) Pronation

23. At what level is high-density lipoprotein (HDL) considered a risk factor in the development of cardiovascular disease?
    A) $<200$ mg $\cdot$ dL$^{-1}$
    B) $<110$ mg $\cdot$ dL$^{-1}$
    C) $<60$ mg $\cdot$ dL$^{-1}$
    D) $<40$ mg $\cdot$ dL$^{-1}$

24. Which of the following health history combinations would place an individual into the MODERATE-RISK category for coronary artery disease (CAD)?
    A) HDL $<50$ mg $\cdot$ dL$^{-1}$; current smoker; female waist-to-hip ratio $<0.86$
    B) HDL $>60$ mg $\cdot$ dL$^{-1}$; current smoker; male waist girth $>102$ cm
    C) HDL $<40$ mg $\cdot$ dL$^{-1}$; current smoker; BMI $<28$
    D) HDL $>60$ mg $\cdot$ dL$^{-1}$; current smoker; fasting blood glucose $>100$

25. What could be an alternative to the contraindicated, high-risk yoga plough (supine legs overhead) exercise?
    A) Squats to 90 degrees
    B) Flexion with rotation
    C) Double knee to chest
    D) Lateral neck stretches

26. Which of the following water-soluble vitamins must be consumed on a daily basis?
    A) Vitamins A and C
    B) Vitamins A, D, E, and K
    C) Vitamins B complex and C
    D) Vitamins A, B complex, D, and K

27. Which of the following is NOT true regarding the psychological benefits of regular exercise in the elderly?
    A) Self-concept
    B) Life satisfaction
    C) Stimulate appetite
    D) Self-efficacy

28. What is angina pectoris?
    A) Discomfort associated with myocardial ischemia
    B) Discomfort associated with hypertension
    C) Discomfort associated with heartburn
    D) Discomfort associated with papillary necrosis

29. To determine program effectiveness, psychological theories provide a conceptual framework for assessment and _____.
    A) Management of programs or interventions
    B) Application of cognitive-behavioral or motivational principles
    C) Measurement
    D) All of the above

30. Information gathered by way of an appropriate health screening allows the personal trainer to develop specific exercise programs that are appropriate to the individual needs and goals of the client. This is called the _____.
    A) Physical Activity Readiness Questionnaire (PAR-Q)
    B) Heart rate (HR)
    C) Exercise prescription
    D) Graded exercise test (GXT)

31. To maximize safety during a physical fitness assessment, which of the following items should be addressed?
    A) Hospital emergency room contact information
    B) Cardiopulmonary resuscitation (CPR) training of the assessment administrator
    C) Emergency plan
    D) All of the above

32. HR can be measured by counting the number of pulses in a specified time period at one of several locations, including the radial and carotid arteries. Which of the following is a special precaution when taking the carotid pulse?
    A) When the HR is measured by palpation, the first two fingers should be used and not the thumb, because the thumb has its own pulse.
    B) HR taken during exercise sometimes exceed 200 bpm, making it too difficult to count at the carotid artery.
    C) If the HR is taken at the carotid artery, do not press too hard or a reflex slowing of the heart can occur and cause dizziness.
    D) The HR should never be taken at the carotid artery.

33. When exercise training children, _____.
    A) Exercise programs should increase physical fitness in the short term and strength and power in the long term.
    B) Strength training should be avoided for safety reasons.
    C) Increasing the rate of training intensity more than approximately 10% per week increases the likelihood of overuse injuries of bone.
    D) Children with exercise-induced asthma are often unable to lead active lives.

34. Which of the following risk factors for the development of CAD has the greatest likelihood of being influenced by regular exercise?
    A) Smoking
    B) Cholesterol
    C) Type 1 diabetes
    D) Hypertension

35. At minimum, professionals performing fitness assessments on others should possess which combination of the following?
    A) CPR and American College of Sports Medicine (ACSM) Certified Personal Trainer (CPT)
    B) Advanced cardiac life support and ACSM Health Fitness Specialist (HFS)
    C) Advanced cardiac life support and ACSM Clinical Exercise Specialist
    D) Only physicians can perform fitness assessments.

36. Which of the following components of the exercise prescription work inversely with each other?
    A) Intensity and duration
    B) Mode and intensity
    C) Mode and duration
    D) Mode and frequency

37. Which of the following types of muscle stretching can cause residual muscle soreness, is time consuming, and typically requires a partner?
    A) Static
    B) Ballistic
    C) Proprioceptive neuromuscular facilitation (PNF)
    D) All of the above

38. Failure of a CPT to perform in a generally acceptable standard is called _____.
    A) Malpractice
    B) Malfeasance
    C) Negligence
    D) None of the above

39. Most sedentary people who begin an exercise program are likely to stop within _____.
    A) 1–2 d
    B) 3–6 wk
    C) 1 mo
    D) 3–6 mo

40. Reasons for fitness testing of the older adult include _____.
    A) Evaluation of progress
    B) Exercise prescription
    C) Motivation
    D) All of the above

41. Feeling good about being able to perform an activity or skill, such as finally being able to run a mile or to increase the speed of walking a mile, is an example of an _____.
    A) Extrinsic reward
    B) Intrinsic reward
    C) External stimulus
    D) Internal stimulus

42. An important safety consideration for exercise equipment in a fitness center includes _____.
    A) Flexibility of equipment to allow for different body sizes
    B) Ability of equipment to restrict range of motion (ROM)
    C) Affordability of equipment to allow for changing out equipment periodically
    D) Mobility of equipment to allow for easy rearrangement

43. The ACSM recommendation for intensity, duration, and frequency of cardiorespiratory exercise for apparently healthy individuals includes _____.
    A) Intensity of 60%–90% maximal heart rate ($HR_{max}$), duration of 20–60 min, and frequency of 3–5 d a week
    B) Intensity of 85%–90% $HR_{max}$, duration of 30 min, and frequency of 3 d a week
    C) Intensity of 50%–70% $HR_{max}$, duration of 15–45 min, and frequency of 5 d a week
    D) Intensity of 60%–90% $HR_{max}$ reserve, duration of 20–60 min, and frequency of 7 d a week

44. A method of strength and power training that involves an eccentric loading of muscles and tendons followed immediately by an explosive concentric contraction is called _____.
    A) Plyometrics
    B) Periodization
    C) Supersets
    D) Isotonic reversals

45. Which of the following personnel is responsible for program design as well as implementation of that program?
    A) Administrative assistant
    B) Personal trainer
    C) Manager or director
    D) Health fitness specialist

46. What is the purpose of agreements, releases, and consent forms?
    A) To inform the client of participation risks, as well as the rights of the client and the facility
    B) To inform the client what he or she can and cannot do in the facility
    C) To define the relationship between the facility operator and the personal trainer
    D) Body composition, flexibility, cardiorespiratory fitness, and muscular fitness

47. After 30 yr of age, skeletal muscle strength begins to decline, primarily because of which of the following?
    A) A gain in fat tissue
    B) A gain in lean tissue
    C) A loss of muscle mass caused by a loss of muscle fibers
    D) Myogenic precursor cell inhibition

48. The Health Belief Model assumes that people will engage in a behavior, such as exercise, when _____.
    A) There is a perceived threat of disease.
    B) External motivation is provided.
    C) Optimal environmental conditions are met.
    D) Internal motivation outweighs external circumstances.

49. The informed consent document _____.
    A) Is a legal document
    B) Provides immunity from prosecution
    C) Provides an explanation of the test to the client
    D) Legally protects the rights of the client

50. A measure of muscular endurance is _____.
    A) One repetition maximum
    B) Three-repetition maximum
    C) Number of curl-ups in 1 min
    D) Number of curl-ups in 3 min

51. If a client exercises too much without rest days or develops a minor injury and does not allow time for the injury to heal, what can occur?
    A) An overuse injury
    B) Shin splints
    C) Sleep deprivation
    D) Decreased physical conditioning

52. The ACSM recommends that exercise intensity be prescribed within what percentage of oxygen uptake reserve ($\dot{V}O_{2max}R$) range?
    A) 30% and 50%
    B) 50% and 70%
    C) 40%–60% and 89%
    D) 75% and 100%

53. The ACSM recommends how many repetitions (reps) of each exercise for muscular strength and endurance?
    A) 5–6 reps
    B) 8–12 reps
    C) 12–20 reps
    D) More than 20 reps

54. Which of the following are changes seen as a result of regular chronic exercise?
    A) Decreased HR at rest
    B) Increased stroke volume at rest
    C) No change in CO at rest
    D) All of the above

55. While assessing the behavioral changes associated with an exercise program, which of the following would be categorized under the cognitive process of the Transtheoretical Model?
    A) Stimulus control
    B) Reinforcement management
    C) Self-reevaluation
    D) Self-liberation

56. Fitness assessment is an important aspect of the training program because it provides information for which of the following?
    A) Developing the exercise prescription
    B) Evaluating proper nutritional choices
    C) Diagnosing musculoskeletal injury
    D) Developing appropriate billing categories

57. For individuals undertaking nonmedically supervised weight loss initiatives to reduce energy intake, the ACSM recommends weight loss of approximately _____.
    A) 1–2 lb $\cdot$ wk$^{-1}$ (0.5–1 kg)
    B) 5–8 lb $\cdot$ wk$^{-1}$ (2.3–4 kg)
    C) 8–10 lb $\cdot$ wk$^{-1}$ (4–4.5 kg)
    D) 10–15 lb $\cdot$ wk$^{-1}$ (4.5–7 kg)

58. Which of the following assumes that a person will adopt appropriate health behaviors if he or she feels the consequences are severe and feel personally vulnerable?
    A) Learning theories
    B) Health Belief Model
    C) Transtheoretical Model
    D) Stages of Motivational Readiness

59. Identify the appropriate self-directed evaluation tool used as a quick health screening before beginning any exercise program.
    A) Minnesota Multiphasic Personality Inventory (MMPI)
    B) Ratings of Perceived Exertion (RPE-Borg scale)
    C) PAR-Q
    D) Exercise Electrocardiogram (E-ECG)

60. You have examined your patient's health screening documents and obtained physiologic resting measurements and you decide to proceed with a single session of fitness assessments. Identify the recommended order of administration.
    A) Flexibility, cardiorespiratory fitness, body composition, and muscular fitness
    B) Flexibility, body composition, muscular fitness, and cardiorespiratory fitness
    C) Body composition, cardiorespiratory fitness, muscular fitness, and flexibility

61. Implementing emergency procedures must include the fitness center's _____.
    A) Management
    B) Staff
    C) Clients
    D) Management and staff

62. Which of the following is a possible medical emergency that a client can experience during an exercise session?
    A) Hypoglycemia
    B) Hypotension
    C) Hyperglycemia
    D) All of the above

63. In commercial settings, clients should be more extensively screened for potential health risks. The information solicited should include which of the following?
    A) Personal medical history
    B) Present medical status
    C) Medication
    D) All of the above

64. Generally, low-fit or sedentary persons may benefit from _____.
    A) Shorter duration, higher intensity, and higher frequency of exercise
    B) Longer duration, higher intensity, and higher frequency of exercise
    C) Shorter duration, lower intensity, and higher frequency of exercise
    D) Shorter duration, higher intensity, and lower frequency of exercise.

65. What is the planning tool that addresses the organization's short- and long-term goals; identifies the steps needed to achieve the goals; and gives the time line, priority, and allocation of resources to each goal?
    A) Financial plan
    B) Strategic plan
    C) Risk management plan
    D) Marketing plan

66. Producing red blood cells, protecting organs and tissues, and providing support for the body are all functions of what tissue?
    A) Collagen
    B) Muscle
    C) Tendon
    D) Bones

67. Through which valve in the heart does blood flow when moving from the right atrium to the right ventricle?
    A) Bicuspid valve
    B) Tricuspid valve
    C) Pulmonic valve
    D) Aortic valve

68. Which of the following is considered an abnormal curve of the spine with lateral deviation of the vertebral column in the frontal plane?
    A) Lordosis
    B) Scoliosis
    C) Kyphosis
    D) Primary curve

69. Which of the following will increase stability?
    A) Lowering the center of gravity
    B) Raising the center of gravity
    C) Decreasing the base of support
    D) Moving the center of gravity farther from the edge of the base of support

70. Which of the following muscle groups is most likely weak when slapping of the foot occurs during heel strike and/or increased knee and hip flexion during swing are observed in running?
    A) Gluteus medius and minimus
    B) Quadriceps femoris
    C) Plantarflexors
    D) Dorsiflexors

71. Modifiable primary risk factors for CAD include _____.
    A) Hypertension, dyslipidemia, advancing age, and tobacco smoking
    B) Homocysteine, lipoprotein (a), C-reactive protein, and gender
    C) Obesity, diabetes mellitus (DM), tobacco smoking, and sedentary lifestyle
    D) Tobacco smoking, dyslipidemia, hypertension, and homocysteine

72. Many of the major health organizations in the United States recommend a minimum of _____ min of physical activity on most days of the week to achieve significant health benefits and protection from chronic diseases, such as coronary heart disease.
    A) 30
    B) 60
    C) 10
    D) 90

73. Which of the following is an example of increasing self-efficacy by setting several short-term goals to attain a long-term goal?
    A) An application of cognitive-behavioral principles
    B) Shaping
    C) A component of antecedent control
    D) An explanatory theory

74. Establishing specific expectations of what you are willing to do as a counselor and staying focused on exercise and physical activity issues and behavioral skills related to exercise are strategies for handling which type of participant?
    A) Dissatisfied participant
    B) Needy participant
    C) Hostile participant
    D) Shy participant

75. Adults age physiologically at individual rates. Therefore, adults of any specified age will vary widely in their physiologic responses to exercise testing. Special considerations should be given to the older adult when giving a fitness test because:
    A) Age may be accompanied by deconditioning and disease
    B) Age automatically predisposes the older adult to clinical depression and neurologic diseases
    C) The older adult cannot be physically stressed beyond 75% of age-adjusted maximum heart rate
    D) The older adult is not as motivated to exercise as a younger person.

76. Which of the following adaptations would NOT be expected to occur as a result of long-term aerobic training?
    A) Decrease in resting HR ($HR_{rest}$)
    B) Increase in resting stroke volume
    C) Increase in resting CO
    D) Increase in $HR_{max}$

77. Compared with running, swimming will result in _____ even if exercise intensity is the same.
    A) A higher HR
    B) A lower HR
    C) A lower CO
    D) A higher CO

78. An increase in both systolic BP (SBP) and diastolic BP (DBP) at rest and during exercise often accompanies aging. BP usually increases because of _____.
    A) Increased arterial compliance and decreased arterial stiffness
    B) Decreased arterial compliance and increased arterial stiffness
    C) Decrease in both arterial compliance and arterial stiffness
    D) Increase in both arterial compliance and arterial stiffness

79. Which condition is commonly associated with a progressive decline in bone mineral density and calcium content in postmenopausal women?
    A) Osteoarthritis
    B) Osteoporosis
    C) Arthritis
    D) Epiphysitis

80. Which of the following is a result of an older person participating in an exercise program?
    A) Overall improvement in the quality of life and increased independence
    B) No changes in the quality of life but an increase in longevity
    C) Increased longevity but a loss of bone mass
    D) Loss of bone mass with a concomitant increase in bone density

81. In response to regular resistance training, _____.
    A) Older men and women demonstrate similar or even greater strength gains when compared with younger individuals.
    B) Younger men have greater gains in strength than older men.
    C) Younger women have greater gains in strength than older women.
    D) Younger men and women demonstrate similar or greater strength gains compared with older persons.

82. Which of the following statements about confidentiality is NOT correct?
    A) All records must be kept by the program director/manager under lock and key.
    B) Data must be available to all individuals who need to see it.
    C) Data should be kept on file for at least 1 yr before being discarded.
    D) Sensitive information (e.g., participant's name) needs to be protected.

83. Which of the following statements best describes capital budgets?
    A) Include the costs of equipment and building or facility expense
    B) Include the costs to operate a program
    C) Are not necessary with fitness programs
    D) Are included as part of the balance sheet in financial reports

84. Emergency procedures and safety planning should address which of the following?
    A) Injury prevention
    B) Basic principles for exercise training
    C) Metabolic calculations
    D) Common exercise scenarios

85. What is the most appropriate action in assisting a person having a seizure?
    A) Hold the person down so that he or she does not hurt himself or herself.
    B) Do not restrain the person but be sure that he or she is in a safe area.
    C) Place a wedge in the person's mouth so that he or she does not swallow the tongue.
    D) Ignore the person and allow the seizure to pass.

86. Within a skeletal muscle fiber, large amounts of calcium are stored in the _____.
    A) Nuclei
    B) Mitochondria
    C) Myosin
    D) Sarcoplasmic reticulum

87. The amount of blood ejected from the heart per minute is referred to as _____.
    A) Stroke volume
    B) HR
    C) CO
    D) End-diastolic volume

88. A male client is 42 yr old. His father died of a heart attack at age 62 yr. He has a consistent resting BP (measured over 6 wk) of 132/86 mm Hg and a total serum cholesterol of 5.4 mmol · L$^{-1}$. Based on his CAD risk stratification, which of the following activities is appropriate?
    A) Maximal assessment of cardiorespiratory fitness without a physician supervising
    B) Submaximal assessment of cardiorespiratory fitness without a physician supervising
    C) Vigorous exercise without a prior medical assessment
    D) Vigorous exercise without a prior physician-supervised exercise test

89. The definition of cardiorespiratory fitness is _____.
    A) The maximal force that a muscle or muscle group can generate in a single effort
    B) The coordinated capacity of the heart, blood vessels, respiratory system, and tissue metabolic systems to take in, deliver, and use oxygen
    C) The ability to sustain a held maximal force or to continue repeated submaximal contractions
    D) The functional ROM about a joint

90. The primary effects of chronic exercise training on blood lipids include _____.
    A) Decreased TG and increased HDL
    B) Decreased total cholesterol and low-density lipoproteins (LDL)
    C) Decreased HDL and increased LDL
    D) Decreased total cholesterol and increased HDL

91. A transient deficiency of blood flow to the myocardium resulting from an imbalance between oxygen demand and oxygen supply is known as _____.
    A) Infarction
    B) Angina
    C) Ischemia
    D) Thrombosis

92. Special precautions for patients with hypertension include all of the following EXCEPT _____.
    A) Avoiding muscle strengthening exercises that involve low resistance
    B) Avoiding activities that involve the Valsalva maneuver
    C) Monitoring for arrhythmias in a person taking diuretics
    D) Avoiding exercise if resting SBP is >200 mm Hg or DBP is >115 mm Hg

93. A 62-yr-old, obese factory worker complains of pain in his right shoulder on arm abduction; on evaluation, decreased ROM and strength are noted. You also notice that he is beginning to use accessory muscles to substitute movements and to compensate. These symptoms may indicate _____.
    A) A referred pain from a herniated lumbar disk
    B) Rotator cuff strain or impingement
    C) Angina
    D) Advanced stages of multiple sclerosis

94. Which of the following statements regarding cool-down is FALSE?
    A) The emphasis should be large muscle activity performed at a low-to-moderate intensity.
    B) Increasing venous return should be a priority during cool-down.
    C) The potential for improving flexibility may be improved during cool-down as compared with warm-up.
    D) Between 1 and 2 min are recommended for an adequate cool-down.

95. A personal trainer should modify exercise sessions for participants with hypertension by _____.
    A) Shortening the cool-down to <5 min
    B) Eliminating resistance training completely
    C) Prolonging the cool-down
    D) Implementing high-intensity (>85% of heart rate reserve [HRR]), short-duration intervals

96. The Health Belief Model assumes that people will engage in a given behavior, such as increasing their level of daily activity, when _____.
    A) There is a perceived threat of disease.
    B) There is the belief of susceptibility to disease.
    C) The risk of disease is nonthreatening to the individual.
    D) Only A and B of the above.

97. A 35-yr-old woman reduced her caloric intake by 1,200 kcal · wk$^{-1}$. How much weight will she lose in 26 wk?
    A) 8.9 lb
    B) 12.0 lb
    C) 26.0 lb
    D) 34.3 lb

98. From question 97, how much weight will she lose in 26 wk if she integrated a 1-mi walk three times per week into her weight loss program?
    A) 3 lb
    B) 6 lb
    C) 11 lb
    D) 15 lb

99. The metabolic syndrome includes dyslipidemia, insulin resistance, elevated BP, and what other component?
    A) Amenorrhea
    B) Laxative use
    C) Abdominal obesity
    D) 25.0 BMI

100. Which of the following is a FALSE statement regarding an informed consent?
    A) The informed consent is not a legal document.
    B) The informed consent does not provide legal immunity to a facility or individual in the event of injury to an individual.
    C) Negligence, improper test administration, inadequate personnel qualifications, and insufficient safety procedures are all items that are expressly covered by the informed consent.
    D) The consent form does not relieve the facility or individual of the responsibility to do everything possible to ensure the safety of the individual.

# CPT EXAMINATION ANSWERS AND EXPLANATIONS

**1—D.** Water exercise

Water exercise has gained in popularity because the buoyancy properties of water help to reduce the potential for musculoskeletal injury and may even allow injured people an opportunity to exercise without further injury. Various activities may be offered in a water-exercise class. Walking, jogging, and dance activity all may be adapted for water. Water-exercise classes typically should combine the benefits of the buoyancy properties of water with the resistive properties of water. In this regard, both an aerobic stimulus as well as activity to enhance muscular strength and endurance may be provided.

**2—C.** Preparation

Preparation is an individual who is planning for or irregularly exercising, whereas the stage of action represents a person who is currently exercising.

**3—C.** Antihyperlipidemics

Nitrates and nitroglycerine are antianginals (used to reduce chest pain associated with angina pectoris). β-Blockers are antihypertensives (used to reduce BP by inhibiting the action of adrenergic neurotransmitters at the β-receptor, thereby promoting peripheral vasodilation). β-Blockers also are designed to reduce BP by inhibiting the action of adrenergic neurotransmitters at the β-receptors, thereby decreasing CO. Antihyperlipidemics control blood lipids, especially cholesterol and LDL. Aspirin helps lower blood platelet coagulation making the blood less "sticky."

**4—C.** TG

Dietary fats include TG, sterols (*e.g.*, cholesterol), and phospholipids. TG represent more than 90% of the fat stored in the body. A TG is a glycerol molecule connected to three fatty acid molecules. The fatty acids are identified by the amount of "saturation" or the number of single or double bonds that link the carbon atoms. Saturated fatty acids only have single bonds. Monounsaturated fatty acids have one double bond, and polyunsaturated fatty acids have two or more double bonds.

**5—B.** Hamstrings

An adequate ROM or joint mobility is requisite for optimal musculoskeletal health. Specifically, limited flexibility of the low back and hamstring regions may relate to an increased risk for development of chronic low back pain and disability. Activities that will enhance or maintain musculoskeletal flexibility should be included as a part of a comprehensive preventive or rehabilitative exercise program.

**6—A.** Macrominerals

Minerals are inorganic substances that perform various functions in the body. Many play an important role in assisting enzymes (or coenzymes) that are necessary for the proper functioning of body systems. They also are found in cell membranes, hormones, muscles, and connective tissues as well as electrolytes in body fluids. Minerals are considered to be either macrominerals (needed in relatively large doses), such as calcium, phosphorus, magnesium, potassium, sulfur, sodium, and chloride, or microminerals (needed in very small amounts), such as iron, zinc, selenium, manganese, molybdenum, iodine, copper, chromium, and fluoride.

**7—C.** Transverse

The body has three cardinal planes, and each individual plane is perpendicular to the other two. Movement occurs along these planes. The sagittal plane divides the body into right and left parts, and the midsagittal plane is represented by an imaginary vertical plane passing through the midline of the body, dividing it into right and left halves. The frontal plane is represented by an imaginary vertical plane passing through the body, dividing it into front and back halves. The transverse plane represents an imaginary horizontal plane passing through the midsection of the body and dividing it into upper and lower portions.

**8—C.** Omission

*Negligence* is a failure to conform one's conduct to a generally accepted standard or duty. *Gross negligence* (also referred to as reckless conduct or willful/wanton conduct) is a conscious, voluntary act (commission), or failure to act (omission), in reckless disregard of the legal duty and of the consequences to the plaintiff. In this situation, the trainer failed to spot (omission) the client, which resulted in injury.

**9—D.** 140/90 mm Hg

To be classified as hypertensive, the SBP must equal or exceed 140 mm Hg or the diastolic pressure must equal or exceed 90 mm Hg as measured on two separate occasions, preferably days apart. An elevation of either the systolic or diastolic pressure is classified as hypertension.

**10—D.** Action

People in the action stage are at the greatest risk of relapse. Instruction about avoiding injury, exercise boredom, and burnout is important for those who have recently begun an exercise program. Providing social support and praise are the most important contributors to maintained activity. Planning for high-risk, relapse situations (*e.g.*, vacations, sickness, bad weather, increased demands on time) is also important. The exercise professional can emphasize that a short lapse in activity can be a learning opportunity and is not failure. Planning can help to develop coping strategies and to eliminate the "all-or-none" thinking sometimes typical of people who have missed several exercise sessions and think they need to give it up.

**11—C.** Heat exhaustion and heat stroke

Heat exhaustion and heat stroke are serious conditions that result from a combination of the metabolic heat generated from exercise accompanied by dehydration and electrolyte loss from sweating. Signs and symptoms include uncoordinated gait, headache, dizziness, vomiting, and elevated body temperature. If these conditions are present, exercise must be stopped. Attempts to rehydrate, perhaps intravenously, should be attempted, and the body must be cooled by any means possible. The person should be placed in the supine position with the feet elevated.

**12—B.** Internally rotates the radius

*Rotation* is a movement of long bones about their long axis. Angular movements decrease or increase the joint angle produced by the articulating bones. The four types of angular movements are flexion (a movement that decreases the joint angle, bringing the bones closer together), extension (the movement opposite to flexion decreasing the joint angle between two bones), abduction (the movement of a body part away from the midline in a lateral direction), and adduction (the opposite of abduction, the movement toward the midline of the body).

**13—A.** 10 W

This question does not require the use of a metabolic formula because it is asking for the subject's work rate. The steps to answering this question are as follows: Write down the known values and convert those values to the appropriate units — 5 RPM $\times$ 6 m = 30 m $\cdot$ min$^{-1}$ (each revolution

on a Monark cycle ergometer = 6 m); 2.0 kp = 2.0 kg. Write down the formula for work rate: Work rate = force $\times$ distance/time. Substitute the known values for the variable name: Work rate = 2.0 kg $\times$ 30 m $\cdot$ min$^{-1}$; Work rate = 60 kg $\cdot$ m $\cdot$ min$^{-1}$. The question asks for watts, so divide the work rate (kg $\cdot$ m $\cdot$ min$^{-1}$) by 6.

$$W = kg \cdot m \cdot min^{-1}/6$$
$$= 600 \ kg \cdot m \cdot min^{-1}/6$$
$$= 10$$

**14—B.** Body composition

Body composition refers to the relative proportions of fat and fat-free (lean) tissue in the body. To determine the relative proportion of fat mass or fat-free mass, each is divided into the total body mass.

**15—A.** 161 kcal

There are 4 kcal $\cdot$ g$^{-1}$ of carbohydrate and protein and 9 kcal $\cdot$ g$^{-1}$ of fat.

5 g $\times$ 9 kcal = 45 kcal from fat
3 g $\times$ 4 kcal = 12 kcal from protein
26 g $\times$ 4 kcal = 104 kcal from carbohydrate

Total calories in the bar is 161 kcal. Fiber is a carbohydrate but, because it is not absorbed, there are no absorbable carbohydrates and it should not be used in determining calorie content of food.

**16—B.** Reinforcement

*Reinforcement* is the positive or negative consequence for performing or not performing a behavior. *Positive consequences* are rewards that motivate behavior. This can include both intrinsic and extrinsic rewards. *Intrinsic rewards* are the benefits gained because of the rewarding nature of the activity. *Extrinsic or external rewards* are the positive outcomes received from others, which may include encouragement and praise or material reinforcements such as T-shirts and money.

**17—C.** Increased heart rate at submaximal workload

Compared with a cool and dry environment, a higher metabolic cost exists at submaximal workloads when exercising in the heat and humidity. Thus, the exercise prescription should be altered by lowering the work intensity. Evaporation of sweat cools the skin; therefore, wiping away sweat would decrease evaporative cooling and heat loss. Heat loss by convection, such as that which occurs when a breeze is created by running, can be beneficial but not unless the workload of activity is reduced. It is necessary in the heat and humidity to become acclimated to the environment; it will not occur by being sedentary.

**18—C.** No change

CO does not change significantly, primarily because the person is performing the same amount of work and, thus, responds with the same CO. It should be noted, however, that the same CO is now being generated with a lower HR and higher stroke volume compared with when the person was untrained.

**19—D.** Osteoporosis

Every population that has been studied exhibits a decline in bone mass with aging. Therefore, bone loss is considered by most clinicians to be an inevitable consequence of aging. *Osteoporosis* refers to a condition that is characterized by a decrease in bone mass and density, producing bone porosity and fragility, and it refers to the clinical condition of low bone mass and the accompanying increase in susceptibility to fracture from minor trauma. The age at which bone loss begins and the rate at which it occurs vary greatly between males and females. Risk factors for age-related bone loss and development of clinical osteoporosis include being a white or Asian female, being thin-boned or petite, having a low peak bone mass at maturity, having a family history of osteoporosis, premature or surgically induced menopause, alcohol abuse and/or cigarette smoking, sedentary lifestyle, and inadequate dietary calcium intake.

**20—B.** Outcomes

Outcomes are designed to measure the success of a program based on the outcome for a patient or client. Outcome studies require quantifiable data that can be analyzed — data that study the success of a program in terms of quantifiable measures (*e.g.*, change in body composition). Measuring client satisfaction, level of change, length of time for change to occur, or percentage of clients who reach their goals are other examples of outcomes. Outcomes can be very helpful in marketing programs as well as in comparing one facility with another.

**21—B.** 12 and 16

Although some learning is required on the part of the participant, the rating of perceived exertion (RPE) should be considered an adjunct to HR measures. The RPE can be used as a reliable barometer of exercise intensity. The RPE is particularly useful when participants are incapable of monitoring their pulse accurately or when medications such as β-blockers alter the HR response to exercise. The ACSM recommends an exercise intensity

that will elicit an RPE within a range of 12–16 on the original Borg scale of 6–20.

**22—A.** Medial rotation

*Rotation* is the turning of a bone around its own longitudinal axis or around another bone. Rotation of the anterior surface of the bone toward the midline of the body is *medial rotation*, whereas rotation of the same bone away from the midline is *lateral rotation*. *Supination* is a specialized rotation of the forearm that results in the palm of the hand being turned forward (anteriorly). *Pronation* (the opposite of supination) is the rotation of the forearm that results in the palm of the hand being directed backward (posteriorly).

**23—D.** $<40$ mg $\cdot$ dL$^{-1}$

Risk factors that contribute to the development of CAD include age (men, $>45$ yr; women, $>55$ yr), a family history of myocardial infarction (MI) or sudden death (male first-degree relatives $<55$ yr and female first-degree relatives $<65$ yr), cigarette smoking, hypertension (arterial BP $>140/90$ mm Hg measured on two separate occasions), hypercholesterolemia (total cholesterol $>200$ mg $\cdot$ dL$^{-1}$ or 5.2 mmol $\cdot$ L$^{-1}$, or HDL $<35$ mg $\cdot$ dL$^{-1}$ or 0.9 mmol $\cdot$ L$^{-1}$), and DM in individuals older than 30 yr or in individuals who have had Type 1 diabetes more than 15 yr or Type 2 diabetes in individuals older than 35 yr. Other risk factors contribute to the development of CAD but are not primary risk factors.

**24—C.** HDL $<40$ mg $\cdot$ dL$^{-1}$; current smoker; BMI $<28$

The low-risk category is asymptomatic and has one or no major risk factor for CAD. A person is placed in the moderate-risk category if he or she has two or more major risk factors for CAD. A person in the high-risk category is someone with signs, symptoms of, or known cardiac disease, pulmonary disease, and metabolic disease. If a person has high serum HDL cholesterol ($>60$ mg $\cdot$ dL$^{-1}$), subtract one risk factor from the sum of positive risk factors because high HDL levels decrease the risk of CAD.

**25—C.** Double knee to chest

Double knee to chest stretches are safe alternative to the plough. Squats to 90 degrees and lateral neck stretches are considered safe alternative exercises to full squats and full neck rolls, respectively. Flexion with rotation is considered a contraindicated high-risk exercise and is not recommended. An alternative to flexion with rotation is supine curl-ups with flexion followed by rotation.

**26—C.** Vitamins B complex and C
Fat-soluble vitamins are composed of vitamins A, D, E, and K and are stored in body fat after consumption. Vitamins C and B complex are water-soluble vitamins, must be consumed on a regular basis, and excess amounts are excreted. Water-soluble vitamins are found in citrus fruits, broccoli, cauliflower, brussel sprouts, whole grain breads and cereals, and organ meats. They serve as antioxidants as well as coenzymes in carbohydrate metabolism, metabolic pathways, amino acid metabolism, and nucleic acid metabolism.

**27—C.** Stimulate appetite
Older people who exercise regularly report greater life satisfaction (older people who exercise regularly have a more positive attitude toward their work and generally are in better health than sedentary persons), greater happiness (strong correlations have been reported between the activity level of older adults and self-reported happiness), higher self-efficacy (older persons taking part in exercise programs commonly report that they can do everyday tasks more easily than before they began exercising), improved self-concept and self-esteem (older adults improve their score on self-concept questionnaires following participation in an exercise program), and reduced psychological stress (exercise is effective in reducing psychological stress without unwanted side effects).

**28—A.** Discomfort associated with myocardial ischemia
*Angina pectoris* is a heart-related chest pain caused by ischemia, which is insufficient blood flow that results from a temporary or permanent reduction of blood flow in one or more coronary arteries. Angina-like symptoms often are felt in the chest area, neck, shoulder, or arm.

**29—B.** Application of cognitive-behavioral or motivational principles
Psychological theories are the foundation for effective use of strategies and techniques of effective counseling and motivational skill building for exercise adoption and maintenance. Theories provide a conceptual framework for development, rather than management, of programs or interventions. Psychological theories facilitate evaluation of program effectiveness, not just measurement of outcomes. Within the field of behavioral change, a theory is a set of assumptions that accounts for the relationships between certain variables and the behavior of interest.

**30—A.** PAR-Q
A well-designed health screening provides the exercise leader or HFS with information that can lead to identification of those individuals for whom exercise is contraindicated. From that information, a proper exercise prescription also can be developed. The PAR-Q is a commonly used health screening tool. A GXT can be useful to measure the HR response.

**31—D.** All of the above
Regularly scheduled practices of responses to emergency situations, including a minimum of one announced and one unannounced drill, should take place. Emergency plans should include written, posted emergency plans, and posted emergency numbers. Contact information for the nearest hospital emergency room may be included in the emergency plan. Maintenance of certifications, such as CPR training, is an accepted professional practice.

**32—C.** If the HR is taken at the carotid artery, do not press too hard or a reflex slowing of the heart can occur and cause dizziness.
If HR is taken at the carotid artery, take care not to press too hard or a reflex slowing of the heart may occur and cause dizziness. Using the thumb to count the carotid pulse may result in an inaccurate count, but this is less of a safety concern than causing dizziness by pressing too hard. HR exceeding 200 bpm are no more difficult to count at the carotid artery than at other sites.

**33—C.** Increasing the HR of training intensity more than approximately 10% per week increases the likelihood of overuse injuries of bone.
Increasing the rate of progression of training more than approximately 10% per week is a risk factor for overuse injuries of bone. Exercise programs for children and adolescents should increase physical fitness in the short term and lead to adoption of a physically active lifestyle in the long term. Strength training in youth carries no greater risk of injury than comparable strength training programs in adults if proper instruction, exercise prescription, and supervision are provided. Children who have exercise-induced asthma often are physically unfit because of restriction of activity imposed by the child, parents, or physicians.

**34—D.** Hypertension
Regular exercise will decrease SBP and DBP. Exercise has no effect on age and family history of heart disease and no direct effect on cigarette smoking, although some individuals may choose to quit smoking after beginning

to exercise. Regular endurance exercise does increase HDL but it has limited influence on total cholesterol. Exercise has no direct effect on Type 1 diabetes but it can promote weight loss and improve glucose tolerance for those with Type 2 diabetes.

**35—A.** CPR and ACSM CPT
At minimum, professionals performing fitness assessments on others should possess CPR and ACSM CPT certification.

**36—A.** Intensity and duration
Intensity and duration of exercise must be considered together and are inversely related. Similar improvements in aerobic fitness may be realized if a person exercises at a low intensity for a longer duration or at a higher intensity for less time.

**37—C.** PNF
Three different stretching techniques typically are practiced and have associated risks and benefits. Static stretching is the most commonly recommended approach to stretching. It involves slowly stretching a muscle to the point of individual discomfort and holding that position for a period of 10–30 s. Minimal risk of injury exists and it has been shown to be effective. Ballistic stretching uses repetitive bouncing-type movements to produce muscle stretch. These movements can produce residual muscle soreness or acute injury. PNF stretching alternates contraction and relaxation of both agonist and antagonist muscle groups. This technique is effective but it can cause residual muscle soreness and is time consuming. Additionally, a partner typically is required, and the potential for injury exists when the partner-assisted stretching is applied too vigorously.

**38—C.** Negligence
Legal issues abound for fitness professionals involved in exercise testing, exercise prescription, and program administration. Legal concerns can develop with the instructor–client relationship, the exercises involved, the exercise setting, the purpose of the programs and exercises used, and the procedures used by the staff. A tort law is simply a type of civil wrong. *Negligence* is the failure to perform on the level of a generally accepted standard. Fitness professionals have certain documented and understood responsibilities to ensure the client's safety and to succeed in reaching predetermined goals. If these responsibilities are not followed, it is possible that a person could be considered negligent.

**39—D.** 3–6 mo
Most sedentary people are not motivated to initiate exercise programs and, if exercise is initiated, they are likely to stop within 3–6 mo. In general, participants in earlier stages benefit most from cognitive strategies, such as listening to lectures and reading books without the expectation of actually engaging in exercise, whereas individuals in later stages depend more on behavioral techniques, such as reminders to exercise and developing social support to help them establish a regular exercise habit and be able to maintain it.

**40—D.** All of the above
Fitness testing is conducted in older adults for the same reasons as in younger adults, including exercise prescription, evaluation of progress, motivation, and education.

**41—B.** Intrinsic reward
Reinforcement is the positive or negative consequence for performing or not performing a behavior. Positive consequences are rewards that motivate behavior. This can include both intrinsic and extrinsic rewards. Intrinsic rewards are the benefits gained because of the rewarding nature of the activity. Extrinsic or external rewards are the positive outcomes received from others, which may include encouragement and praise or material reinforcements such as T-shirts and money.

**42—A.** Flexibility of equipment to allow for different body sizes.
Creating a safe environment in which to exercise is a primary responsibility for any fitness facility. In developing and operating facilities and equipment for use by exercisers, the managers and staff are obligated to meet a standard of care for exerciser safety. The equipment to be used not only includes testing, cardiovascular, strength, and flexibility pieces but also rehabilitation, pool, locker room, and emergency equipment. You must evaluate a number of criteria when selecting equipment. These criteria include correct anatomic positioning, ability to adjust to different body sizes, quality of design and materials, durability, repair records, and then price.

**43—A.** Intensity of 60%–90% $HR_{max}$, duration of 20–60 min, and frequency of 3–5 d a week
The ability to take in and to use oxygen depends on the health and integrity of the heart, lungs, and circulatory systems. Efficiency of the aerobic metabolic pathways also is necessary to optimize cardiorespiratory fitness.

The degree of improvement that may be expected in cardiorespiratory fitness relates directly to the frequency, intensity, duration, and mode or type of exercise. Maximal oxygen uptake may improve between 5% and 30% with training. The exercise prescription can be altered for different populations to achieve the same results. However, for an apparently healthy person, the ACSM recommends an intensity of 60%–90% $HR_{max}$, duration of 20–60 min, and frequency of 3–5 d a week.

**44—A.** Plyometrics
*Plyometrics* is a method of strength and power training that involves an eccentric loading of muscles and tendons followed immediately by an explosive concentric contraction. This stretch-shortening cycle may allow an enhanced generation of force during the concentric (shortening) phase. Most well-controlled studies have shown no significant difference in power improvement when comparing plyometrics with high-intensity strength training. The explosive nature of this type of activity may increase the risk for musculoskeletal injury. Plyometrics should not be considered a practical resistance exercise alternative for health/fitness applications but may be appropriate for select athletic or performance needs.

**45—C.** Manager or director
The characteristics of a good manager or director include designing programs and monitoring the implementation of programs. He or she also guides the staff or clients through the program. He or she is a good communicator who also purchases equipment and supplies. A good manager monitors the safety of the program or facility and surveys clients and staff to assess the success and value of the program.

**46—A.** To inform the client of participation risks, as well as the rights of the client and the facility
Agreements, releases, and consents are documents that clearly describe what the client is participating in, the risks involved, and the rights of the client and the facility. If signed by the client, he or she is accepting some of the responsibility and risk by participating in this program. All fitness facilities are strongly encouraged to have program or service agreements and informed consents drafted by a lawyer for their protection.

**47—C.** A loss of muscle mass caused by a loss of muscle fibers
After 30 yr of age, skeletal muscle strength begins to decline. However, the loss of strength

is not linear, with most of the decline occurring after 50 yr of age. By 80 yr of age, strength loss usually is in the range of 30%–40%. The loss of strength with aging results primarily from a loss of muscle mass, which, in turn, is caused by both the loss of muscle fibers and the atrophy of the remaining fibers.

**48—A.** There is a perceived threat of heart disease. The Health Belief Model assumes that people will engage in a behavior (*e.g.*, exercise) when there exist a perceived threat of disease and a belief of susceptibility to disease and the threat of disease is severe. This model also incorporates cues to action as critical to adopting and maintaining behavior. The concept of self-efficacy (confidence) is also added to this model. Motivation and environmental considerations are not a part of the Health Belief Model.

**49—C.** Provides an explanation of the test to the client
Informed consent is not a legal document. It does not provide legal immunity to a facility or individual in the event of injury to a client nor does it legally protect the rights of the client. It simply provides evidence that the client was made aware of the purposes, procedures, and risks associated with the test or exercise program. The consent form does not relieve the facility or individual of the responsibility to do everything possible to ensure the safety of the client. Negligence, improper test administration, inadequate personnel qualifications, and insufficient safety procedures all are items that are not expressly covered by informed consent. Because of the limitations associated with informed consent documents, legal counsel should be sought during the development of the document.

**50—C.** Number of curl-ups in 1 min
Three common assessments for muscular endurance include the bench press, for upper body endurance (a weight is lifted in cadence with a metronome or other timing device; the total number of lifts performed correctly and in time with the cadence); the push-up, for upper body endurance (the client assumes a standardized beginning position with the body held rigid and supported by the hands and toes for men and the hands and knees for women; the body is lowered to the floor, then pushed back up to the starting position; the score is the total number of properly performed push-ups completed without a pause by the client, with no time limit); and the curl-up (crunch), for abdominal muscular endurance (the client

begins in the bent-knee sit-up with knees at 90 degrees, the arms at the side, and palms facing down with middle fingers touching masking tape. A second piece of tape is placed 10-cm apart. OR set a metronome to 50 bpm and the client performs slow, controlled curl-ups to lift the shoulder blades off the mat with the trunk making a 30-degree angle, in time with the metronome at a rate of 25 per minute done for 1 min. OR the client performs as many curl-ups as possible in 1 min).

**51—A.** An overuse injury
Overuse injuries become more common when people participate in more cardiovascular exercise by increasing time, duration, or intensity too quickly. A client exercises too much without time for rest and recovery or develops a minor injury and does not reduce or change that exercise allowing the injury to heal.

**52—C.** 40%–60% and 89%
Several methods are available to define exercise intensity objectively. The ACSM recommends that exercise intensity be prescribed within a range of 64%–70% and 94% of $HR_{max}$ or between 40%–60% and 89% of oxygen uptake reserve ($VO_{2max}R$). Lower intensities will elicit a favorable response in individuals with very low fitness levels. Because of the variability in estimating $HR_{max}$ from age, it is recommended that, whenever possible, an actual $HR_{max}$ from a GXT be used. Factors to consider when determining appropriate exercise intensity include age, fitness level, medications, overall health status, and individual goals.

**53—B.** 8–12
The ACSM recommends that one set of 8–12 reps of each exercise should be performed to volitional fatigue for healthy individuals. Choose a range of reps between 3 and 20 (*i.e.*, 3–5, 8–10, 10–15) that can be performed at a moderate rep duration (~3 s concentric, ~3 s eccentric) based on age, fitness level, assessment, and ability. The ACSM recommends exercising each muscle group 2–3 non-consecutive days per week.

**54—D.** All of the above
The effects of regular (chronic) exercise can be classified or grouped into those that occur at rest, during moderate (or submaximal) exercise, and during maximal effort work. For example, you can measure an untrained individual's $HR_{rest}$, train the person for several weeks or months, and then measure $HR_{rest}$ again to see what change has occurred. $HR_{rest}$

declines with regular exercise, probably because of a combination of decreased sympathetic tone, increased parasympathetic tone, and decreased intrinsic firing rate of the sinoatrial node. Stroke volume increases at rest as a result of increased time for ventricular filling and an increased myocardial contractility. Little or no change occurs in CO at rest, because the decline in HR is compensated for by the increase in stroke volume.

**55—C.** Self-reevaluation
Key components of the Transtheoretical Model are the processes of behavioral change. These processes include five cognitive processes (consciousness raising, dramatic relief, environmental reevaluation, self-reevaluation, and social liberation) and five behavioral processes (counterconditioning, helping relationships, reinforcement management, self-liberation, and stimulus control).

**56—A.** Developing the exercise prescription
The purpose of the fitness assessment is to develop a proper exercise prescription (the data collected through appropriate fitness assessments assist the HFS in developing safe, effective programs of exercise based on the individual client's current fitness status), to evaluate the rate of progress (baseline and follow-up testing indicate progression toward fitness goals), and to motivate (fitness assessments provide information needed to develop reasonable, attainable goals). Progress toward or attainment of a goal is a strong motivator for continued participation in an exercise program.

**57—A.** 1–2 lb · wk$^{-1}$ (0.5–1 kg)
The goal of the exercise component of a weight reduction program should be to maximize caloric expenditure. Frequency, intensity, and duration must be manipulated in conjunction with a dietary regimen in an attempt to create a caloric deficit of 500–1,000 kcal · d$^{-1}$. The recommended maximal rate for weight loss is 1–2 lb · wk$^{-1}$.

**58—B.** Health Belief Model
The *Health Belief Model* is a theoretical framework to help explain and predict interventions to increase physical activity. The model originated in the 1950s based on work by Rosenstock. Learning theories assume that an overall complex behavior arises from many small simple behaviors. By reinforcing partial behaviors and modifying cues in the environment, it is possible to shape the desired behavior.

**59—C.** PAR-Q

The PAR-Q is a screening tool for self-directed exercise programming. The MMPI is a psychological scale. The RPE-Borg scale is used to measure or to rate perceived exertion during exercise or during an exercise test. The E-ECG would involve continuous electrical heart monitoring during exercise stress test used in a clinical setting when deemed appropriate by a physician.

**60—C.** Body composition, cardiorespiratory fitness, muscular fitness, and flexibility

To get the best and most accurate information, the following order of testing is recommended: resting measurements (*e.g.*, HR, BP, blood analysis), body composition, cardiorespiratory fitness, muscular fitness, and flexibility. Some methods of body composition assessment are sensitive to hydration status and some tests of cardiorespiratory and muscular fitness may affect hydration, so it is inappropriate to administer those before the body composition assessment. Assessing cardiorespiratory fitness often uses measures of HR. Some tests of muscular fitness and flexibility affect HR so they are inappropriate to administer before cardiorespiratory fitness testing, because the elevated HR from those assessments may, in turn, affect the cardiorespiratory fitness testing results.

**61—D.** Management and staff

When an emergency or injury occurs, safe and effective management of the situation will assure the best care for the individual. Implementing emergency procedures is an important part of the training of the staff. In-services, safety plans, and emergency procedures should be a part of the staff training. In addition, all exercise staff should be CPR certified and knowledgeable of first aid. Therefore, the fitness center management and staff all are included in the implementation of an emergency plan.

**62—D.** All of the above

Possible medical emergencies during exercise include heat exhaustion or heat stroke, fainting, hypoglycemia, hyperglycemia, simple or compound fractures, bronchospasm, hypotension or shock, seizures, bleeding, and other cardiac symptoms.

**63—D.** All of the above

Different types of health screenings are used for various purposes. In commercial settings, clients should be screened more extensively for potential health risks. At minimum, a personal medical history should be taken. In addition, present medical status should be examined and questions asked regarding the use of medications (both prescription and over-the-counter).

**64—C.** Shorter duration, lower intensity, and higher frequency of exercise

The number of times per day or per week that a person exercises is interrelated with both the intensity and the duration of activity. Generally, sedentary persons or those with poor fitness may benefit from multiple short-duration, low-intensity exercise sessions per day. Individual goals, preferences, limitations, and time constraints also will determine frequency and the relationship between duration, frequency, and intensity.

**65—B.** Strategic plan

The strategic plan addresses strategic decisions of the organization in defining short-and long-term goals and serves as the overarching planning tool. Health and fitness programs, financial plans, risk management efforts, and marketing plans only address subsegments within the overall strategic plan.

**66—D.** Bones

The bones of the skeletal system act as levers for changing the magnitude and direction of forces that are generated by the skeletal muscles attaching to the bones. The bones of the skeletal system provide structural support for the body through their arrangement in the axial and appendicular skeletal divisions. The axial skeleton forms the longitudinal axis of the body and it supports and protects organs as well as provides attachment for muscles. The appendicular skeleton provides for attachment of the limbs to the trunk. Blood cells are formed in bone marrow.

**67—B.** Tricuspid valve

Blood from the peripheral anatomy flows to the heart through the superior and inferior venae cavae into the right atrium. From the right atrium, the blood passes through the tricuspid valve to the right ventricle, then out through the pulmonary semilunar valve to the pulmonary arteries, and then to the lungs to be oxygenated. The tricuspid valve is so named because of the three cusps, or flaps, of which it is made. The bicuspid valve is a similar valve, having only two cusps; it is found between the left atrium and left ventricle (LV). Blood leaving the LV will pass through the aortic semilunar valve to the ascending aorta and then out to the systemic circulation.

**68—B.** Scoliosis

The vertebral column serves as the main axial support for the body. The adult vertebral column exhibits four major curvatures when viewed from the sagittal plane. *Scoliosis* is an abnormal lateral deviation of the vertebral column. *Kyphosis* is an abnormal increased posterior curvature, especially in the thoracic region. *Lordosis* is an abnormal, exaggerated anterior curvature in the lumbar region. A primary curve refers to the thoracic and sacral curvatures of the vertebral column that remain in the original fetal positions.

**69—A.** Lowering the center of gravity

Lowering the center of gravity will increase stability. Stability would also be increased by increasing the size of the base of support, by moving the center of gravity closer to the center of the base of support, or both.

**70—D.** Dorsiflexors

Dorsiflexor weakness leads to foot drop during heel strike. To ensure that the toe does not catch the walking surface, knee and hip flexion increases during swing. Weakness in the plantarflexors reduces push-off and, thereby, step length. Weakness in the gluteus medius and minimus decreases their stabilizing function during stance and can lead to increased lateral shift in the pelvis. Quadriceps weakness can lead to forward lean of the trunk or knee hyperextension.

**71—C.** Obesity, DM, tobacco smoking, and sedentary lifestyle

The primary modifiable risk factors for CAD are tobacco smoking, dyslipidemia, hypertension, sedentary lifestyle, obesity, and DM. The primary nonmodifiable risk factors for CAD are advance age, male gender, and family history. Emerging risk factors for CAD are numerous and include, for example, homocysteine, fibrinogen tissue plasminogen activator, lipoprotein (a), and C-reactive protein.

**72—A.** 30

Research has shown that 30 min of moderate-intensity physical activity per day, when performed on most if not all days of the week, will convey significant protection against the major killers in modern society (*e.g.*, cardiovascular disease, some forms of cancer).

**73—A.** An application of cognitive-behavioral principles

Applications of cognitive-behavioral principles are the methods used within programs to improve motivational skills as suggested by the assessment. For example, setting several small short-term goals to attain a long-term goal is likely to increase self-efficacy as the person successfully reaches each short-term goal on the way to attaining the long-term goal.

**74—B.** Needy participant

Despite the best efforts, working with some individuals is difficult. Issues related to interaction with the exercise professional must be resolved before exercise goals can be achieved. The needy person wants more support than can be given. It is important, then, to establish specific expectations of what is possible and to remain focused on the exercise or physical activity issues and behavioral skills related to those issues. Often, a primary goal of the needy individual is to gain attention. It is important to remember that the exercise professional is not a trained counselor, and, in some cases, it may be appropriate to refer that person for additional help.

**75—A.** Age may be accompanied by deconditioning and disease

Age is often accompanied by deconditioning and disease and these factors must be taken into consideration when selecting appropriate fitness test protocols. In addition, adaptation to a specific workload is often prolonged in older adults (a prolonged warm-up, followed by small increments in workload are recommended). Test stages in graded exercise tests should be prolonged, lasting at least 3 min, to allow the participant to reach steady state. An appropriate test protocol should be selected to accommodate these special needs.

**76—C.** Increase in resting CO

At rest, CO is not affected by training status. The amount of blood needed to sustain the body's functions at rest does not differ between those who are trained and those who are sedentary.

**77—B.** A lower HR

At any given intensity, HR will be lower during swimming than exercise performed in a standing position, such as running, because of postural differences. While swimming, the body is in a prone position so that the heart's pumping action does not have to overcome the full effects of gravity. Thus, even at rest, stroke volume is at its maximal value. Because of the higher stroke volume evident during submaximal swimming compared with running, the same CO can be achieved with a lower HR during swimming.

**78—B.** Decreased arterial compliance and increased arterial stiffness
A decrease in arterial compliance and an increase in arterial stiffness with age can result in elevated SBP and DBP both at rest and during exercise.

**79—B.** Osteoporosis
Advancing age brings a progressive decline in bone mineral density and calcium content. This loss is accelerated in women immediately after menopause. As a result, older adults are more susceptible to osteoporosis and bone fractures.

**80—A.** Overall improvement in the quality of life and increased independence
Most older adults are not sufficiently active. This population can benefit greatly from regular participation in a well-designed exercise program. Benefits of such a program include increased fitness, improved health status (reduction in risk factors associated with various diseases), increased independence, and overall improvement in the quality of life.

**81—A.** Older men and women demonstrate similar or even greater strength gains when compared with younger individuals.
Muscle strength peaks in the mid-20s for both genders and remains fairly stable through the mid-40s. Muscle strength declines by approximately 15% per decade in the sixth and seventh decades and by approximately 30% per decade thereafter. However, older men and women demonstrate similar or even greater strength gains when compared with younger individuals in response to resistance training. These strength gains are related to improved neurologic function and, to a lesser extent, increased muscle mass.

**82—C.** Data should be kept on file for at least 1 yr before being discarded.
There is no accepted minimal or maximal amount of time that data should be stored. Clearly, however, data must be stored in a confidential (lock-and-key) manner and discretion must be used when sharing data.

**83—A.** Include the costs of equipment and building or facility expense
*Capital budgets* refer to the budgeting of program implementation or facility. How much does it cost to start the program and to implement the first stage? Capital budgets usually include equipment, facility expense, staffing, initial marketing, and so on in the start-up. Operating a program is part of the operating budget, not the capital budget. Capital budgets are critical in determining whether to start a program. Capital budgets are not included in the balance sheet.

**84—A.** Injury prevention
Injury prevention often is overlooked, but it is an important part of a facility's emergency procedures and safety program. All exercise professionals should understand how to avoid emergencies. Basic principles for exercise training are important for general day-to-day operations but not for emergency procedures.

**85—B.** Do not restrain the person but be sure that he or she is in a safe area.
Most people having seizures display convulsing actions. With a convulsing seizure, the safest action is to not restrain the person and to let the convulsion pass. It is not safe to hold the person down or try to wedge anything into the victim's mouth. Make the area safe for the person by clearing any objects that he or she may contact.

**86—D.** Sarcoplasmic reticulum
Within skeletal muscle fibers, the endoplasmic (sarcoplasmic) reticulum is particularly well developed so that it can store large amounts of calcium. When the motor neuron excites the membrane (sarcolemma) of the fiber, calcium is released from the sarcoplasmic reticulum, which triggers the fiber to twitch or contract.

**87—C.** CO
Under resting conditions, CO, the amount of blood ejected by the heart per minute, is $5 \text{ L} \cdot \text{min}^{-1}$. As described previously, CO is a function of stroke volume multiplied by HR. In an untrained person, CO can increase to $25–30 \text{ L} \cdot \text{min}^{-1}$ during maximal effort exercise. In a well-trained endurance athlete, maximal CO can be as high as $35–40 \text{ L} \cdot \text{min}^{-1}$.

**88—B.** Submaximal assessment of cardiorespiratory fitness without a physician supervising
The patient has only one risk factor, hypercholesterolemia, with total serum cholesterol $>5.2 \text{ mmol} \cdot \text{L}^{-1}$. He is, however, classified as "older" for exercise purposes because he is older than 40 yr of age. Consequently, it is recommended that he should have medical clearance and an exercise test before engaging in vigorous exercise and that a physician should supervise any maximal assessment of cardiorespiratory fitness.

**89—B.** The coordinated capacity of the heart, blood vessels, respiratory system, and tissue metabolic systems to take in, deliver, and use oxygen

The maximal force that a muscle or muscle group can generate in a single effort is the definition of *muscular strength*. The ability to sustain a held maximal force or to continue repeated submaximal contractions is the definition of *muscular endurance*. The functional ROM about a joint is the definition of *flexibility*. The coordinated capacity of the heart, blood vessels, respiratory system, and tissue metabolic systems to take in, deliver, and use oxygen is the definition of *cardiorespiratory fitness*.

**90—A.** Decreased TG and increased HDL
Chronic exercise training has its greatest benefit on lowering TG and increasing HDL. Changes in total cholesterol or LDL cholesterol are influenced more by dietary habits and body weight than by exercise training.

**91—C.** Ischemia
Myocardial ischemia occurs when the oxygen supply does not meet oxygen demand resulting from decreased blood flow to the myocardium. This is usually owing to atherosclerotic lesions reducing blood flow or coronary artery spasm, both of which are the result of atherosclerosis. This process often leads to angina (symptoms) or MI caused by a thrombosis.

**92—A.** Avoiding muscle strengthening exercises that involve low resistance
Low-resistance, muscle-strengthening exercises can be performed by those diagnosed with hypertension if they follow appropriate lifting techniques and avoid the Valsalva maneuver. In addition, hemodynamic parameters (HR and BP) and medications should be controlled.

**93—B.** Rotator cuff strain or impingement
The subdeltoid bursa, supraspinatus muscle, and nerves become impinged between the coracoid and acromion process with shoulder abduction. The resulting pain leads to decreased ROM, disuse, and muscle atrophy. Such impingement of the rotator cuff is common in assembly line workers performing repetitive overhead tasks.

**94—D.** Between 1 and 2 min are recommended for an adequate cool-down.
The primary purpose of cool-down is to increase venous return, and this is accomplished by low-intensity, large-muscle activity. This type of activity also aids the removal of lactic acid. Evidence of an effective cool-down is an HR of <100 bpm and a SBP within 10 mm Hg of preexercise levels. Between 5 and 10 min will allow these changes to occur and provide time for some attention to flexibility exercises. The potential for improving flexibility is increased when the body is warm and the muscles and connective tissue are more pliable as is the case after (vs. before) exercise.

**95—C.** Prolonging cool-down
A prolonged cool-down of 5–10 min will enhance venous return and the hypotensive effects that are associated with many antihypertensive medications.

**96—D.** Only A and B of the above.
The Health Belief Model assumes that people will engage in a given behavior, such as increasing daily levels of activity, when there is a perceived threat of disease, a belief that they are susceptible to disease, and that the threat is severe. The individual will take action depending on whether the benefits of the activity outweigh the barriers. Self-efficacy (self-confidence) also plays a major role of the Health Belief Model.

**97—A.** 8.9 lb
No metabolic formula is needed. The steps are as follows:
a. Multiply the number of calories per week she is eliminating by the number of weeks:

$$1{,}200 \text{ kcal} \cdot \text{wk}^{-1} \times 26 \text{ wk} = 31{,}200 \text{ total kcal}$$

b. Now divide by 3,500 to get the total pounds she will lose:

$$31{,}200 \div 3{,}500 \text{ total kcal} = 8.9 \text{ or about } 9 \text{ lb over } 26 \text{ wk}$$

**98—C.** 11 lb
No metabolic formula is needed. The steps are as follows:
a. One mile of walking or running expends about 100 kcal. Because she walks 1 mile three times per week, she expends about 300 kcal · wk⁻¹. Multiply 300 kcal by 26 wk to determine the total amount of calories she expends by walking:

$$300 \text{ kcal} \cdot \text{wk}^{-1} \times 26 \text{ wk} = 7{,}800 \text{ kcal}$$

b. Divide 7,800 kcal by 3,500 to see how many pounds of fat this represents:

$$7{,}800 \text{ kcal} \div 3{,}500 = 2.22 \text{ lb or about } 2 \text{ lb}$$

So she would lose about 11 lb (9 lb from question 22 + 2 lb from adding the walking) over 26 wk if she incorporated walking into her weight loss program.

**99—C.** Abdominal obesity

Abdominal obesity is the major component of the metabolic syndrome and is a better predictor of CAD. Amenorrhea is part of the Female Athlete Triad. Laxative use is common in bulimia.

**100—C.** Negligence, improper test administration, inadequate personnel qualifications, and insufficient safety procedures are all items that are expressly covered by the informed consent. Negligence, improper test administration, inadequate personnel qualifications, and insufficient safety procedures are all items that are expressly NOT covered by the informed consent. The informed consent is also not a legal document; it does not provide legal immunity to a facility or individual in the event of injury to a person and it does not relieve the facility or individual of the responsibility to do everything possible to ensure the safety of an individual.

## CPT EXAMINATION QUESTIONS BY DOMAIN

Use the following table as a guide to assist you in your studying process. It is important to note that some questions can be classified as testing multiple domains by the knowledge, skills, and abilities (KSAs).

| Domain Number | I | II | III | IV |
|---|---|---|---|---|
| Domain Name | Initial Client Consultation and Assessment | Exercise Programming and Implementation | Exercise Leadership and Client Education | Legal, Professional, Business, and Marketing |
| Percentage of Test Questions | 26% | 26% | 27% | 20% |
| Question Numbers | 9, 23, 24, 26, 28, 30, 32, 34, 40, 50, 56, 59, 60, 63, 67, 70, 71, 76, 87, 89 | 1, 3, 4, 5, 6, 7, 12, 13, 14, 15, 17, 18, 19, 21, 36, 43, 47, 52, 53, 57, 66, 72, 75, 77, 86, 90, 91, 92, 93, 94, 97, 98, 99 | 2, 10, 11, 16, 22, 25, 27, 33, 37, 39, 41, 48, 54, 55, 58, 62, 64, 68, 69, 73, 78, 79, 80, 81, 85, 88, 95, 96 | 8, 20, 29, 31, 35, 38, 42, 44, 45, 46, 49, 51, 61, 65, 74, 82, 83, 84, 100 |

# ACSM Certified Health Fitness Specialist (HFS)

MEIR MAGAL, PhD, FACSM, ACSM-CES, *Associate Editor*

HFS

*Note: HFS certification candidates should also review the case studies found in Part 1, ACSM Certified Personal Trainer (CPT).*

## DOMAIN I: HEALTH AND FITNESS ASSESSMENT

**CASE STUDY HFS.I**

Author: **Julie J. Downing, PhD, FACSM**
Author's Certifications: **ACSM-CPT, ACSM-HFD**

You are a health fitness specialist at a 5,000-member athletic club in your city. A member, Giselle, has been working out at the club for nearly 5 yr but has never taken advantage of the fitness testing or exercise prescription services that the club offers. She is frustrated that she is gaining weight, is not fitting into her clothes well, does not have good energy, fatigues quicker than she used to with exertion, can't seem to run as fast, and is going through perimenopause. She has decided that she wants guidance from you.

Giselle is a nonsmoking, 44-yr-old Caucasian female who currently weighs 135 lb (she weighed 125 lb 1 yr ago) and is 5 ft 5 in tall with a waist circumference of 30.5 in and a hip circumference of 38 in. Her resting blood pressure (BP) has always been ideal, and you measured it recently at 112/68 mm Hg. Her resting heart rate ($HR_{rest}$) averages 54 bpm when taken first thing in the morning and her fasting blood glucose is 80 mg $\cdot$ dL$^{-1}$. Her total cholesterol, triglycerides, low-density lipoprotein (LDL) cholesterol, and total cholesterol/high-density lipoprotein (HDL) ratio numbers are on the higher side of normal, and her HDL-cholesterol value is 45 mL $\cdot$ dL$^{-1}$. Both her mother (age 72 yr) and father (age 71 yr) are obese and on lipid-lowering and BP medications but have no symptoms of cardiovascular disease. Her father has Type 2 diabetes. Giselle runs 3 times a week for 50 min, does Vinyasa yoga twice weekly for an hour, road bikes once weekly for 2 h, and plays tennis once weekly for 90 min. In the winter, she cross-country skis twice weekly in place of the tennis and road biking. She parents two very young children and works full-time.

You have her complete a health history questionnaire, determine her long- and short-term goals, and answer questions that she has pertaining to the upcoming assessments/program. Once you determine that she is clear to participate in fitness testing by stratifying her risk, you have her complete your club's informed consent form for fitness testing and obtain the following data:

1. Cardiorespiratory fitness assessment — Because she runs regularly, you choose to have Giselle perform the 1.5-mile run test. It takes her 10 min and 9 s to complete the test. You measure her BP at rest before she warms up for the 1.5-mi run test and find it to be 112/68 mm Hg.
2. Body composition — You elect to use the 3-site Jackson-Pollock formula to determine body composition from skinfold thickness. For the triceps skinfold, you get 18 mm; for suprailiac, you get 16 mm; and for thigh, you get 26 mm.
3. Muscular flexibility — You have Giselle perform the sit-and-reach, trunk flexion test. She obtains a score of 15 in.

4. Muscular endurance — You have her perform two tests: push-ups from the knees performed consecutively without rest and curl-ups (crunch) until either Giselle reaches 75 curl-ups or the cadence is broken. Metronome for curl-ups is set at 40 bpm. She does 20 push-ups and 60 curl-ups.

5. Muscular strength — Giselle performs upper body (bench press) and lower body (leg press) exercises. She lifts 65 lb (one repetition maximum [1-RM]) on the bench press and 170 lb (1-RM) on the leg press.

## MULTIPLE-CHOICE QUESTIONS FOR CASE HFS.I

1. What order MUST fitness assessments be administered when there are multiple tests?
   A) Resting values, muscular strength and endurance, flexibility, cardiorespiratory fitness, body composition
   B) Resting values, body composition, flexibility, cardiorespiratory fitness, muscular strength and endurance
   C) Resting values, body composition, cardiorespiratory fitness, muscular strength and endurance, flexibility
   D) Resting values including body composition first; although the order of the cardiorespiratory, muscular strength and endurance, and flexibility are not established, there must be sufficient time allowed for heart rate (HR) and BP to return to baseline between tests.

2. What is her relative maximal volume of oxygen consumed per unit of time ($\dot{V}O_{2max}$) as estimated by the 1.5-mi run test and what percentile does this put her in?
   A) 31 mL $\cdot$ kg$^{-1}$ $\cdot$ min$^{-1}$, 35th percentile
   B) 38 mL $\cdot$ kg$^{-1}$ $\cdot$ min$^{-1}$, 75th percentile
   C) 42 mL $\cdot$ kg$^{-1}$ $\cdot$ min$^{-1}$, 90th percentile
   D) 51 mL $\cdot$ kg$^{-1}$ $\cdot$ min$^{-1}$, 99th percentile

3. What is her body mass index (BMI) and what category does that put her in?
   A) 22.5 kg $\cdot$ m$^{-2}$, Normal
   B) 49.5 kg $\cdot$ m$^{-2}$, Obesity class III
   C) 19.5 kg $\cdot$ m$^{-2}$, Normal
   D) 37.0 kg $\cdot$ m$^{-2}$, Obesity class II

4. Using the Jackson-Pollock body density formula and the population-specific percent body fat formula, what is her body fat percentage and what percentile does this put her in?
   A) 16% body fat, ~94th percentile
   B) 20% body fat, 80th percentile
   C) 26% body fat, ~47th percentile
   D) 29% body fat, ~32nd percentile

5. Which of the following statements best characterize Giselle's muscular endurance scores and need for work?
   A) Push-ups = Excellent and Curl-ups = >90th percentile, work on strength
   B) Push-ups = Very good and Curl-ups = >90th percentile, work on strength
   C) Both Push-ups = Need improvement and Curl-ups = 20th percentile, BOTH strength and muscular endurance need work
   D) Push-ups = Very good and Curl-ups = 80th percentile, work on muscular endurance only

6. What are Giselle's muscular strength percentiles for bench and leg press respectively? Does she have good balance between upper and lower body strength based on these percentiles?
   A) 35th and 65th percentiles, NO — not balanced
   B) 22nd and 49th percentiles, NO — not balanced
   C) 35th and 35th percentiles, YES — perfect balance
   D) 25th and 30th percentiles, YES — near balanced

7. The sit-and-reach test is the best measure of flexibility in which muscle group?
   A) Calf
   B) Hamstrings
   C) Low back
   D) Upper back

8. What risk category did Giselle's waist circumference fall into?
   A) Very low
   B) Low
   C) High
   D) Very high

9. What does waist circumference alone evaluate the risk of?
   A) Health risk
   B) Heart disease only
   C) Cancer only
   D) Hypertension only

10. When you measured Giselle's BP at rest to be 112/68 mm Hg, how did you determine the systolic and diastolic values based on Korotkoff sounds?

A) Diastolic is first of two Korotkoff sounds and systolic is point before no more Korotkoff sounds.

B) Systolic is 10 mm Hg above first Korotkoff sound and diastolic is point before no more Korotkoff sounds.

C) Systolic is first of two Korotkoff sounds and diastolic is 10 mm Hg below last Korotkoff sound.

D) Systolic is first of two Korotkoff sounds and diastolic is point before no more Korotkoff sounds.

## DISCUSSION QUESTIONS FOR CASE HFS.I

1. Which is better to determine body composition and risk of chronic disease, anthropometric data such as BMI, circumferences, and skinfolds OR densitometry data such as hydrodensitometry (underwater weighing) or plethysmography?

2. What do you think is the reason for the 10-lb weight gain in the past year for Giselle? What suggestions will you offer to her in order to lose the weight, have more energy, fit into her clothes better, run faster, and feel better about herself? What can she work on based on all of her initial fitness assessment data?

## DOMAIN II: EXERCISE PRESCRIPTION AND IMPLEMENTATION

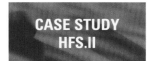
**CASE STUDY HFS.II**

Author: **Shawn Drake, PT, PhD**
Authors Certifications: **ACSM-RCEP, ACSM-PD**

Ms. Smith is a 66-yr-old, married female who worked at a local grocery store for 25 yr. She is not involved in an exercise program but would like to start exercising after her health care provider encouraged her to lose weight. She has been contemplating this decision for approximately 6 wk but is now sure that she wants to begin the exercise program. She states that she can come to the facility three times per week for 1 hr each visit. All participants of your exercise facility must have an initial exercise test and you are the Health Fitness Specialist (HFS) performing the test.

Ms. Smith states that she has a past medical history of a heart murmur and hypertension. She stated that she smoked cigarettes for 20 yr but quit 10 yr ago after her father passed away. Her mother has a history of diabetes mellitus.

On today's visit, her $HR_{rest}$ was 85 bpm and her resting BP was 168/92 mm Hg. She weighs 271 lb and is 64 in tall. You measured her body composition with the Bod Pod, which reported her percent fat to be 38. Her fasting blood lipid profile were measured as follows: total cholesterol = 190 mg $\cdot$ dL$^{-1}$; HDL-C = 30 mg $\cdot$ dL$^{-1}$; LDL = 110 mg $\cdot$ dL$^{-1}$; triglycerides = 232 mg $\cdot$ dL$^{-1}$.

Ms. Smith completed the Balke Treadmill exercise test in 10:00 ($\dot{V}O_{2max}$ = 27.8 mL $\cdot$ kg$^{-1}$ $\cdot$ min$^{-1}$). Her max HR reached 165 bpm and her maximum BP was 198/100 mm Hg. Other health-related physical fitness parameters included: sit and reach at 32 cm (the sit-and-reach box has a zero point at 23 cm), 5 curl-ups, and 0 push-ups.

## MULTIPLE-CHOICE QUESTIONS FOR CASE STUDY HFS.II

1. Based on Ms. Smith's history, what level of risk would you classify Ms. Smith for atherosclerotic cardiovascular disease?
   A) Low
   B) Moderate
   C) High
   D) Unknown

2. Based on Ms. Smith's curl-up score, which fitness category would she be?
   A) Well above average
   B) Above average
   C) Average
   D) Below average

3. Based on Ms. Smith's sit-and-reach score (cm), which fitness category would she be ranked for trunk forward flexion (assume the sit-and-reach box has a zero point at 23 cm)?
   A) Excellent
   B) Very good
   C) Good
   D) Fair

4. Based on Ms. Smith's cardiovascular assessment (Balke Treadmill), which fitness category would she be ranked for maximal aerobic power?
   A) Excellent
   B) Very good

   C) Good
   D) Fair

5. What is Ms. Smith's target $\dot{V}O_2R$ if prescribing a 60% intensity level?
   A) $16.7 \text{ mL} \cdot \text{kg}^{-1} \cdot \text{min}^{-1}$
   B) $18.1 \text{ mL} \cdot \text{kg}^{-1} \cdot \text{min}^{-1}$
   C) $20.4 \text{ mL} \cdot \text{kg}^{-1} \cdot \text{min}^{-1}$
   D) $23.3 \text{ mL} \cdot \text{kg}^{-1} \cdot \text{min}^{-1}$

6. How many kilocalories would Ms. Smith burn if exercising at the 60% intensity level for 30 min?
   A) 259 kcal
   B) 300 kcal
   C) 327 kcal
   D) 502 kcal

7. According to the Transtheoretical Model of Behavior Change, what stage of change is Ms. Smith?
   A) Precontemplation
   B) Contemplation
   C) Preparation
   D) Action

## DISCUSSION QUESTIONS FOR CASE STUDY HFS.II

1. Implement a weight management program and design an exercise prescription for Ms. Smith using the FITT framework (frequency, intensity, time, and type) based on her current health/fitness status and her time commitment.

2. Should Ms. Smith consult a physician prior to beginning her exercise program if she will begin at a moderate-intensity level? Is it necessary for Ms. Smith to have a graded exercise test (GXT) prior to initiating a moderate-intensity exercise program? If so, is it necessary that a physician supervise the GXT?

# DOMAIN III: COUNSELING AND BEHAVIORAL STRATEGIES

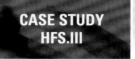
**CASE STUDY HFS.III**

Author: **Brian Coyne, MEd**
Author's Certifications: **ACSM-RCEP, ACSM/NCPAD-CIFT**

Mr. Felden is a 39-yr-old black male who enters your fitness center and asks about joining the facility and starting an exercise program. He is married and the father of three children (two boys, one girl) whom he says he has a hard time keeping up with. During your initial interview with Mr. Felden, he states his weight has fluctuated over the last couple of years with different diets he has tried; the most he has weighed is 268 lb. His height is 68 in; his current weight is 265 lb.

HFS

During your interview with Mr. Felden, he states he was told he has high BP, prediabetes, high cholesterol, and a family history of cardiovascular disease with his father having had a heart attack at the age of 50 yr. Mr. Felden has brought his latest laboratory results with him (total cholesterol = 242 mg · dL$^{-1}$, LDL = 134 mg · dL$^{-1}$, HDL = 41 mg · dL$^{-1}$, triglycerides = 184 mg · dL$^{-1}$). He also states he is a former smoker and drinks one to two 12 oz beers per day. His current medications include aspirin, lisinopril, and simvastatin.

In the past, Mr. Felden played high school football and rugby in college so he is familiar with strength training. After college, Mr. Felden tried to jog to get in shape but did not really enjoy doing it on his own. Prior to marrying his wife, they exercised together and did so until the last trimester of his wife's first pregnancy. Since then, he has done minimal physical activity but is now worried about his health.

His wife has encouraged him in the past few years to become physically active on a regular basis, but he has only played in college alumni rugby games, which have become harder to play in each year. This year, he has decided not to play because it is in 2 wk, and he cannot keep up with his children running around the yard. He states he becomes very short of breath chasing his children around the yard.

At this point, Mr. Felden is very adamant about starting an exercise program. He does not know how he will fit it into his current lifestyle though. Mr. Felden works up to 50 h · wk$^{-1}$, is tired when he gets home from work, and does not even feel like walking the family dog with his wife and/or children. Mr. Felden usually eats dinner, sits on the sofa, and watches TV after dinner before going to bed. He is able to sleep in his bed but only sleeps a few hours at a time before waking up. When he gets up in the morning, Mr. Felden does not feel well rested.

## MULTIPLE-CHOICE QUESTIONS FOR CASE STUDY HFS.III

1. What would be the first questionnaire you ask Mr. Felden to complete before allowing him to exercise in your facility?
   A) Informed consent
   B) Physical Activity Readiness Questionnaire (PAR-Q)
   C) SF-36 Quality of Life survey
   D) DASI (Duke Activity Score Index)

2. What else would you ask of Mr. Felden before he starts his exercise program in your facility?
   A) What medications he is currently taking
   B) Prior medications he is no longer taking
   C) His level of motivation
   D) How consistently he takes his medications

3. What positive risk factors does Mr. Felden have?
   A) HDL
   B) Stress
   C) Hypertension
   D) Exercise history

4. What is one cardiovascular fitness assessment you would have Mr. Felden perform before prescribing him an exercise program?
   A) Submaximal exercise test with electrocardiogram (ECG) monitoring
   B) Maximal exercise test without EKG monitoring
   C) 1-RM squat
   D) 1.5-mi walk/run

5. Based on Mr. Felden past exercise history and using Prochaska's Stages of Change model, what stage do you think Mr. Felden is in?
   A) Precontemplation
   B) Contemplation
   C) Preparation
   D) Action

6. How would you first suggest moving Mr. Felden toward compliance using the health beliefs model?
   A) Provide him with a schedule of all group exercise classes offered at the fitness center.
   B) Encourage him to schedule exercise into his daily routine.
   C) Set goals that will take him 3 mo to attain with consistent adherence to the prescribed lifestyle modifications.
   D) Ask him how he plans to implement the lifestyle modifications he desires to make and understand the benefit of a regular exercise program.

7. What risk factors would you focus on initially to see positive change in?
   A) BP
   B) Cholesterol levels
   C) Weight
   D) Sedentary lifestyle

8. How would you help facilitate Mr. Felden's motivation to continue exercising each week?
   A) Set 3-mo goals and remind him of them each week.
   B) Set monthly goals and remind him of them each week.
   C) Set weekly goals that are attainable but take some effort to attain.
   D) Set daily goals.

9. What short-term exercise goal would you have for Mr. Felden during his exercise program?
   A) 60 min of moderate aerobic exercise per day by the end of 3 wk
   B) At least $3 \, d \cdot wk^{-1}$ of exercise the first 3 wk of his program
   C) 20 min vigorous activity per day, 3 times a week by the end of 4 wk
   D) 5 d of moderate physical activity in the first week of his program

## DISCUSSION QUESTIONS FOR CASE STUDY HFS.III

1. How would you create an environment that enabled Mr. Felden to examine his motives for coming to see you?

2. What tools could you use to increase the likelihood of his success?

3. How would you assist Mr. Felden's in incorporating his family into his exercise program and adherence to the program?

# DOMAIN IV: LEGAL/PROFESSIONAL

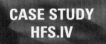

**CASE STUDY HFS.IV**

Author: **Matthew W. Parrott, PhD**
Author's Certifications: **ACSM-HFD**

You have recently been hired as the fitness director at a midsize (~35,000 ft²) health and fitness facility. The grand opening for the facility is scheduled in 1 mo from today. The general manager has asked you to hire all of the positions necessary for the operation of a successful and profitable fitness department. As fitness director, you will be the direct supervisor for all of the employees you hire and will be responsible for their payroll, schedules, and productivity.

In addition, you have been asked to set up the fitness evaluation policies and procedures for your employees to follow.

## MULTIPLE-CHOICE QUESTIONS FOR CASE STUDY HFS.IV

1. Which position will you most likely compensate with commission rather than hourly wage?
   A) Massage therapists
   B) Personal trainers
   C) Weight floor personnel
   D) A and B only
   E) All of the above

2. Rather than hiring a number of part-time staff for weight floor supervision, you have elected to hire two full-time staff. How many hours of overtime must you pay an employee who works 52 h during a given week?
   A) 12
   B) 17
   C) 22
   D) 0

3. How will you decide the pay rate for various positions you are hiring?
   A) Arbitrarily
   B) Based on what you were paid when you had the position
   C) Perform a job pricing analysis
   D) Based on national/state normative statistics
   E) C and D

4. Why would you decide to institute performance-based pay for a given position?
   A) Decreased employee morale
   B) Increased employee turnover
   C) Decreased employee retention
   D) Increased employee productivity

5. Which of the following should be included as part of the fitness testing program?
   A) Informed consent
   B) Pretest evaluation (risk stratification)
   C) Flexibility assessment
   D) All of the above

6. Which of the following strategies would result in the most organized fitness testing program?
   A) Memorize the protocol and perform all fitness testing personally.
   B) Assign your most talented personal trainer the task of fitness testing for all members.
   C) Create a handbook outlining testing protocols and train your staff accordingly.
   D) Memorize body composition analyses because that's the most important fitness test to the members.

7. Which strategy would be the best way to ensure fitness testing confidentiality while maintaining accurate recordkeeping?
   A) Create a hardcopy of fitness test results and place it in a file cabinet in the fitness testing room.
   B) Create an electronic file of fitness test results and save the file on a password-protected computer.
   C) Hand the member a copy of his or her results and keep no other records of the test.
   D) Share results verbally with the member, then, destroy the hard copy of results.

8. Which of the following is NOT a pretest instruction you would provide to the client?
   A) Wear comfortable, loose-fitting clothing.
   B) Avoid strenuous physical activity the day of the assessment.
   C) Avoid caffeine the day of the assessment.
   D) Avoid hydration the day of the assessment.

9. Which of the following is one of your primary goals for the fitness assessment program?
   A) Present a professional image of the organization.
   B) Provide member with fitness evaluation against normative data.
   C) Establish a friendly relationship, thereby enhancing retention.
   D) All of the above.

10. What is the primary advantage to hiring personal trainers as independent contractors versus employees?
   A) Reduced tax liability for the club
   B) Increased professionalism in the fitness department
   C) Independent contractors are usually better trainers
   D) Better long-term retention of training staff

## DISCUSSION QUESTION FOR CASE STUDY HFS.IV

1. Write a sample job description for a personal trainer in a commercial fitness setting. Be sure to include any or all pertinent components to hiring for this position.

# DOMAIN V: MANAGEMENT

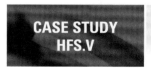

**CASE STUDY HFS.V**

Author: **Frederick Klinge, MBA**
Author's Certifications: **ACSM-HFS**

You are the fitness director and group exercise coordinator for a large, successful multipurpose health/fitness center that has recently purchased another local fitness center that declared bankruptcy a few months ago. The newly acquired club has 1,100 active memberships, and it is your understanding that the facility has the capacity to handle 2,800–3,000 memberships.

The newly acquired club is a 35,000 ft² fitness-only facility. Your company is planning a gradual renovation of the acquired club while keeping the facility operational. The overall condition of the facility is good and the activity areas and equipment are up-to-date and fully functional. The facility is located in a middle-class residential neighborhood with a median household annual income of $57,000. Other health/fitness businesses in the local area include a 25-yr-old YMCA (average monthly dues rate of $55) and three newer 24/7 gyms (average monthly dues rate of $29).

You have been assigned the task of revitalizing the group exercise program of the newly acquired club. The previous group exercise program consisted of basic step aerobics, kick-boxing, body sculpting, and a circuit training class using a 10-piece selectorized weight machine circuit. Due to staffing cutbacks, the previous management discontinued group exercise classes on Friday, Saturday, and Sunday, and there are currently 22 classes per week. The group exercise studio is spacious and is in good shape. The renovation project will include upgrading the studio's sound system and installing a new state-of-the-art studio floor surface.

An important part of your task is putting together a staff for the new group exercise program, including the hiring of a group exercise coordinator for the new club.

## MULTIPLE-CHOICE QUESTIONS FOR CASE STUDY HFS.V

1. You have received approval to offer 60 classes per week and you plan to use a mix of current instructors from your club as well as new hires. A recent analysis of your facility's group exercise staff indicates the average per-class pay rate is $23. Annual performance evaluations are performed for all instructors, and you strictly adhere to a 3% merit raise policy. You have been asked by the company controller to submit a pro forma projection for annual group exercise instructor wages. Given the information earlier, what is the most accurate payroll expense projection for the first 12 mo of operation for the group exercise program at the new club?
   A) $26,312
   B) $27,101
   C) $71,760
   D) $73,913
   E) $84,920

2. Hearing protection safety is an important topic when training new group exercise instructors. Part of your New Instructor Orientation program for the newly acquired club should list which maximum class decibel level?
   A) 75 dB
   B) 90 dB
   C) 105 dB
   D) Sound level should be determined by the group exercise instructor depending on the demographic makeup of each class.
   E) None of the above

3. The group exercise studio will be one of most highly used spaces in the newly acquired facility. The new group exercise program will include boot camp classes, low-impact aerobics, yoga classes, body sculpting, and sports performance classes. Selected ancillary equipment may include which of the following?
   A) Step benches
   B) Spin class cycles

   C) Medicine balls
   D) Strength bands
   E) All of the above

4. You will be hiring a full-time group exercise coordinator to supervise the group exercise program at the new facility. According to _____, what is the recommended formal education for a group exercise coordinator in the health/fitness industry?
   A) High School diploma or general education development (GED) equivalent
   B) 2 yr post–high school education in fitness, health, recreation, or related field from an accredited college or university
   C) 4-yr degree in fitness, exercise science, or related field
   D) No formal education is recommended for the position, only a professional certification combined with at least 3 yr of experience as a group exercise instructor.

5. Your company follows a strict policy of "safety first" when it comes to member participation in programs. When selecting exercises appropriate for a group or individuals, which of the following are important considerations?
   A) Selected exercises should be an effective way to increase flexibility, strength, coordination, balance, or cardiovascular endurance.
   B) Demonstration of exercise modifications is necessary to accommodate all participant skill levels and abilities.
   C) Exercises must be safe for the 25–45-yr-old age demographic because this group compromises the majority of most group exercise classes.
   D) A and B

6.  You are responsible for instructing the new club's group exercise coordinator on how to perform employee performance evaluations. When it comes to performance evaluations, an important objective is _____.
    A)  To look for opportunities to keep the meeting social in nature, allowing for a relaxed communication environment.
    B)  To base most of your management feedback on what is planned and expected of the employee for the upcoming year.
    C)  To bridge the gap between present and ideal performance.
    D)  To compare an employee's performance to other employees performing the same job function.

7.  To assure success of the group exercise program at the new facility, it is important to be consistent with process evaluation on the program. Which of the following statements is true regarding program process evaluation?
    A)  Process evaluation assesses effectiveness by measuring whether program goals and objectives have been met.

B)  Process evaluation can demonstrate whether procedures were followed and whether they were appropriate and effective.
C)  A cost-benefit analysis should part of any process evaluation.
D)  The first step of a process evaluation is always reviewing the program goals and objectives.

8.  It is very important for the new club to retain as many existing members as possible. You need to solicit input and feedback from existing members regarding the quality of the existing group exercise program, what the members like about the program, what they don't like about the program. Methods for acquiring this type of information include _____.
    A)  Target Market Surveys
    B)  Health Screening and Fitness Assessments
    C)  Participant Surveys
    D)  Health Care Usage Reports

## DISCUSSION QUESTIONS FOR CASE STUDY HFS.V

1.  It is important to engage the club members and group exercise participants and get them involved in the new program format. The new club has a Web site, and your company has had success in marketing programs via Web-based social media platforms like Facebook, Twitter, blogs, etc. What some creative ways to use social media and other Web-based programs to promote your new group exercise program?

2.  Keeping track of group exercise class participation numbers an important source of information for ongoing program evaluation. Discuss methods of tracking class participation and organizing class participation information for effective program analysis.

HFS

# HFS CASE STUDIES ANSWERS AND EXPLANATIONS

## CASE STUDY HFS.I

### Multiple-Choice Answers for Case Study HFS.I

**1—D.** Resting values including body composition first although the order of the cardiorespiratory, muscular strength and endurance, and flexibility are not established, there must be sufficient time allowed for HR and BP to return to baseline between tests.

*ACSM's Guideline for Exercise Testing and Prescription*, 9th edition (*GETP9*), Chapter 4 states: "When multiple tests are to be administered, the organization of the testing session can be very important, depending on what physical fitness components are to be evaluated. Resting measurements such as heart rate (HR), blood pressure (BP), height, weight, and body composition should be obtained first. Research has not established an optimal testing order for multiple health-related components of fitness (*i.e.*, cardiorespiratory [CR] endurance, muscular fitness, body composition, and flexibility), but sufficient time should be allowed for HR and BP to return to baseline between tests conducted serially."

*Resource:* Pescatello LS, senior editor. *ACSM's Guidelines for Exercise Testing and Prescription.* 9th ed. Baltimore (MD): Lippincott Williams and Wilkins; 2014.

**2—D.** $51 \text{ mL} \cdot \text{kg}^{-1} \cdot \text{min}^{-1}$, 99th percentile

*ACSM's GETP9*, Chapter 4, Table 4.8 states that a Balke treadmill time of 25:00, a 12-min run distance of 1.74 mile, or a 1.5-mile run time of 10:09 gives a $\dot{V}O_{2max}$ of $51 \text{ mL} \cdot \text{kg}^{-1} \cdot \text{min}^{-1}$ and a 99th percentile ranking. There is also a formula available to calculate $\dot{V}O_{2max}$ from the 1.5-mi run test: $\dot{V}O_{2max}$ $(\text{mL} \cdot \text{kg}^{-1} \text{ min}^{-1}) = 3.5 + (483/\text{Time})$. Time must be in the nearest hundredth of a minute so 10:09 would be 10.15 because 9 s/60 s = 0.15. So, $\dot{V}O_{2max} = 3.5 + (383/10.15) = 51 \text{ mL} \cdot \text{kg}^{-1} \cdot \text{min}^{-1}$.

*Resource:* Pescatello LS, senior editor. *ACSM's Guidelines for Exercise Testing and Prescription.* 9th ed. Baltimore (MD): Lippincott Williams and Wilkins; 2014.

**3—A.** $22.5 \text{ kg} \cdot \text{m}^{-2}$, Normal

*ACSM GETP9*, Chapter 4 contains the BMI formula of kilogram body weight divided by height in meters squared. MATH WORK: 135 lb/2.2 = 61.4 kg. Five feet 5 in tall is 65 in × .0254,

which is the conversion from inches to meters = 1.651 m tall. Squaring 1.651 = 2.726, so taking 61.4/2.726 = 22. 5 $\text{kg} \cdot \text{m}^{-2}$. In *ACSM's GETP9*, Chapter 4, Table 4.1 lists classifications for BMI and disease risk. The 49.5 is incorrect because pounds was used for weight instead of kilograms. The 19.5 is incorrect because lb is divided by 2.54 instead of 2.2. Finally, 37.0 is wrong as well because the meters are not squared.

*Resource:* Pescatello LS, senior editor. *ACSM's Guidelines for Exercise Testing and Prescription.* 9th ed. Baltimore (MD): Lippincott Williams and Wilkins; 2014.

**4—C.** 26% body fat, ~47th percentile

*ACSM's GETP9*, Chapter 4, Box 4.3 contains the 3-site Jackson-Pollack body density formula for women using triceps, suprailiac, and thigh:

Body Density = $1.099421 - 0.0009929$ (sum of 3 skinfolds) + $0.0000023$ (sum of 3 skinfolds)$^2$ − $0.0001392$ (age)

The population-specific formula for body fat percentage for Caucasian females age 18–59 yr found in Table 4.4 of *ACSM's GETP9* is:

Percent Body Fat = (496/Body Density) − 451

With data: Body Density = $1.099421 - 0.0009929$ (60) + $0.0000023$ (60)$^2$ − $0.0001392$ (44) = 1.040022

With data: Percent Body Fat = (496/Body Density) − 451= 25.9% round to 26%

In Table 4.6 of *ACSM's GETP9*, the percentile classification for women age 40–49 yr with 26% fat is ~47th percentile.

*Resource:* Pescatello LS, senior editor. *ACSM's Guidelines for Exercise Testing and Prescription.* 9th ed. Baltimore (MD): Lippincott Williams and Wilkins; 2014.

**5—B.** Push-ups = Very good and Curl-ups = >90th percentile, work on strength

*ACSM's GETP9*, Chapter 4, Table 4.11 contains categories for women age 40–49 yr for push-ups, whereas partial curl-up categories are in Table 4.12. Because her muscular strength percentiles were 35th and 65th and her muscular endurance categories came out at very good (20 push-ups is between the range of 15–23) and over the 90th percentile (60 curl-ups), it is evident that Giselle needs to focus more on her muscular strength than her muscular endurance at this point. She should retest these values periodically with you her HFS.

*Resource:* Pescatello, LS, senior editor. *ACSM's Guidelines for Exercise Testing and Prescription.* 9th ed. Baltimore (MD): Lippincott Williams and Wilkins; 2014.

**6—A.**  35th and 65th percentiles, NO — not balanced

*ACSM's GETP9*, Chapter 4, Table 4.9 includes percentiles for women age 40–49 yr for bench press and Table 4.10 has her leg press percentiles. Giselle's 1-RM for bench press was 65 lb so divide 65 by 135, which is her body weight, to get a ratio of 0.48, which you find in Table 4.9 puts her into the 35th percentile. Her 1-RM for leg press was 170 lb so divide 170 by 135 body weight to get a ratio of 1.26, which puts her in the 65th percentile. If you answered B as the correct answer, you were accidently looking at the age 30–39 percentile column. Be careful when looking up data on tables, always double check your work as you do NOT want to give your clients misinformation.

*Resource:* Pescatello LS, senior editor. *ACSM's Guidelines for Exercise Testing and Prescription.* 9th ed. Baltimore (MD): Lippincott Williams and Wilkins; 2014.

**7—B.**  Hamstrings

*ACSM GETP9*, Chapter 4 states that "the sit-and-reach test has been used commonly to assess low back and hamstring flexibility; however, its relationship to predict the incidence of low back pain is limited. The sit-and-reach test is suggested to be a better measure of hamstring flexibility than low back flexibility."

*Resource:* Pescatello LS, senior editor. *ACSM's Guidelines for Exercise Testing and Prescription.* 9th ed. Baltimore (MD): Lippincott Williams and Wilkins; 2014.

**8—B.**  Low

*ACSM's GETP9*, Chapter 4, Table 4.3 shows that a waist circumference between 28.5–35.0 in (70–89 cm) falls into a low-risk category.

*Resource:* Pescatello LS, senior editor. *ACSM's Guidelines for Exercise Testing and Prescription.* 9th ed. Baltimore (MD): Lippincott Williams and Wilkins; 2014.

**9—A.**  Health risk

*ACSM's GETP9*, Chapter 4 states that "waist circumference can be used alone as an indicator of health risk because abdominal obesity is the primary issue. Research has demonstrated that waist circumference thresholds effectively identify individuals at increased health risk across the different BMI categories."

*Resource:* Pescatello LS, senior editor. *ACSM's Guidelines for Exercise Testing and Prescription.* 9th ed. Baltimore (MD): Lippincott Williams and Wilkins; 2014.

**10—D.**  Systolic is first of two Korotkoff sounds and diastolic is point before no more Korotkoff sounds.

*ACSM's GETP9* states that "systolic BP is the point at which the first of two or more Korotkoff sounds is heard and diastolic BP is the point before the disappearance of Korotkoff sounds. Prior to this make sure that you've inflated cuff pressure to 20 mm Hg above first Korotkoff sound and slowly release pressure at rate equal to 2–5 mm Hg $\cdot$ s$^{-1}$."

*Resource:* Pescatello LS, senior editor. *ACSM's Guidelines for Exercise Testing and Prescription.* 9th ed. Lippincott Williams and Wilkins; 2014.

## Discussion Question Answers for Case Study HFS.I

1. Outline of discussion under body composition
   a. Define anthropometric and densitometry.
   b. Determine margins of error with each technique.
   c. Cost, complexity, calibration, amount of time-required for each technique
   d. Correlation of each to disease
   e. Pros and cons of each technique
2. Outline
   a. Suggest to Giselle that she see her gynecologist to check various hormone levels to make sure that she does not have some sort of hormonal abnormality going on.
   b. Discuss energy balance with Giselle. She exercises quite a lot and is still gaining weight so perhaps it is her diet that needs the major overhaul.
   c. Talk about healthy snacks and total kilocalories eaten each day and total kilocalories burned off each day via resting metabolic rate and physical activity.
   d. Perhaps you need to refer her to a registered dietician who is comfortable working with active individuals.
   e. Perhaps Giselle needs to add two components into her training plan that are lacking: (a) speed work or higher intensity running

days and (b) strength training. The only strength she gets now is in her Vinyasa yoga classes. The increased muscle mass may help her increase her metabolic rate, which would burn more kilocalories and hopefully she will fit into her clothes better, which will hopefully help her self-esteem. The speed work will help her to regain her running speed and may also help with self-efficacy.

f. You could calculate an ideal body weight at the 75th percentile for Giselle ($\sim$21%).

g. Discuss losing weight gradually, no more than $1–2$ lb $\cdot$ wk$^{-1}$ and not getting her weight or body fat too low.

## CASE STUDY HFS.II

### Multiple-Choice Answers for Case Study HFS.II

**1—C.**  High

According to ACSM risk classification, Ms. Smith has a known heart murmur, which is a major sign that is suggestive of cardiovascular, pulmonary, or metabolic disease. See Figure 2.3 in *ACSM's GETP9* for logic model for classification for risk.

*Resource:* Pescatello LS, senior editor. *ACSM's Guidelines for Exercise Testing and Prescription.* 9th ed. Baltimore (MD): Lippincott Williams and Wilkins; 2014.

**2—D.**  Below average

Using Table 4.12 in *ACSM's GETP9*, Ms. Smith would be ranked in the below average (30th percentile) category for curl-ups.

*Resource:* Pescatello LS, senior editor. *ACSM's Guidelines for Exercise Testing and Prescription.* 9th ed. Baltimore (MD): Lippincott Williams and Wilkins; 2014.

**3—A.**  Excellent

Rationale: Using Table 4.16 in *ACSM's GETP9*, normative data would rank Ms. Smith in the excellent fitness category for trunk forward flexion. Because a sit-and-reach box that has a zero point at 23 cm, subtract 3 cm from each value in Table 4.16. The excellent category is 35 cm, but 3 cm should be subtracted ($35$ cm $−$ $3$ cm $=$ $32$ cm). Therefore, 32 cm would be ranked as excellent.

*Resource:* Pescatello LS, senior editor. *ACSM's Guidelines for Exercise Testing and Prescription.* 9th ed. Baltimore (MD): Lippincott Williams and Wilkins; 2014.

**4—C.**  Good

Rationale: Using Table 4.8 in *ACSM's GETP9*, Ms. Smith would be ranked in the "good" category (65%) for maximal aerobic power.

*Resource:* Pescatello LS, senior editor. *ACSM's Guidelines for Exercise Testing and Prescription.* 9th ed. Baltimore (MD): Lippincott Williams and Wilkins; 2014.

**5—B.**  18.1 mL $\cdot$ kg$^{-1}$ $\cdot$ min$^{-1}$

Rationale: $\dot{V}O_2R = [(\dot{V}O_{2max} − \dot{V}O_{2rest}) \times$ % intensity desired] $+ \dot{V}O_{2rest}$

$\dot{V}O_2R = [(27.8$ mL $\cdot$ kg$^{-1}$ $\cdot$ min$^{-1}$ $− 3.5$ mL $\cdot$ kg$^{-1}$ $\cdot$ min$^{-1}$) $\times 0.60] + 3.5$ mL $\cdot$ kg$^{-1}$ $\cdot$ min$^{-1}$

$\dot{V}O_2R = [14.58$ mL $\cdot$ kg$^{-1}$ $\cdot$ min$^{-1}$] $+ 3.5$ mL $\cdot$ kg$^{-1}$ $\cdot$ min$^{-1}$

$\dot{V}O_2R = 18.1$ mL $\cdot$ kg$^{-1}$ $\cdot$ min$^{-1}$

*Resource:* Pescatello LS, senior editor. *ACSM's Guidelines for Exercise Testing and Prescription.* 9th ed. Baltimore (MD): Lippincott Williams and Wilkins; 2014.

**6—C.**  327 kcal

Rationale:

Convert pounds to kilograms: 271 lb $\times$ 0.454 $= 123.0$ kg

18.1 mL $\cdot$ kg$^{-1}$ $\cdot$ min$^{-1}$ $\times$ 123 kg $\times$ 1L/1,000 mL $= 2.23$ L $\cdot$ min$^{-1}$

2.23 L $\cdot$ min$^{-1}$ $\times$ 4.9 kcal $\cdot$ L$^{-1}$ $= 10.9$ kcal $\cdot$ min$^{-1}$

10.9 kcal $\cdot$ min$^{-1}$ $\times$ 30 min $= 327$ kcal

**7—C.**  Preparation

Rationale: Ms. Smith is currently preparing to begin her program. She is not currently active but intends to become active in the next 6 mo. She has started to make small steps toward behavior change by completing her initial exercise test. Once she begins her exercise program, she will move into the "action" stage of change.

HFS

## Discussion Question Answers for Case Study HFS.II

1. The HFS should choose an effective behavior weight loss program as recommended by ACSM's Position Stand, "Appropriate Physical Activity Intervention Strategies for Weight Loss and Prevention of Weight Regain for Adults" (2009). An effective behavior weight loss program includes moderate-intensity physical activity for 150–250 min · wk$^{-1}$ with an energy equivalent of 1,200–2,000 kcal · wk$^{-1}$ along with moderate diet restrictions that lead to negative energy balance. Diet restrictions should follow basic nutritional guidelines as set forth by and United States Department of Agriculture (USDA) Dietary Guidelines for Americans. Although resistance training may not be an effective means for reducing percent fat, other health benefits such as decreased chronic disease risk factors are plausible.

   The exercise prescription should address the five components of fitness (cardiopulmonary endurance, muscular strength, muscular endurance, body composition, and flexibility). Body composition is addressed by tracking the kcal per session and dietary intake. For this client, cardiopulmonary endurance and muscular strength/endurance will be key components of the exercise prescription to enhance weight loss and reduce chronic disease risk. Ms. Smith needs to maintain her current flexibility levels. An initial exercise prescription example is shown in the following table. The client wishes only to exercise three times a week for 1 h.

|  | Frequency | Intensity | Time | Type |
|---|---|---|---|---|
| Cardio-pulmonary endurance | Three times a week | 60% | 30 min (intermittent) | Bike/treadmill |
| Muscular strength/endurance | Two times a week | 50% of 1-RM | 1 × 10 reps of at least eight different muscle groups | Thera-Band, free weights (1–3 lb) |
| Flexibility | Two times a week | Mild discomfort | 3 × 30 s hold | Static stretching |

A typical daily exercise program would include a 5–10 min warm-up, 30–40 min of exercise followed by 5–10 min of cool-down. Exercise should be kept at low intensities to avoid delayed onset muscle soreness and to increase exercise adherence. As exercise sessions increase in duration and the client has success with her current program, discuss advantages of increasing number of days per week in the exercise program. This program should progress to reach the target of 250 min · wk$^{-1}$ of moderate intensity of aerobic exercise.

2. Yes, current American College of Sports Medicine (ACSM) recommendations state that individuals at high risk with symptoms or diagnosed disease should consult with their physician prior to initiating an exercise program. An exercise test is recommended prior to starting her exercise program and a physician should supervise the exercise test (both submaximal or maximal test).

## CASE STUDY HFS.III

## Multiple-Choice Answers for Case Study HFS.III

**1—B.**  PAR-Q

After having the client sign an informed consent, you would have him complete a PAR-Q to assist you in gaining more about his recent history (physical activity, medical) and assist you in risk stratifying him. This questionnaire can also be used to identify how lifestyle modifications can benefit his risk of mortality.

*Resource:* Pescatello LS, senior editor. *ACSM's Guidelines for Exercise Testing and Prescription.* 9th ed. Baltimore (MD): Lippincott Williams and Wilkins; 2014.

**2—A.**  What medications he is currently taking

Current medications are important to know prior to allowing Mr. Felden to start exercise. They may have an influence on his exercise tolerance, HR, and BP. Motivation is also important; however, it is not something you should need to ask him because he came to your fitness center wanting to start an exercise program. This shows that he has a certain level of motivation. Mr. Felden's motivation level can be gleaned through conducting a motivational interviewing activity with him during his initial interview. His motivation level will also be monitored during the early stages of his exercise program.

HFS

**3—C.**   Hypertension

HDL are not low at 41 mg · dL$^{-1}$; thus, they are not a positive risk factor. Stress is not discussed earlier, so it cannot be assumed although there is a chance it plays a factor in cardiovascular risk. His sedentary behavior would be a positive risk factor; however, his exercise history is not.

*Resource:* Pescatello LS, senior editor. *ACSM's Guidelines for Exercise Testing and Prescription.* 9th ed. Baltimore (MD): Lippincott Williams and Wilkins; 2014.

**4—D.**   1.5-mi walk/run

Mr. Felden does not need to do a submaximal exercise test with EKG monitoring. A maximal exercise test without EKG monitoring would not be done (especially with his family history).

*Resource:* Pescatello LS, senior editor. *ACSM's Guidelines for Exercise Testing and Prescription.* 9th ed. Baltimore (MD): Lippincott Williams and Wilkins; 2014.

**5—C.**   Preparation

Mr. Felden is past the precontemplation and contemplation stages. He has acted on his thoughts and has inquired about joining the fitness center. Using active listening techniques and proper communication techniques with Mr. Felden, you understand that he is preparing to act on his thoughts.

*Resource:* Pecatello LS, senior editor. *ACSM's Guidelines for Exercise Testing and Prescription.* 9th ed. Baltimore (MD): Lippincott Williams and Wilkins; 2014.

**6—D.**   Ask him how he plans to implement the lifestyle modifications he desires to make and understand the benefit of a regular exercise program.

Mr. Felden is preparing to make changes to his lifestyle and discussed what he wanted to do. At this point, it is important for him to have an idea of how he will integrate those modifications into his lifestyle. Once completing this, it would be good to encourage Mr. Felden to schedule exercise into his daily routine. Through all of this, Mr. Felden should understand the benefit compared to the cost of the exercise program.

*Resource:* Pescatello LS, senior editor. *ACSM's Guidelines for Exercise Testing and Prescription.* 9th ed. Baltimore (MD): Lippincott Williams and Wilkins; 2014.

**7—D.**   Sedentary lifestyle

Consistent exercise will be the easiest risk factor to see an improvement in at the start of his program. It hopefully will have a positive impact on his weight, if he does not increase his caloric intake to make up for the calories burned during physical activity/exercise. His high BP is being treated with medication, and hopefully in the future, the dosage can be decreased or the medication can be stopped. Improvements in BP from exercise programs can take up to 6 mo to see noticeable change. His high cholesterol levels are being treated with medications. Exercise will have a beneficial effect on this as well, but the noticeable differences will not be seen without dietary modifications as well.

*Resource:* Pescatello LS, senior editor. *ACSM's Guidelines for Exercise Testing and Prescription.* 9th ed. Baltimore (MD): Lippincott Williams and Wilkins; 2014.

**8—C.**   Set weekly goals that are attainable but take some effort to attain.

Detailed Answer: Short-term goals are easier for clients to attain. Getting a client to make lifestyle modifications is usually easier when he or she has relatively easy short-term goals to attain. The goals take effort; however, they are something he or she can attain and move forward with success. Long-term goals can be set, but they should not initially be the focus of his or her lifestyle modification program. Daily goals are good, but it takes much effort by the practitioner and client's part to set daily goals; also, the client may not be seeing the practitioner on a daily basis. With any goal setting, there should be someone that the client reports to monitor progress.

*Resource:* Pescatello LS, senior editor. *ACSM's Guidelines for Exercise Testing and Prescription.* 9th ed. Baltimore (MD): Lippincott Williams and Wilkins; 2014.

**9—B.**   At least 3 d · wk$^{-1}$ of exercise the first 3 wk of his program

A moderate-intensity exercise program is usually easier for clients to become accustomed to. One of the keys of behavior modification is setting goals that are attainable that allow for progress to be made. Expecting too much at the beginning of an exercise program can set up the client for potential failure. Too vigorous an exercise program initially can hinder a client's adherence to the exercise program.

*Resource:* Pescatello LS, senior editor. *ACSM's Guidelines for Exercise Testing and Prescription.* 9th ed. Baltimore (MD): Lippincott Williams and Wilkins; 2014.

## Discussion Question Answers for Case Study HFS. III

1. He needs to reiterate to himself why he started his exercise program. Mr. Felden should understand his internal motivation to start the exercise program. If he is being truthful with himself, he can use the medical diagnoses he is at risk for as motivators. Mr. Felden should be afraid to get diabetes.

2. Mr. Felden could use a calendar or daily planner to schedule his exercise time each day. He could also create a checklist for each day that includes an exercise session on most, if not all, days of the week. The exercise practitioner could also use educational materials and statistical data to help demonstrate and encourage Mr. Felden to believe that there is a need for him to continue his exercise program.

3. Encouraging Mr. Felden to take walks with his family and their dog would be a good way to incorporate daily exercise into his lifestyle. Also incorporating the family with the exercise program would allow them to help motivate him. On the days when Mr. Felden does not feel like walking or exercising, his family could be his external motivation.

   In order to promote exercise outside of a fitness center and to promote increased physical activity during the day, Mrs. Felden and the children can also encourage Mr. Felden to play games with the children. This would increase his overall activity and potentially help increase his compliance to the exercise program.

   Promote good communication between Mr. Felden, his wife, and their children to facilitate an increase in physical activity in the household.

## CASE STUDY HFS.IV

## Multiple-Choice Answers for Case Study HFS.IV

1—**D.** A and B Only

2—**A.** 12

3—**E.** C and D

4—**D.** Increased employee productivity

5—**D.** All of the above

6—**C.** Create a handbook outlining testing protocols and train your staff accordingly.

7—**B.** Create an electronic file of fitness test results and save the file on a password-protected computer.

8—**D.** Avoid hydration the day of the assessment.

9—**D.** All of the above.

10—**A.** Reduced tax liability for the club

## Discussion Question Answer for Case Study HFS.IV

1. Outline
   - Date
   - Job title
   - Department
   - Reporting relationship
   - Exempt status
   - Salary range
   - Work schedule
   - Job summary
     — Describe duties and responsibilities
   - Job requirements
     — Education, experience, certifications, skills
   - Physical environment and working conditions

## CASE STUDY HFS.V

## Multiple-Choice Answers for Case Study HFS.V:

1—**D.** $73,913

   *Resource:* American College of Sports Medicine. *ACSM's Resource Manual for Guidelines for Exercise Testing and Prescription.* 7th ed. Baltimore (MD): Lippincott Williams and Wilkins; 2014.

*Resource:* American College of Sports medicine. *ACSM's Health/Fitness Facility Standards and Guidelines.* 3rd ed. Champaign (IL): Human Kinetics; 2007. p. 36.

2—**E.** None of the above

   *Resource:* American College of Sports Medicine. *ACSM's Health/Fitness Facility Standards and Guidelines.* 3rd ed. Champaign (IL): Human Kinetics. 2007. p. 41.

HFS

**3—B.** Spin class cycles

> *Resource:* American College of Sports Medicine. *ACSM's Health/Fitness Facility Standards and Guidelines.* 3rd ed. Champaign (IL): Human Kinetics. 2007. p. 27. Table 5.2

**4—D.** No formal education is recommended fo the position, only a professional certification combined with at least 3 yr of experience as a group exercise instructor.

> *Resource:* American College of Sports Medicine. *ACSM's Resource Manual for Guidelines for Exercise Testing and Prescription.* 7th ed. Baltimore (MD): Lippincott Williams and Wilkins; 2014.

**5—C.** Exercises must be safe for the 25–45-yr-old age demographic because this group compromises the majority of most group exercise classes.

> *Resource:* American College of Sports Medicine. *ACSM's Resource Manual for Guidelines for Exercise Testing and Prescription.* 7th ed. Baltimore (MD): Lippincott Williams and Wilkins; 2014.

**6—B.** To base most of your management feedback on what is planned and expected of the employee for the upcoming year.

> *Resource:* American College of Sports Medicine. *ACSM's Resource Manual for Guidelines for Exercise Testing and Prescription.* 7th ed. Baltimore (MD): Lippincott Williams and Wilkins; 2014.

**7—B.** Process evaluation can demonstrate whether procedures were followed and whether they were appropriate and effective.

> *Resource*: ACSM's Resource Manual for Guidelines for Exercise Testing and Prescription. 4th ed., page 606

**8—C** Participant Surveys

> *Resource:* ACSM's Resource Manual for Guidelines for Exercise Testing and Prescription. 4th ed., pages 603–604

## Discussion Question Answers for Case Study HFS.V

1. Enlist or recruit a high-level staff member; for example, club general manager, to participate in a "challenge" promotion featuring the group exercise program. The general manager (GM) will participate in every group exercise class on the club schedule, then blog about his or her class experience on the club Web site. In each class the GM attends, a club gift certificate drawing is held for class participants.

Develop a Facebook promotion strategy for the group exercise program. Feature special classes and guest instructors. Solicit member comments and feedback regarding classes that the club offers.

Members love to read their names and see their photos on Facebook. Using group exercise class instructors, plan a "photo-taking initiative" featuring photos of members enjoy different class activities. Post these photos on Facebook and on the club Web site homepage. Make sure to get the proper permissions to use member likeness for club promotional efforts. This language can often be included in membership application form. Ensure that membership staff explains the photo permission clause and provides a decline option for member.

Group exercise coordinator takes on the daily responsibility of tweeting about the group exercise program on Twitter. It is important to be consistent with Twitter tweets, recommend at least one per day. The group exercise coordinator should understand company marketing strategy and professionalism guidelines when creating tweet information. Group exercise coordinator should work closely with membership and marketing departments, welcoming input for Twitter information. Promote the group exercise Twitter account on the club Web site homepage and create signage promoting the Twitter initiative, displayed in the group exercise activity areas.

2. Use a separate software package (*e.g.*, Les Mills Club Count software) that provides class scheduling and participation analysis capability. Some software packages can import member information from club management software systems and also export class schedule templates to URL Web sites.

Use existing club management software module that allows for separate group exercise class check-in information — participate checks into class via computer terminal connected to club management software systems. This information can then be exported to separate spreadsheet for analysis.

Each participant signs a class participation sheet made available near the entry of the exercise area. The instructor performs a head count prior to class starting and these two numbers are compared/averaged.

Class attendance numbers are input into an Excel (or similar software program) spreadsheet for analysis. It is important to analyze average class attendance figures, determining if participation meets a predetermined minimum attendance requirements. It is also important to set minimum attendance requirements based on the type of class (*e.g.*, mind/body, spinning, boot camp, step) and then adjust minimum attendance requirements based on seasonal participation patterns.

*Note: HFS certification candidates should also review the knowledge, skills, and abilities (KSAs) found in Part 1, ACSM Certified Personal Trainer (CPT).*

## DOMAIN I: HEALTH AND FITNESS ASSESSMENT

| A. Implement assessment protocols and preparticipation health screening procedures to maximize participant safety and minimize risk. | | |
|---|---|---|
| **Knowledge or Skill Statement** | **Explanation/Examples** | **Resources** |
| **Knowledge** of preactivity screening procedures and tools that provide accurate information about the individual's health/medical history, current medical conditions, risk factors, sign/symptoms of disease, current physical activity habits, and medications | • Consider self-guided methods.<br>• Cardiovascular disease (CVD) risk factor assessment<br>• Medical evaluation<br>• Exercise history | *ACSM's Guidelines for Exercise Testing and Prescription* (GETP), 9th edition (7)<br>• Tables 2.1, 2.2, and 2.4<br>• Figures 2.1–2.4 |
| **Knowledge** of the key components included in informed consent and health/medical history | • Content and extent may vary.<br>• Participant should be familiar with the purpose and the risks of the procedures.<br>• The form should be explained verbally. | *ACSM's Guidelines for Exercise Testing and Prescription* (GETP), 9th edition (7)<br>• Figure 3.1<br>*ACSM'S Health-Related Physical Fitness Assessment Manual*, 4th edition (4)<br>• Chapter 2 |
| **Knowledge** of the limitations of informed consent and health/medical history | • The participant is playing a major role in the informed consent process. He or she must be liable and responsible for informing the health fitness specialist (HFS) of any problems experienced (past, present, and during the assessment) that may increase the risk of the test or prohibit participation. | *ACSM's Health-Related Physical Fitness Assessment Manual*, 4th edition (4)<br>• Chapter 2 |

| B. Determine participant's readiness to take part in a health-related physical fitness assessment and exercise program. | | |
|---|---|---|
| **Knowledge or Skill Statement** | **Explanation/Examples** | **Resources** |
| **Knowledge** of risk factor thresholds for American College of Sports Medicine (ACSM) risk stratification including genetic and lifestyle factors related to the development of cardiovascular disease (CVD) | • Consider positive and negative risk factors. | *ACSM's Guidelines for Exercise Testing and Prescription* (GETP), 9th edition (7)<br>• Table 2.3 |

## B. Determine participant's readiness to take part in a health-related physical fitness assessment and exercise program. (cont.)

| Knowledge or Skill Statement | Explanation/Examples | Resources |
|---|---|---|
| **Knowledge** of the major signs or symptoms suggestive of cardiovascular, pulmonary, and metabolic disease | • Consider nine major signs and/or symptoms. <br> • Be aware of clarifications/significance. | *ACSM's Guidelines for Exercise Testing and Prescription* (GETP), 9th edition (7) <br> • Table 2.2 |
| **Knowledge** of cardiovascular risk factors or conditions that may require consultation with medical personnel prior to exercise testing or training (*e.g.*, inappropriate changes in resting heart rate and/or blood pressure [BP]; new onset discomfort in chest, neck, shoulder, or arm; changes in the pattern of discomfort during rest or exercise, fainting, dizzy spells, claudication) | • Consider nine major signs and/or symptoms. <br> • Be aware of clarifications/significance. <br> • Be aware of the different termination criteria based on signs and symptoms. | *ACSM's Guidelines for Exercise Testing and Prescription* (GETP), 9th edition (7) <br> • Table 2.2 <br> • Boxes 4.5 and 5.2 <br> • Table 10.1 |
| **Knowledge** of the pulmonary risk factors or conditions that may require consultation with medical personnel prior to exercise testing or training (*e.g.*, asthma, exercise-induced asthma/bronchospasm, extreme breathlessness at rest or during exercise, chronic bronchitis, emphysema) | • Nine major signs and/or symptoms <br> • Be aware of clarifications/significance. <br> • Be aware of spirometry-related measures. | *ACSM's Guidelines for Exercise Testing and Prescription* (GETP), 9th edition (7) <br> • Tables 2.2, 3.4, and 10.1 |
| **Knowledge** of the metabolic risk factors or conditions that may require consultation with medical personnel prior to exercise testing or training (*e.g.*, obesity, metabolic syndrome, diabetes or glucose intolerance, hypoglycemia) | • Be aware of conditions that may postpone or terminate an exercise session. | *ACSM's Guidelines for Exercise Testing and Prescription* (GETP), 9th edition (7) <br> • Tables 10.2 and 10.3 <br> • Chapter 10 |
| **Knowledge** of the musculoskeletal risk factors or conditions that may require consultation with medical personnel prior to exercise testing or training (*e.g.*, acute or chronic pain, osteoarthritis, rheumatoid arthritis, osteoporosis, inflammation/pain, low back pain) | • Be aware of common signs and symptoms that are associated with these conditions. | *ACSM's Guidelines for Exercise Testing and Prescription* (GETP), 9th edition (7) <br> • Chapter 10 |
| **Knowledge** of ACSM risk classification categories and their implications for medical clearance before administration of an exercise test or participation in an exercise program | • Be aware of the differences between low, moderate, and high risk classifications. <br> • Be aware of conditions that may require exercise testing in asymptomatic participants prior to the commencement of an exercise program. | *ACSM's Guidelines for Exercise Testing and Prescription* (GETP), 9th edition (7) <br> • Tables 2.1 and 2.3 |
| **Knowledge** of risk factors that may be favorably modified by physical activity habits | • Consider the benefits of regular physical activity and/or exercise. | *ACSM's Guidelines for Exercise Testing and Prescription* (GETP), 9th edition (7) <br> • Box 1.2 |

HFS

## B. Determine participant's readiness to take part in a health-related physical fitness assessment and exercise program. (cont.)

| Knowledge or Skill Statement | Explanation/Examples | Resources |
|---|---|---|
| **Knowledge** of medical terminology including but not limited to total cholesterol (TC), high-density lipoprotein cholesterol (HDL-C), low-density lipoprotein cholesterol (LDL-C), triglycerides, impaired fasting glucose, impaired glucose tolerance, hypertension, atherosclerosis, myocardial infarction, dyspnea, tachycardia, claudication, syncope, and ischemia | • Consider key medical terms that influence health and may affect exercise prescription and outcome. | *ACSM's Resource Manual for Guidelines for Exercise Testing and Prescription*, 7th edition (8)<br>• Chapters 6, 7, and 13<br>*ACSM's Guidelines for Exercise Testing and Prescription* (GETP), 9th edition (7)<br>• Table 2.2 |
| **Knowledge** of recommended plasma cholesterol levels for adults based on National Cholesterol Education Program (NCEP)/Adult Treatment Panel (ATP) Guidelines. | • Adapted from the "Third Report of the Expert Panel on Detection, Evaluation, and Treatment of High Blood Cholesterol in Adults," ATP III outlines the NCEP's recommendations for cholesterol testing and management.<br>• Guideline may be adjusted periodically. | *ACSM's Guidelines for Exercise Testing and Prescription* (GETP), 9th edition (7)<br>• Table 3.2 |
| **Knowledge** of recommended BP levels for adults based on National High Blood Pressure Education Program Guidelines | • Adapted from "The Seventh Report of the Joint National Committee on Prevention, Detection, Evaluation, and Treatment of High Blood Pressure (JNC7)."<br>• Guideline may be adjusted periodically. | *ACSM's Guidelines for Exercise Testing and Prescription* (GETP), 9th edition (7)<br>• Table 3.1 |
| **Knowledge** of medical supervision recommendations for cardiorespiratory fitness testing | • When recommended to have a medical doctor (MD) supervision during a test, one should be in close proximity and readily available. | *ACSM's Guidelines for Exercise Testing and Prescription* (GETP), 9th edition (7)<br>• Chapter 2<br>• Figure 2.4 |
| **Knowledge** of the components of a health history questionnaire (*e.g.*, past and current medical history, family history of cardiac disease, orthopedic limitations, prescribed medications, activity patterns, nutritional habits, stress and anxiety levels, and smoking and alcohol use) | • This process should be thorough and include past and present items. | *ACSM's Guidelines for Exercise Testing and Prescription* (GETP), 9th edition (7)<br>• Box 3.1 |
| **Skill** in risk classification of participants using CVD risk factor thresholds, major signs or symptoms suggestive of cardiovascular, pulmonary, or metabolic disease and/or the presence of known cardiovascular, pulmonary, and metabolic disease status | • Consider positive and negative risk factors.<br>• Consider nine major signs and/or symptoms and be aware of clarifications/significance of each chapter.<br>• Differentiate between low, moderate, and high risk classifications. | *ACSM's Guidelines for Exercise Testing and Prescription* (GETP), 9th edition (7)<br>• Tables 2.2 and 2.3<br>• Figure 2.3 |
| **Skill** in reviewing preactivity screening documents to determine the need for medical clearance prior to exercise and to select appropriate physical fitness assessment protocols | • Review, when applied, self-guided or professionally guided screening forms.<br>• Consider risk classification.<br>• Consider various physical fitness assessment protocols such as body composition, cardiorespiratory fitness, muscular strength and muscular endurance, and flexibility. | *ACSM's Guidelines for Exercise Testing and Prescription* (GETP), 9th edition (7)<br>• Chapter 2<br>• Figures 2.3 and 2.4<br>• Chapter 4 |

HFS

## C.    Select and prepare physical fitness assessments for healthy participants and those with controlled disease.

| Knowledge or Skill Statement | Explanation/Examples | Resources |
|---|---|---|
| **Knowledge** of the physiological basis of the major components of physical fitness — cardiorespiratory fitness, body composition, flexibility, muscular strength, and muscular endurance | • If detailed exercise physiology review is warranted, review Chapter 3 of *ACSM's Resource Manual for Guidelines for Exercise Testing and Prescription*, 7th edition. | *ACSM's Guidelines for Exercise Testing and Prescription* (GETP), 9th edition (7)<br>• Chapter 4 |
| **Knowledge** of selecting the most appropriate testing protocols for each participant based on preliminary screening data | • Consider specific fitness goals.<br>• Consider injury history. | *ACSM's Guidelines for Exercise Testing and Prescription* (GETP), 9th edition (7)<br>• Chapter 4 |
| **Knowledge** of calibration techniques and proper use of fitness testing equipment | • To ensure the accuracy of the collected data, devices and related equipment (stationary bikes, treadmills, etc.) must be calibrated prior to the testing session.<br>• Review equipment manuals for specifics. | *ACSM's Health-Related Physical Fitness Assessment Manual*, 4th edition (4)<br>• Chapter 1<br>*ACSM's Resource Manual for Guidelines for Exercise Testing and Prescription*, 7th edition (8)<br>• Chapter 20 |
| **Knowledge** of the purpose and procedures of fitness testing protocols for the components of health-related fitness | • Review pretest instruction and follow appropriate test order.<br>• Be aware of different modes to measure the components of health-related physical fitness. | *ACSM's Guidelines for Exercise Testing and Prescription* (GETP), 9th edition (7)<br>• Chapter 4 |
| **Knowledge** of test termination criteria and proper procedures to be followed after discontinuing health fitness tests | • These indications apply for exercise tests but could also be applied for any health-related physical fitness components tests. | *ACSM's Guidelines for Exercise Testing and Prescription* (GETP), 9th edition (7)<br>• Box 4.5 |
| **Knowledge** of fitness assessment sequencing | • These may apply to related forms, equipment to be used, and environmental conditions. | *ACSM's Guidelines for Exercise Testing and Prescription* (GETP), 9th edition (7)<br>• Chapter 4 |
| **Knowledge** of the effects of common medications and substances on exercise testing (*e.g.*, antianginals, antihypertensives, antiarrhythmics, bronchodilators, hypoglycemics, psychotropics, alcohol, diet pills, cold tablets, caffeine, nicotine) | • For each class of common medication and substances, recognize drug name and related brand and effect on heart rate, blood pressure, electrocardiogram (ECG), and exercise capacity. | *ACSM's Guidelines for Exercise Testing and Prescription* (GETP), 9th edition (7)<br>• Appendix A |
| **Knowledge** of the physiologic and metabolic responses to exercise testing associated with each chronic diseases and conditions (*e.g.*, heart disease, hypertension, diabetes mellitus, obesity, pulmonary disease) | • Review pathophysiology, exercise responses, and the effects of exercise training for each chronic condition. | *ACSM's Exercise Management for Persons with Chronic Diseases and Disabilities*, 3rd edition (2)<br>• Parts II–IV |
| **Skill** in analyzing and interpreting information obtained from assessment of the components of health-related fitness | • Use appropriate criterion-referenced and normative standard tables to analyze and interpret data. | *ACSM's Guidelines for Exercise Testing and Prescription* (GETP), 9th edition (7)<br>• Tables 4.1–4.3, 4.5–4.6, 4.8–4.13, and 4.15–4.17 |
| **Skill** in modifying protocols and procedures for testing children, adolescents, older adults, and individuals with special considerations | • Be aware of the differences between testing an apparently healthy population and healthy population with special considerations. | *ACSM's Guidelines for Exercise Testing and Prescription* (GETP), 9th edition (7)<br>• Chapter 8 |

HFS

## D.  Conduct and interpret cardiorespiratory fitness assessments.

| Knowledge or Skill Statement | Explanation/Examples | Resources |
|---|---|---|
| **Knowledge** of common submaximal and maximal cardiorespiratory assessment protocols | • Be aware of the pros and cons of using different modes of exercise and different protocols to determine cardiorespiratory performance. | *ACSM's Health-Related Physical Fitness Assessment Manual,* 4th edition (4)<br>• Chapters 7 and 8 |
| **Knowledge** of blood pressure (BP) measurement techniques | • Be aware of different conditions and considerations that may affect resting BP measurements such as body posture, appropriate cuff size, etc. | *ACSM's Health-Related Physical Fitness Assessment Manual,* 4th edition (4)<br>• Chapter 3 |
| **Knowledge** of Korotkoff sounds for determining systolic BP (SBP) and diastolic BP (DBP) | • Be aware of the significance and the difference between the 4th (true DBP) and the 5th (clinical DBP) Korotkoff sounds in respect to resting and exercise measurements. | *ACSM's Health-Related Physical Fitness Assessment Manual,* 4th edition (4)<br>• Box 3.1 |
| **Knowledge** of the BP response to exercise | • Be aware of abnormal responses to exercise such as a drop in SBP and substantial increase in DBP.<br>• Be aware of the significance of rate-pressure product. | *ACSM's Guidelines for Exercise Testing and Prescription* (GETP), 9th edition (7)<br>• Chapter 6 |
| **Knowledge** of techniques of measuring heart rate (HR) and HR response to exercise | • Be aware of the two common anatomical palpation sites.<br>• Be aware of the wide interindividual variability with respect to HR responses during exercise and therefore the potential inaccuracy in predicting maximal heart rate ($HR_{max}$). | *ACSM's Resource Manual for Exercise Testing and Prescription,* 7th edition (8)<br>• Chapter 20<br>*ACSM's Guidelines for Exercise Testing and Prescription* (GETP), 9th edition (7)<br>• Chapter 6 |
| **Knowledge** of the rating of perceived exertion (RPE) | • Be aware of the limitation of the RPE scale.<br>• Similar to HR responses to exercise, the RPE scale presents a wide interindividual variability and therefore should be used with caution. | *ACSM's Guidelines for Exercise Testing and Prescription* (GETP), 9th edition (7)<br>• Chapter 4<br>• Table 4.7 |
| **Knowledge** of HR, BP, and RPE monitoring techniques before, during, and after cardiorespiratory fitness testing | • Be aware that there are several techniques to measure HR.<br>• BP should be measured at the horizontal level of the heart.<br>• The subjective measure of perceived exertion may be influenced by many factors and therefore should be used with caution. | *ACSM's Guidelines for Exercise Testing and Prescription* (GETP), 9th edition (7)<br>• Chapter 4<br>• Table 4.4 |
| **Knowledge** of the anatomy and physiology of the cardiovascular and pulmonary systems | • This information could also be found in any undergraduate or graduate level exercise physiology textbook. | *ACSM's Resource Manual for Exercise Testing and Prescription,* 7th edition (8)<br>• Chapters 1 and 3 |
| **Knowledge** of cardiorespiratory terminology including angina pectoris, tachycardia, bradycardia, arrhythmia, and hyperventilation | • These terms could be found in any other reputable clinical exercise physiology textbook. | *Clinical Exercise Physiology,* 2nd edition (12)<br>• Glossary, pp. 593–610 |

HFS

## D.  Conduct and interpret cardiorespiratory fitness assessments. (cont.)

| Knowledge or Skill Statement | Explanation/Examples | Resources |
|---|---|---|
| **Knowledge** of the pathophysiology of myocardial ischemia, myocardial infarction (MI), stroke, hypertension, and hyperlipidemia | • Be familiar with the different stages (significance) and progression of atherosclerosis.<br>• Be aware of the intimate relationship that each condition often has with one another. | *ACSM's Resource Manual for Exercise Testing and Prescription*, 7th edition (8)<br>• Chapter 6 |
| **Knowledge** of the effects of myocardial ischemia, MI, hypertension, claudication, and dyspnea on cardiorespiratory responses during exercise | • Be aware of the multifaceted relationship between atherosclerosis and these conditions. | *ACSM's Exercise Management for Persons with Chronic Diseases and Disabilities*, 3rd edition (2)<br>• Chapters 6, 14, and 15 |
| **Knowledge** of oxygen consumption dynamics during exercise (*e.g.*, HR, stroke volume, cardiac output, ventilation, ventilatory threshold) | • This information could also be found in any undergraduate or graduate level exercise physiology textbook. | *ACSM's Resource Manual for Exercise Testing and Prescription*, 7th edition (8)<br>• Chapter 3<br>*ACSM's Guidelines for Exercise Testing and Prescription* (GETP), 9th edition (7)<br>• Chapter 6<br>• Box 6.1 |
| **Knowledge** of methods of calculating maximal volume of oxygen consumed per unit of time ($\dot{V}O_{2max}$) | • Be aware that there are several methods of calculating $\dot{V}O_{2max}$. Each of the methods provides some pros and cons in respect to the level of difficulty and accuracy of performing the test. | *ACSM's Health-Related Physical Fitness Assessment Manual*, 4th edition (4)<br>• Chapters 7 and 8 |
| **Knowledge** of cardiorespiratory responses to acute graded exercise of conditioned and unconditioned participants | • This information could be found in any other reputable exercise physiology textbook. | *Exercise Physiology: Integrating Theory and Application* (19)<br>• Chapter 5 |
| **Skill** in interpreting cardiorespiratory fitness test results | • Consider the pros and cons of each method in respect to the level of difficulty and accuracy of the results. | *ACSM's Health-Related Physical Fitness Assessment Manual*, 4th edition (4)<br>• Chapters 7 and 8 |
| **Skill** in locating anatomic landmarks for palpation of peripheral pulses and BP | • Palpate for the brachial artery prior to attempting to measure BP. | *ACSM's Resource Manual for Guidelines for Exercise Testing and Prescription*, 7th edition (8)<br>• Chapters 1 and 20 |
| **Skill** in measuring HR, BP, and RPE at rest and during exercise | • Consider the order of measurements during a submaximal or maximal graded exercise test. | *ACSM's Resource Manual for Guidelines for Exercise Testing and Prescription*, 7th edition (8)<br>• Chapter 20<br>*ACSM's Guidelines for Exercise Testing and Prescription* (GETP), 9th edition (7)<br>• Chapter 4<br>• Table 4.7 |
| **Skill** in determining cardiorespiratory fitness based on submaximal exercise test results | • Consider the pros and cons of using different modes of exercise and different protocols to determine cardiorespiratory fitness. | *ACSM's Health-Related Physical Fitness Assessment Manual*, 4th edition (4)<br>• Chapter 7 |

HFS

## E.   Conduct assessments of muscular strength, muscular endurance, and flexibility.

| Knowledge or Skill Statement | Explanation/Examples | Resources |
|---|---|---|
| **Knowledge** of common muscular strength, muscular endurance, and flexibility assessment protocols | • Be aware of the pros and cons of using different common muscular strength, muscular endurance, and flexibility assessment protocols. | *ACSM's Health-Related Physical Fitness Assessment Manual,* 4th edition (4)<br>• Chapters 5 and 6 |
| **Knowledge** of interpreting muscular strength, muscular endurance, and flexibility assessments | • Use appropriate criterion-referenced and normative standard tables to analyze and interpret data. | *ACSM's Health-Related Physical Fitness Assessment Manual,* 4th edition (4)<br>• Chapters 5 and 6 |
| **Knowledge** of relative strength, absolute strength, and one repetition maximum (1-RM) estimation | • Be aware that there are other methods of measuring strength using both static and isokinetic assessments. | *ACSM's Resource Manual for Guidelines for Exercise Testing and Prescription,* 7th edition (8)<br>• Chapter 31 |
| **Knowledge** of the anatomy of bone, skeletal muscle, and connective tissues | • Be aware of the relationship these different systems have in respect to human movement. | *ACSM's Resource Manual for Guidelines for Exercise Testing and Prescription,* 7th edition (8)<br>• Chapter 1<br>*ACSM's Health-Related Physical Fitness Assessment Manual,* 4th edition (4)<br>• Chapter 5 |
| **Knowledge** of muscle action terms including anterior, posterior, inferior, superior, medial, lateral, supination, pronation, flexion, extension, adduction, abduction, hyperextension, rotation, circumduction, agonist, antagonist, and stabilizer | • Be aware of the different joints in the body in respect to planes and axes of rotation and associated movements.<br>• Be aware of the different roles performed by each muscle. | *ACSM's Resource Manual for Guidelines for Exercise Testing and Prescription,* 7th edition (8)<br>• Chapter 1<br>• Table 1.5<br>*Basic Biomechanics,* 6th edition (16)<br>• Chapter 6 |
| **Knowledge** of the planes and axes in which movement action occurs | • Be aware that the starting position for recognizing planes and axis of all movements in the human body is the anatomical position. | *ACSM's Resource Manual for Guidelines for Exercise Testing and Prescription,* 7th edition (8)<br>• Chapter 1<br>• Figure 1.2 |
| **Knowledge** of the interrelationships among center of gravity, base of support, balance, stability, posture, and proper spinal alignment | • This information could be found in any other reputable biomechanics textbook. | *Basic Biomechanics,* 6th edition (16)<br>• Chapters 9 and 13 |
| **Knowledge** of the normal curvatures of the spine and common assessments of postural alignment | • Be aware of the difference between primary and secondary spinal curves.<br>• This information could be found in any other reputable biomechanics textbook. | *Basic Biomechanics,* 6th edition (16)<br>• pp. 283–284 |
| **Knowledge** of the location and function of the major muscles (*e.g.,* pectoralis major, trapezius, latissimus dorsi, biceps, triceps, rectus abdominis, internal and external obliques, erector spinae, gluteus maximus, quadriceps, hamstrings, adductors, abductors, and gastrocnemius) | • Be aware of the relationship between muscles location, line of pull, and specific movements. | *ACSM's Resource Manual for Guidelines for Exercise Testing and Prescription,* 7th edition (8)<br>• Chapter 1<br>• Figures 1.29 and 1.30 |

HFS

## E.    Conduct assessments of muscular strength, muscular endurance, and flexibility. (cont.)

| Knowledge or Skill Statement | Explanation/Examples | Resources |
|---|---|---|
| **Knowledge** of the major joints and their associated movement | • Be aware of each joint's classification and the relationship to planes and axes. | *ACSM's Resource Manual for Guidelines for Exercise Testing and Prescription*, 7th edition (8)<br>• Chapter 1<br>• Tables 1.3 and 1.4 |
| **Skill** in identifying the major bones, muscles, and joints | • Be aware of the adjacent bones, muscles, and joints. | *ACSM's Resource Manual for Guidelines for Exercise Testing and Prescription*, 7th edition (8)<br>• Chapter 1<br>• Figures 1.23, 1.29, and 1.30<br>• Table 1.5 |
| **Skill** in conducting assessments of muscular strength, muscular endurance and flexibility (*e.g.*, 1-RM, hand grip dynamometer, push-ups, curl-ups, sit-and-reach) | • Be aware of the pros and cons of using different common muscular strength, muscular endurance, and flexibility tests. | *ACSM's Health-Related Physical Fitness Assessment Manual*, 4th edition (4)<br>• Chapters 5 and 6 |
| **Skill** in estimating 1-RM using lower resistance (2–10 RM) | • Consider the advantages and disadvantages of using an estimation rather than measuring 1-RM. | *Designing Resistance Training Programs*, 3rd edition (13)<br>• Chapter 5 |
| **Skill** in interpreting results of muscular strength, muscular endurance, and flexibility assessments | • Use appropriate criterion-referenced and normative standard tables to analyze and interpret data. | *ACSM's Health-Related Physical Fitness Assessment Manual*, 4th edition (4)<br>• Chapters 5 and 6 |

## F.    Conduct anthropometric and body composition assessments.

| Knowledge or Skill Statement | Explanation/Examples | Resources |
|---|---|---|
| **Knowledge** of the advantages, disadvantages, and limitations of body composition techniques (*e.g.*, air displacement plethysmography [BOD POD], duel-energy X-ray absorptiometry [DEXA], hydrostatic weighing, skinfolds, and bioelectrical impedance) | • Be aware of the pros and cons of each method in respect to the level of difficulty and accuracy of the results. | *ACSM' Health-Related Physical Fitness Assessment Manual*, 4th edition (4)<br>• Chapter 4 |
| **Knowledge** of the standardized descriptions of circumference and skinfold sites | • Be familiar with the differences between circumference and skinfold measurement in respect to accuracy, significance, and use. | *ACSM's Health-Related Physical Fitness Assessment Manual*, 4th edition (4)<br>• Chapter 4<br>*ACSM's Guideline for Exercise Testing and Prescription* (GETP), 9th edition (7)<br>• Chapter 4 |
| **Knowledge** of procedures for determining body mass index (BMI) and taking skinfold and circumference measurements | • Be aware of the pros and cons of each method in respect to the level of difficulty and accuracy of the results. | *ACSM's Health-Related Physical Fitness Assessment Manual*, 4th edition (4)<br>• Chapter 4<br>*ACSM's Guidelines for Exercise Testing and Prescription* (GETP), 9th edition (7)<br>• Chapter 4 |

HFS

## F. Conduct anthropometric and body composition assessments. (cont.)

| Knowledge or Skill Statement | Explanation/Examples | Resources |
|---|---|---|
| **Knowledge** of the health implications of variation in body fat distribution patterns and the significance of BMI, waist circumference, and waist-to-hip ratio | • Be aware of the relationship between BMI, waist circumference, and the related disease risk. | *ACSM's Guidelines for Exercise Testing and Prescription* (GETP), 9th edition (7)<br>• Chapter 4 |
| **Skill** in locating anatomic landmarks for skinfold and circumference measurements | • Consider the anatomic landmarks differences between skinfold and circumference sites. | *ACSM's Guidelines for Exercise Testing and Prescription* (GETP), 9th edition (7)<br>• Chapter 4<br>• Boxes 4.1 and 4.2 |
| **Skill** in interpreting the results of anthropometric and body composition assessments | • Consider the process of calculating skinfold measurement, specifically, body density conversion to percent body fat. | *ACSM's Guidelines for Exercise Testing and Prescription* (GETP), 9th edition (7)<br>• Chapter 4<br>• Tables 4.3 and 4.5 |

## DOMAIN II: EXERCISE PRESCRIPTION AND IMPLEMENTATION

### A. Review preparticipation health screening including self-guided health questionnaires and appraisals, exercise history, and physical fitness assessments.

| Knowledge or Skill Statement | Explanation/Examples | Resources |
|---|---|---|
| **Skill** in synthesizing prescreening results and reviewing them with participants | • Be aware of the major changes to the preparticipation procedures in this edition of Guidelines for Exercise Testing and Prescription (GETP) when compared to previous publications of American College of Sports Medicine (ACSM). | *ACSM's Guidelines for Exercise Testing and Prescription* (GETP), 9th edition (7)<br>• Tables 2.1–2.4<br>• Figures 2.1–2.4 |

### B. Determine safe and effective exercise programs to achieve desired outcomes and goals.

| Knowledge or Skill Statement | Explanation/Examples | Resources |
|---|---|---|
| **Knowledge** of strength, cardiovascular, and flexibility-based exercise | • Be aware of the basic components of an exercise training session; quantity of exercise; and frequency, intensity, time, and type, volume and progression (FITT-VP) principles. | *ACSM's Guidelines for Exercise Testing and Prescription* (GETP), 9th edition (7)<br>• Chapter 7 |
| **Knowledge** of the benefits and precautions associated with exercise training in apparently healthy participants and those with controlled disease | • Be familiar with the benefits of regular physical activity and/or exercise.<br>• Be familiar with the risk that is associated with physical activity and/or exercise. | *ACSM's Guidelines for Exercise Testing and Prescription* (GETP), 9th edition (7)<br>• Chapter 1<br>• Box 1.2<br>• Tables 1.3–1.6 |
| **Knowledge** of program development for specific client needs (*e.g.*, sport-specific training, performance, health, lifestyle, functional ability, balance, agility, aerobic, anaerobic) | • Consider client-specific fitness goals (health and performance related).<br>• Collect baseline and follow-up data in order to provide individualized and appropriate exercise prescription. | *ACSM's Guidelines for Exercise Testing and Prescription* (GETP), 9th edition (7)<br>• Chapter 4 |
| **Knowledge** of the six motor skill–related physical fitness components: agility, balance, coordination, reaction time, speed, and power | • Be aware of the fundamental differences between health-related physical fitness components and skill-related physical fitness components. | *ACSM's Guidelines for Exercise Testing and Prescription* (GETP), 9th edition (7)<br>• Chapter 1<br>• Box 1.1 |

## B.  Determine safe and effective exercise programs to achieve desired outcomes and goals. (cont.)

| Knowledge or Skill Statement | Explanation/Examples | Resources |
|---|---|---|
| **Knowledge** of the physiologic changes associated with an acute bout of exercise | • Be familiar with changes in heart rate (HR), stroke volume (SV), cardiac output (CO [Q̇]), blood flow, blood pressure, arteriovenous oxygen difference (a-vO2 DIFF), and ventilation.<br>• This information could also be found in any undergraduate or graduate level exercise physiology textbook. | *ACSM's Resource Manual for Guidelines for Exercise Testing and Prescription*, 7th edition (8)<br>• Chapter 3<br>*ACSM's Guidelines for Exercise Testing and Prescription* (GETP), 9th edition (7)<br>• Chapter 6 |
| **Knowledge** of the physiologic adaptations following chronic exercise training | • This information could be found in any reputable exercise physiology textbook.<br>• The adaptations that are associated with chronic exercise training improve physiological function, reduce coronary artery disease (CAD) risk factors, decrease morbidity and mortality rates, and provide other health-related benefits. | *ACSM's Resource Manual for Guidelines for Exercise Testing and Prescription*, 7th edition (8)<br>• Chapter 32<br>*ACSM's Guidelines for Exercise Testing and Prescription* (GETP), 9th edition (7)<br>• Chapter 1<br>• Box 1.2 |
| **Knowledge** of American College of Sports Medicine (ACSM) exercise prescription guidelines for strength, cardiovascular, and flexibility-based exercise for apparently healthy clients, clients with increased risk, and clients with controlled disease | • Be familiar with FITT-VP principles.<br>• The information may apply to apparently healthy population, healthy population with special consideration, and inpatient and outpatient rehabilitation programs. | *ACSM's Guidelines for Exercise Testing and Prescription* (GETP), 9th edition (7)<br>• Chapters 7–9 |
| **Knowledge** of the components and sequencing incorporated into an exercise session (*e.g.*, warm-up, stretching, conditioning or sports-related exercise, cool-down) | • Be aware that these components should be incorporated in some form with aerobic exercise as well as muscular fitness exercise. | *ACSM's Guidelines for Exercise Testing and Prescription* (GETP), 9th edition (7)<br>• Chapter 7 |
| **Knowledge** of the physiological principles related to warm-up and cool-down | • Although both the warm-up and cool-down are often overlooked by many professionals, the physiological principles are important and valid. | *ACSM's Resource Manual for Guidelines for Exercise Testing and Prescription*, 7th edition (8)<br>• Chapter 34 |
| **Knowledge** of the principles of reversibility, progressive overload, individual differences and specificity of training, and how they relate to exercise prescription | • When determining an appropriate exercise prescription, be aware of client/patient goals. Prescribe appropriate exercise and be mindful of attainable goals. | *ACSM's Resource Manual for Guidelines for Exercise Testing and Prescription*, 7th edition (8)<br>• Chapter 31 |
| **Knowledge** of the role of aerobic and anaerobic energy systems in the performance of various physical activities | • Be very familiar with the intricate relationship between the aerobic and anaerobic systems as they relate to the intensity and duration of different physical activities. | *ACSM's Resource Manual for Guidelines for Exercise Testing and Prescription*, 7th edition (8)<br>• Chapter 3 |
| **Knowledge** of the basic biomechanical principles of human movement | • Be familiar with biomechanics and the relationship to activities of daily living (ADL) as well as to sport performance.<br>• This information could also be found in any reputable undergraduate or graduate level biomechanics textbook. | *ACSM's Resource Manual for Guidelines for Exercise Testing and Prescription*, 7th edition (8)<br>• Chapter 2 |

HFS

## B. Determine safe and effective exercise programs to achieve desired outcomes and goals. (cont.)

| Knowledge or Skill Statement | Explanation/Examples | Resources |
|---|---|---|
| **Knowledge** of the psychological and physiological signs and symptoms of overtraining | • Be familiar with differences between overtraining from aerobic exercise vs. resistance exercise. | *ACSM's Resource Manual for Guidelines for Exercise Testing and Prescription*, 7th edition (8)<br>• Chapters 32 and 33 |
| **Knowledge** of the signs and symptoms of common musculoskeletal injuries associated with exercise (*e.g.*, sprain, strain, bursitis, tendonitis) | • Be aware of the differences between musculature and joint-related injuries.<br>• This information could also be found in any reputable undergraduate or graduate athletic training textbook. | *Basic Biomechanics*, 6th edition (16)<br>• Chapter 5 |
| **Knowledge** of the advantages and disadvantages of exercise equipment (*e.g.*, free weights, selectorized machines, cardiovascular equipment) | • Both free weights and exercise machines can be beneficial if used appropriately and when following published guidelines. | *ACSM's Resource Manual for Guidelines for Exercise Testing and Prescription*, 7th edition (8)<br>• Chapter 31 |
| **Skill** in teaching and demonstrating exercises | • Health fitness specialist (HFS) is expected to be able to properly instruct aerobic, resistance, and flexibility exercises. | *ACSM's Guidelines for Exercise Testing and Prescription* (GETP), 9th edition (7)<br>• Chapters 7–9 |
| **Skill** in designing safe and effective training programs | • HFS is expected to be able to take raw data that is collected during exercise tests, interpret the results, and design safe and effective training programs. | *ACSM's Guidelines for Exercise Testing and Prescription* (GETP), 9th edition (7)<br>• Chapters 7–9 |
| **Skill** in implementing exercise prescription guidelines for apparently healthy clients, clients with increased risk, and clients with controlled disease | • HFS is expected to be able to take raw data that is collected during exercise tests, interpret the results, and provide a population specific exercise prescription. | *ACSM's Guidelines for Exercise Testing and Prescription* (GETP), 9th edition (7)<br>• Chapters 7–9 |

## C. Implement cardiorespiratory exercise prescriptions using the frequency, intensity, time, and type (FITT) principle for apparently healthy participants based on current health status, fitness goals, and availability of time.

| Knowledge or Skill Statement | Explanation/Examples | Resources |
|---|---|---|
| **Knowledge** of the recommended FITT framework for the development of cardiorespiratory fitness | • Health fitness specialist (HFS) should be very familiar with the FITT-VP framework, more specifically, the intricate relationship between frequency, intensity, time, and type of exercise. | *ACSM's Guidelines for Exercise Testing and Prescription* (GETP), 9th edition (7)<br>• Chapter 7<br>• Tables 7.5–7.7 |
| **Knowledge** of the benefits, risks, and contraindications of a wide variety of cardiovascular training exercises based on client experience, skill level, current fitness level, and goals | • Consider appropriate risk classification.<br>• Consider individualized and appropriate exercise prescription. | *ACSM's Guidelines for Exercise Testing and Prescription* (GETP), 9th edition (7)<br>• Chapter 1 |
| **Knowledge** of the minimal threshold of physical activity required for health benefits and/or fitness development | • HFS should be aware that FITT-VP principles applies to aerobic, resistance, and flexibility exercises. | *ACSM's Guidelines for Exercise Testing and Prescription* (GETP), 9th edition (7)<br>• Tables 7.5–7.7 |

HFS

**C.    Implement cardiorespiratory exercise prescriptions using the frequency, intensity, time, and type (FITT) principle for apparently healthy participants based on current health status, fitness goals, and availability of time. (cont.)**

| Knowledge or Skill Statement | Explanation/Examples | Resources |
|---|---|---|
| **Knowledge** of determining exercise intensity using heart rate reserve (HRR), oxygen uptake reserve ($\dot{V}O_2R$), peak heart rate ($HR_{peak}$) method, peak volume of oxygen consumed per unit of time ($\dot{V}O_{2peak}$) method, peak metabolic equivalents (MET) method, and the rating of perceived exertion (RPE) scale. | • Be aware that the RPE scale and other measures of perceived effort and/or affective variability should not be used as primary method of prescribing exercise intensity. | *ACSM's Guidelines for Exercise Testing and Prescription* (GETP), 9th edition (7)<br>• Chapter 7<br>• Box 7.2<br>• Table 7.1<br>• Chapter 11 |
| **Knowledge** of the accuracy of HRR, $\dot{V}O_2R$, $HR_{peak}$ method, $\dot{V}O_{2peak}$ method, peak MET method, and the RPE scale | • Be aware of different prediction equation for maximal heart rate ($HR_{max}$)<br>• The HRR or $\dot{V}O_2R$ methods may be preferable when compared to %HR and %$\dot{V}O_2$. | *ACSM's Guidelines for Exercise Testing and Prescription* (GETP), 9th edition (7)<br>• Chapter 7<br>• Table 7.2 |
| **Knowledge** of abnormal responses to exercise (*e.g.*, hemodynamic, cardiac, ventilatory) | • Be aware that these variables play a major role when assessing the therapeutic, diagnostic, and prognostic application of a test. | *ACSM's Guidelines for Exercise Testing and Prescription* (GETP), 9th edition (7)<br>• Box 6.1 |
| **Knowledge** of metabolic calculations (*e.g.*, unit conversions, deriving energy cost of exercise, caloric expenditure) | • Be aware of the different unit conversions.<br>• These formulas are most accurate during a steady state exercise. | *ACSM's Guidelines for Exercise Testing and Prescription* (GETP), 9th edition (7)<br>• Chapter 7<br>• Figure 7.1<br>• Table 7.3 |
| **Knowledge** of calculating the caloric expenditure of an exercise session (kilocalories per session) | • 1 lb (0.45 kg) of fat = 3,500 kcal<br>• Be aware of the MET level equation of calculating caloric expenditure per minute. | *ACSM's Resource Manual for Guidelines for Exercise Testing and Prescription*, 7th edition (8)<br>• Chapter 28 |
| **Knowledge** of methods for establishing and monitoring levels of exercise intensity including heart rate (HR), RPE, and MET. | • Be aware that the RPE scale and other measures of perceived effort and/or affective valence should not be used as primary method of prescribing exercise intensity. | *ACSM's Guidelines for Exercise Testing and Prescription* (GETP), 9th edition (7)<br>• Chapter 7<br>• Box 7.2<br>• Table 7.1<br>• Chapter 11 |
| **Knowledge** of the applications of anaerobic training principles | • Be aware that plyometric training is also considered as a method of anaerobic training. | *ACSM's Resource Manual for Guidelines for Exercise Testing and Prescription*, 7th edition (8)<br>• Chapter 31 |
| **Knowledge** of the anatomy and physiology of the cardiovascular and pulmonary systems including the basic properties of cardiac muscle | • Be aware of the relationship between these two systems in respect to normal function at rest and during exercise.<br>• Be aware of the relationship between these two systems in respect to upper limitation of aerobic performance.<br>• This information could be found in any other reputable exercise physiology textbook. | *ACSM's Resource Manual for Guidelines for Exercise Testing and Prescription*, 7th edition (8)<br>• Chapter 1<br>*Exercise Physiology: Integrating Theory and Application* (19)<br>• Chapters 5 and 6 |

HFS

## C. Implement cardiorespiratory exercise prescriptions using the frequency, intensity, time, and type (FITT) principle for apparently healthy participants based on current health status, fitness goals, and availability of time. (cont.)

| Knowledge or Skill Statement | Explanation/Examples | Resources |
|---|---|---|
| **Knowledge** of the basic principles of gas exchange | • Be familiar with the concept of open-circuit spirometry.<br>• Be familiar with the significance of respiratory exchange ratio (RER) and the relationship to respiratory quotient (RQ). | *ACSM's Guidelines for Exercise Testing and Prescription* (GETP), 9th edition (7)<br>• Chapter 4 |
| **Skill** in determining appropriate exercise frequency, intensity, time, and type for clients with various fitness levels | • Be familiar with the interaction between the different components of FITT-VP principles, specifically, intensity and time (duration) of the activity.<br>• Be aware of different prediction equation for $HR_{max}$.<br>• The HRR or $\dot{V}O_2R$ methods may be preferable when compared to %HR and %$\dot{V}O_2$.<br>• Be aware that the RPE scale and other measures of perceived effort and/or affective valence should not be used as primary method of prescribing exercise intensity. | *ACSM's Guidelines for Exercise Testing and Prescription* (GETP), 9th edition (7)<br>• Chapter 7 |
| **Skill** in determining the energy cost, absolute and relative oxygen costs ($\dot{V}O_2$), and MET levels of various activities and apply the information to an exercise prescription | • Consider the conversions between relative and absolute $\dot{V}O_2$ (mL $\cdot$ kg$^{-1}$ $\cdot$ min$^{-1}$ $\rightarrow$ L $\cdot$ min$^{-1}$ $\rightarrow$ /1000 $\times$ body mass), relative $\dot{V}O_2$, and MET (mL $\cdot$ kg$^{-1}$ $\cdot$ min$^{-1}$ $\rightarrow$ MET $\rightarrow$ /3.5) and vice versa. | *ACSM's Guidelines for Exercise Testing and Prescription* (GETP), 9th edition (7)<br>• Chapter 7<br>• Figure 7.1<br>• Table 7.3 |
| **Skill** in identifying improper technique in the use of cardiovascular equipment | • Consider the client-specific FITT-VP principles.<br>• If needed, consider consulting the specific manual of the cardiovascular exercise equipment. | *ACSM's Guidelines for Exercise Testing and Prescription* (GETP), 9th edition (7)<br>• Chapter 7 |
| **Skill** in teaching and demonstrating the use of various cardiovascular exercise equipment | • Consider the client-specific FITT-VP principles.<br>• If needed, consider consulting the specific manual of the cardiovascular exercise equipment. | *ACSM's Guidelines for Exercise Testing and Prescription* (GETP), 9th edition (7)<br>• Chapter 7 |

HFS

**D. Implement exercise prescriptions using the frequency, intensity, time, and type (FITT) principle for flexibility, muscular strength, and muscular endurance for apparently healthy participants based on current health status, fitness goals, and availability of time.**

| Knowledge or Skill Statement | Explanation/Examples | Resources |
|---|---|---|
| **Knowledge** of the recommended FITT framework for the development of muscular strength, muscular endurance, and flexibility | • Be aware of the differences between prescribing muscular strength and endurance in respect to the number of repetitions and the intensity (% of one repetition maximum [1-RM]). <br>• Be aware of the different types of flexibility exercises. | *ACSM's Guidelines for Exercise Testing and Prescription* (GETP), 9th edition (7) <br>• Chapter 7 <br>• Box 7.4 |
| **Knowledge** of the minimal threshold of physical activity required for health benefits and/or fitness development | • Be aware of the interaction between the intensity and the time of the exercise. <br>• Minimal threshold intensity may vary and be affected by individual's corticotropin-releasing factor level, age, health status, physiologic differences, genetics, habitual physical activity, and social and psychological factors. | *ACSM's Guidelines for Exercise Testing and Prescription* (GETP), 9th edition (7) <br>• Chapter 7 |
| **Knowledge** of safe and effective exercises designed to enhance muscular strength and/or endurance of major muscle groups | • When determining an appropriate exercise prescription, be aware of client/patient goals. <br>• Prescribe appropriate exercise and be mindful of attainable goals. | *ACSM's Resource Manual for Guidelines for Exercise Testing and Prescription*, 7th edition (8) <br>• Chapter 29 |
| **Knowledge** of safe and effective stretches that enhance flexibility | • There are many effective stretching exercises that may involve major muscle groups and/or individual muscles. <br>• Be aware of the differences between static, dynamic, ballistic stretches, and proprioceptive neuromuscular facilitation (PNF). | *Stretching for Functional Flexibility* (9) <br>• Chapter 5 |
| **Knowledge** of indications for water-based exercise (*e.g.*, arthritis, obesity) | • Although aquatic exercise may be appropriate for some populations, there are some notable disadvantages (*i.e.*, non–weight-bearing exercise). | *Therapeutic Exercise: From Theory to Practice* (18) <br>• Table 12.1 |
| **Knowledge** of the types of resistance training programs (*e.g.*, total body, split routine) and modalities (*e.g.*, free weights, variable resistance equipment, pneumatic machines, bands) | • When choosing total body or a variation of a split routine, be mindful of other variables such as number of training sessions per week and frequency of training. <br>• Be aware of the pros and cons of both free weights and variable resistance equipment. | *ACSM's Resource Manual for Guidelines for Exercise Testing and Prescription*, 7th edition (8) <br>• Chapter 31 <br>• Table 31.1 |
| **Knowledge** of acute (*e.g.*, load, volume, sets, repetitions, rest periods, order of exercises) and chronic training variables (*e.g.*, periodization) | • Be aware of the interaction between the number of repetitions and the load. <br>• Be aware of the variation in volume of the training and periodization schedule. | *ACSM's Resource Manual for Guidelines for Exercise Testing and Prescription*, 7th edition (8) <br>• Chapter 31 |
| **Knowledge** of the types of muscle contractions (*e.g.*, eccentric, concentric, isometric) | • Be aware of the pros and cons of using each of the types of muscle contractions. | *ACSM's Resource Manual for Guidelines for Exercise Testing and Prescription*, 7th edition (8) <br>• Chapter 31 |

## D. Implement exercise prescriptions using the frequency, intensity, time, and type (FITT) principle for flexibility, muscular strength, and muscular endurance for apparently healthy participants based on current health status, fitness goals, and availability of time. (cont.)

| Knowledge or Skill Statement | Explanation/Examples | Resources |
|---|---|---|
| **Knowledge** of joint movements (*e.g.*, flexion, extension, adduction, abduction) and the muscles responsible for them | • This information could be found in any other reputable kinesiology or biomechanics textbook. | *Basic Biomechanics*, 6th edition (16) <br>• Chapter 7 <br>• Tables 7.1–7.3 <br>• Chapter 8 <br>• Tables 8.1 and 8.2 <br>• Chapter 9 <br>• Table 9.1 |
| **Knowledge** of acute and delayed onset muscle soreness (DOMS) | • DOMS is related to microtears of myocytes rather than lactate accumulation. <br>• This information could be found in any other reputable exercise physiology textbook. | *Exercise Physiology: Integrating Theory and Application* (19) <br>• Chapter 3 |
| **Knowledge** of the anatomy and physiology of skeletal muscle fiber, the characteristics of fast- and slow-twitch muscle fibers, and the sliding-filament theory of muscle contraction | • This information is fairly extensive and should be covered thoroughly. <br>• This information could be found in any other reputable exercise physiology textbook. | *Exercise Physiology: Integrating Theory and Application* (19) <br>• Chapter 3 |
| **Knowledge** of the stretch reflex, proprioceptors, Golgi tendon organ (GTO), muscle spindles, and how they relate to flexibility | • Be aware of the positive and negative effects that these sensory organs have on the different modes of flexibility training such as static, ballistic and dynamic flexibility, and PNF. <br>• This information could be found in any other reputable exercise physiology, kinesiology, or biomechanics textbook. | *Exercise Physiology: Integrating Theory and Application* (19) <br>• Chapter 3 <br>*Basic Biomechanics*, 6th edition (16) <br>• Chapter 5 |
| **Knowledge** of muscle-related terminology including atrophy, hyperplasia, and hypertrophy | • Be aware of the differences between those terms and the prevalence among humans in response to exercise or lack of it. <br>• This information could be found in any other reputable exercise physiology, kinesiology, or biomechanics textbook. | *Exercise Physiology: Integrating Theory and Application* (19) <br>• Chapter 3 <br>*ACSM's Resource Manual for Guidelines for Exercise Testing and Prescription*, 7th edition (8) <br>• Chapter 31 and Key Terms |
| **Knowledge** of the Valsalva maneuver and its implications during exercise | • This maneuver should not be overlooked. In both apparently healthy and diseased populations, this maneuver could lead to significant and dangerous hemodynamic-related alterations. | *ACSM's Resource Manual for Guidelines for Exercise Testing and Prescription*, 7th edition (8) <br>• Chapter 22 |
| **Knowledge** of the physiology underlying plyometric training and common plyometric exercises (*e.g.*, box jumps, leaps, bounds) | • Plyometric exercises are considered as a form of anaerobic training and can be prescribed as a form of resistance training exercises. <br>• Intensity may be adjusted by varying different components of the same exercise (*i.e.*, the height of the box, one vs. two leg exercise) | *Exercise Physiology: Integrating Theory and Application* (19) <br>• Chapter 3 |

HFS

**D. Implement exercise prescriptions using the frequency, intensity, time, and type (FITT) principle for flexibility, muscular strength, and muscular endurance for apparently healthy participants based on current health status, fitness goals, and availability of time. (cont.)**

| Knowledge or Skill Statement | Explanation/Examples | Resources |
|---|---|---|
| **Knowledge** of the contraindications and potential risks associated with muscular conditioning activities (*e.g.*, straight-leg sit-ups, double-leg raises, squats, hurdler's stretch, yoga plough, forceful back hyperextension, and standing bent-over toe touch, behind neck press/lat pull-down) | • Consider appropriate exercise techniques. | *Advanced Fitness Assessment and Exercise Prescription*, 4th edition (17) <br> • Appendices C and F |
| **Knowledge** of prescribing exercise using the calculated %1-RM | • This knowledge is vital when there is a need to vary the intensity of the exercise such as between different periodization cycles. | *ACSM's Resource Manual for Guidelines for Exercise Testing and Prescription*, 7th edition (8) <br> • Chapters 22 and 31 |
| **Knowledge** of spotting positions and techniques for injury prevention and exercise assistance | • Spotter should be very familiar with the given the exercise. <br> • Spotting is paramount for proper and safe exercise. | *ACSM's Resource Manual for Guidelines for Exercise Testing and Prescription*, 7th edition (8) <br> • Chapter 31 |
| **Knowledge** of periodization (*e.g.*, macrocycles, microcycles, mesocycles) and associated theories | • Be aware of the differences between linear and nonlinear periodization methods. <br> • Be aware of the differences between microcycle, mesocycle, and macrocycle. <br> • Be aware of the relationship between volume, intensity, and the specificity of exercises in relationship to different periodization cycles. | *ACSM's Resource Manual for Guidelines for Exercise Testing and Prescription*, 7th edition (8) <br> • Chapter 31 |
| **Knowledge** of safe and effective Olympic weightlifting exercises | • Consider if these exercises are appropriate for the client. <br> • This information is fairly extensive and should be covered thoroughly. | *Explosive Lifting for Sports—Enhanced Edition* (23) <br> • Chapters 4–9 |
| **Knowledge** of safe and effective core stability exercises (*e.g.*, planks, crunch, bridges, cable twists) | • Consider the use of different aids (*i.e.*, stability and medicine balls). | *Strength Ball Training*, 2nd edition (15) <br> • Chapters 3 and 4 |
| **Skill** in identifying improper technique in the use of resistive equipment (*e.g.*, stability balls, weights, bands, resistance bars, and water exercise equipment) | • Lead and demonstrate the correct technique of using different resistive equipment. | *Advanced Fitness Assessment and Exercise Prescription*, 4th edition (17) <br> • Appendices C and F <br> *Strength Ball Training*, 2nd edition (15) <br> • Chapters 3 and 4 <br> *Therapeutic Exercise: From Theory to Practice* (18) <br> • Table 12.1 |
| **Skill** in teaching and demonstrating appropriate exercises for enhancing musculoskeletal flexibility | • Differentiate between static, dynamic, ballistic stretches, and PNF. | *Stretching for Functional Flexibility* (9) <br> • Chapter 5 |

HFS

## D. Implement exercise prescriptions using the frequency, intensity, time, and type (FITT) principle for flexibility, muscular strength, and muscular endurance for apparently healthy participants based on current health status, fitness goals, and availability of time. (cont.)

| Knowledge or Skill Statement | Explanation/Examples | Resources |
|---|---|---|
| **Skill** in teaching and demonstrating safe and effective muscular strength and endurance exercises (*e.g.*, free weights, weight machines, resistive bands, Swiss balls, body weight, and all other major fitness equipment) | • This information is fairly extensive and should be covered thoroughly.<br>• Lead by example! | *Advanced Fitness Assessment and Exercise Prescription*, 4th edition (17)<br>• Appendices C and F<br>*Strength Ball Training*, 2nd edition (15)<br>• Chapters 3 and 4 |

## E. Establish exercise progression guidelines for resistance, aerobic, and flexibility activity to achieve the goals of apparently healthy participants.

| Knowledge or Skill Statement | Explanation/Examples | Resources |
|---|---|---|
| **Knowledge** of the basic principles of exercise progression | • Regarding cardiovascular exercise prescription, be aware of the different progression stages.<br>• Be aware of different methods to progress resistance exercises (*i.e.*, periodization). | *ACSM's Resource Manual for Guidelines for Exercise Testing and Prescription*, 7th edition (8)<br>• Chapters 30 and 31<br>*ACSM's Guidelines for Exercise Testing and Prescription* (GETP), 9th edition (7)<br>• Chapter 7 |
| **Knowledge** of adjusting the frequency, intensity, time, and type (FITT) framework in response to individual changes in conditioning | • Be familiar with the interaction between the different components of FITT-VP principles. | *ACSM's Resource Manual for Guidelines for Exercise Testing and Prescription*, 7th edition (8)<br>• Chapters 30 and 31<br>*ACSM's Guidelines for Exercise Testing and Prescription* (GETP), 9th edition (7)<br>• Chapter 7 |
| **Knowledge** of the importance of performing periodic reevaluations to assess changes in fitness status | • This information is vital to the adjustment and development of sound exercise prescription as well as short- and long-term goals. | *ACSM's Guidelines for Exercise Testing and Prescription* (GETP), 9th edition (7)<br>• Chapter 4 |
| **Knowledge** of the training principles that promote improvements in muscular strength, muscular endurance, cardiorespiratory fitness, and flexibility | • Be aware of the underlying physiological differences between muscular strength, muscular endurance, and cardiorespiratory fitness.<br>• Be familiar with the interaction between the different components of FITT-VP principles in respect to both resistance and cardiorespiratory exercises. | *ACSM's Resource Manual for Guidelines for Exercise Testing and Prescription*, 7th edition (8)<br>• Chapters 30 and 31<br>*ACSM's Guidelines for Exercise Testing and Prescription* (GETP), 9th edition (7)<br>• Chapter 7 |
| **Skill** in recognizing the need for progression and communicating updates to exercise prescriptions | • Gradual progression may reduce the risk of cardiovascular disease (CVD) and musculoskeletal injury.<br>• Client goals may be more achievable. | "ACSM Position Stand. Quantity and Quality of Exercise for Developing and Maintaining Cardiorespiratory, Musculoskeletal, and Neuromotor Fitness in Apparently Healthy Adults: Guidance for Prescribing Exercise" (14) |

HFS

**F.  Implement a weight management program as indicated by personal goals that are supported by preparticipation health screening, health history, and body composition/anthropometrics.**

| Knowledge or Skill Statement | Explanation/Examples | Resources |
|---|---|---|
| **Knowledge** of exercise prescriptions for achieving weight management, including weight loss, weight maintenance, and weight gain goals | • Consider different weight loss programs/approaches.<br>• Consider client's caloric intake, expenditure, and current body fat percentage. | *ACSM's Resource Manual for Guidelines for Exercise Testing and Prescription*, 7th edition (8)<br>• Chapter 35 |
| **Knowledge** of energy balance and basic nutritional guidelines (*e.g.*, MyPyramid, United States Department of Agriculture [USDA] Dietary Guidelines for Americans) | • Be aware of various diet assessments and their advantages and disadvantages.<br>• The assessment of nutritional status may serve as an important secondary tool to exercise prescription. | *ACSM's Resource Manual for Guidelines for Exercise Testing and Prescription*, 7th edition (8)<br>• Chapter 14 |
| **Knowledge** of weight management terminology including but not limited to obesity, overweight, percent fat, body mass index (BMI), lean body mass (LBM), anorexia nervosa, bulimia, binge eating, metabolic syndrome, body fat distribution, adipocyte, bariatrics, ergogenic aid, fat-free mass (FFM), resting metabolic rate (RMR), and thermogenesis | • Be aware of the differences between the different terms in respect to a description of a disease condition, anthropometric assessment, and/or physiological descriptor. | *ACSM's Resource Manual for Guidelines for Exercise Testing and Prescription*, 7th edition (8)<br>• Chapter 18 and Key Terms<br>• Chapter 35<br>*ACSM's Guidelines for Exercise Testing and Prescription* (GETP), 9th edition (7)<br>• Chapter 10<br>*Exercise Physiology: Integrating Theory and Application* (19)<br>• Chapter 11 |
| **Knowledge** of the relationship between body composition and health | • Be aware of the link between overweight and obesity and other debilitating chronic conditions such as cardiovascular disease (CVD) and diabetes.<br>• Be aware of the link between overweight and obesity and other risk factors such as hypertension. | *ACSM's Guidelines for Exercise Testing and Prescription* (GETP), 9th edition (7)<br>• Chapter 10 |
| **Knowledge** of the unique dietary needs of participant populations (*e.g.*, women, children, older adults, pregnant women) | • In order to fully comprehend this information, the health fitness specialist (HFS) needs to be fully aware of dietary needs of the general population. | "USDA Center for Nutrition Policy and Promotion" (27) |
| **Knowledge** of common nutritional ergogenic aids, their purported mechanisms of action, and associated risks and benefits (*e.g.*, protein/amino acids, vitamins, minerals, herbal products, creatine, steroids, caffeine) | • Many ergogenic aids are effective in improving performance, but many are barred from used in official competition. | *Exercise Physiology: Integrating Theory and Application* (19)<br>• Chapter 14 |
| **Knowledge** of methods for modifying body composition including diet, exercise, and behavior modification | • In many cases and in order to achieve lasting results, modifying body composition requires simultaneous use of diet, exercise, and behavior modification. | *ACSM's Resource Manual for Guidelines for Exercise Testing and Prescription*, 7th edition (8)<br>• Chapters 14, 15, and 44<br>*ACSM's Guidelines for Exercise Testing and Prescription* (GETP), 9th edition (7)<br>• Chapter 10 |

## F.  Implement a weight management program as indicated by personal goals that are supported by preparticipation health screening, health history, and body composition/anthropometrics. (cont.)

| Knowledge or Skill Statement | Explanation/Examples | Resources |
|---|---|---|
| **Knowledge** of fuel sources for aerobic and anaerobic metabolism including carbohydrates, fats, and proteins | • Be aware of the interaction between the different fuel sources in respect to both aerobic and anaerobic exercises.<br>• This information could be found in any other reputable exercise physiology textbook. | *ACSM's Resource Manual for Guidelines for Exercise Testing and Prescription*, 7th edition (8)<br>• Chapter 3<br>*Exercise Physiology: Integrating Theory and Application* (19)<br>• Chapter 2 |
| **Knowledge** of the effects of overall dietary composition on healthy weight management | • The application of "proper diet" may vary based on such factors as age, gender, and activity level (sedentary lifestyle vs. active lifestyle).<br>• This information is fairly extensive and should be covered thoroughly. | *ACSM's Resource Manual for Guidelines for Exercise Testing and Prescription*, 7th edition (8)<br>• Chapter 4 |
| **Knowledge** of the importance of maintaining normal hydration before, during, and after exercise | • There are several ways to assess hydration (*i.e.*, urine color and osmolality).<br>• Be aware of hyponatremia and its association with overhydration. | *Exercise Physiology: Integrating Theory and Application* (19)<br>• Chapter 9 |
| **Knowledge** of the consequences of inappropriate weight loss methods (*e.g.*, saunas, dietary supplements, vibrating belts, body wraps, over exercising, very low calorie diets, electric stimulators, sweat suits, fad diets) | • Proper and substantial weight loss is a long-term process. | *ACSM's Resource Manual for Guidelines for Exercise Testing and Prescription*, 7th edition (8)<br>• Chapter 35 |
| **Knowledge** of the kilocalorie levels of carbohydrate, fat, protein, and alcohol | • Energy content of different nutrients is not equal. | *ACSM's Resource Manual for Guidelines for Exercise Testing and Prescription*, 7th edition (8)<br>• Chapter 4<br>• Table 4.1 |
| **Knowledge** of the relationship between kilocalorie expenditures and weight loss | • Deficit of 3,500 kcal = loss of 1 lb of body mass.<br>• This is common knowledge among exercise scientists. | *Exercise Physiology: Integrating Theory and Application* (19)<br>• Chapter 11 |
| **Knowledge** of published position statements on obesity and the risks associated with it (*e.g.*, National Institutes of Health, American Dietetic Association, American College of Sports Medicine [ACSM]) | • Be aware of the difference between overweight and obesity in respect to the definition of these terms. | *ACSM's Resource Manual for Guidelines for Exercise Testing and Prescription*, 7th edition (8)<br>• Chapter 14<br>*ACSM's Guidelines for Exercise Testing and Prescription* (GETP), 9th edition (7)<br>• Chapter 10 |
| **Knowledge** of the relationship between body fat distribution patterns and health | • Android obesity ("apple shape") vs. gynoid ("pear shape")<br>• Visceral vs. subcutaneous fat distribution | *ACSM's Resource Manual for Guidelines for Exercise Testing and Prescription*, 7th edition (8)<br>• Chapter 35 |

HFS

**F.    Implement a weight management program as indicated by personal goals that are supported by preparticipation health screening, health history, and body composition/anthropometrics. (cont.)**

| Knowledge or Skill Statement | Explanation/Examples | Resources |
|---|---|---|
| **Knowledge** of the physiology and pathophysiology of overweight and obese participants | • Individuals who are overweight and/or obese are often present with comorbidities and/or debilitating orthopedic conditions. | *ACSM's Resource Manual for Guidelines for Exercise Testing and Prescription,* 7th edition (8) <br>• Chapter 14 <br>*ACSM's Exercise Management for Persons with Chronic Diseases and Disabilities,* 3rd edition (2) <br>• Chapter 21 |
| **Knowledge** of the recommended frequency, intensity, time, and type (FITT) framework for participants who are overweight or obese. | • The amount of physical activity may need to be greater than recommended for apparently healthy individuals. <br>• Exercise should be coupled with sound nutritional and behavior change interventions. | *ACSM's Guidelines for Exercise Testing and Prescription* (GETP), 9th edition (7) <br>• Chapter 10 |
| **Knowledge** of comorbidities and musculoskeletal conditions associated with overweight and obesity that may require medical clearance and/or modifications to exercise testing and prescription | • Due to the potential existence of other chronic and orthopedic issues, additional medical intervention may be warranted. | *ACSM's Guidelines for Exercise Testing and Prescription* (GETP), 9th edition (7) <br>• Chapter 10 |
| **Skill** in applying behavioral strategies (*e.g.*, exercise, diet, behavioral modification strategies) for weight management | • Be aware that the appropriate way to lose weight may require some time and may involve additional exercise and/or diet, exercise, and/or behavior modification. | *ACSM's Resource Manual for Guidelines for Exercise Testing and Prescription,* 7th edition (8) <br>• Chapter 35 <br>*ACSM's Guidelines for Exercise Testing and Prescription* (GETP), 9th edition (7) <br>• Chapter 10 |
| **Skill** in modifying exercises for individuals limited by body size | • Exercise prescription may need to be individualized and modified based on abilities and the presence or absence of comorbidities and/or preexisting orthopedic limitations. | *ACSM's Resource Manual for Guidelines for Exercise Testing and Prescription,* 7th edition (8) <br>• Chapter 41 |
| **Skill** in calculating the volume of exercise in terms of kilocalories per session | • Be aware of all the conversions that are at the bottom of the table (Table 7.3). | *ACSM's Guidelines for Exercise Testing and Prescription* (GETP), 9th edition (7) <br>• Table 7.3 |

HFS

## G. Prescribe and implement exercise programs for participants with controlled cardiovascular, pulmonary, and metabolic diseases and other clinical populations.

| Knowledge or Skill Statement | Explanation/Examples | Resources |
|---|---|---|
| **Knowledge** of American College of Sports Medicine (ACSM) risk stratification and exercise prescription guidelines for participants with cardiovascular, pulmonary, and metabolic diseases and other clinical populations | • This information is fairly extensive and should be covered thoroughly. | *ACSM's Guidelines for Exercise Testing and Prescription* (GETP), 9th edition (7)<br>• Chapter 2<br>• Tables 2.2 and 2.3<br>• Figure 2.3<br>• Box 2.2<br>• Chapters 9 and 10 |
| **Knowledge** of ACSM relative and absolute contraindications for initiating exercise sessions or exercise testing and indications for terminating exercise sessions and exercise testing | • Be aware of the difference between relative and absolute contraindications in respect to the benefits vs. risks that are associated with exercise/testing. | *ACSM's Guidelines for Exercise Testing and Prescription* (GETP), 9th edition (7)<br>• Chapter 3<br>• Box 3.5<br>• Chapter 4<br>• Box 4.5 |
| **Knowledge** of physiology and pathophysiology of cardiac disease, arthritis, diabetes mellitus, dyslipidemia, hypertension, metabolic syndrome, musculoskeletal injuries, overweight and obesity, osteoporosis, peripheral artery disease, and pulmonary disease | • Extensive prior knowledge of cardiopulmonary physiology is highly recommended. | *ACSM's Resource Manual for Guidelines for Exercise Testing and Prescription*, 7th edition (8)<br>• Chapter 6<br>*ACSM's Guidelines for Exercise Testing and Prescription* (GETP), 9th edition (7)<br>• Chapter 10 |
| **Knowledge** of the effects of diet and exercise on blood glucose levels in diabetics | • Be aware of special considerations that may affect exercise such as hypoglycemia, blood glucose before, during, and immediately following exercise, hyperglycemia, polyurea, neuropathy, nephropathy, and retinopathy. | *ACSM's Guidelines for Exercise Testing and Prescription* (GETP), 9th edition (7)<br>• Chapter 10 |
| **Knowledge** of the recommended frequency, intensity, time, and type (FITT) principle for the development of cardiorespiratory fitness, muscular fitness, and flexibility for participants with cardiac disease, arthritis, diabetes mellitus, dyslipidemia, hypertension, metabolic syndrome, musculoskeletal injuries, overweight and obesity, osteoporosis, peripheral artery disease, and pulmonary disease | • In order to fully comprehend this information, the health fitness specialist (HFS) needs to be fully aware of FITT-VP principles because they apply to apparently healthy individuals.<br>• This information is fairly extensive and should be covered thoroughly. | *ACSM's Guidelines for Exercise Testing and Prescription* (GETP), 9th edition (7)<br>• Chapter 10 |
| **Skill** in progressing exercise programs, according to the FITT principle, in a safe and effective manner | • Rate of progression in both aerobic and strength exercises should be individualized. | *ACSM's Guidelines for Exercise Testing and Prescription* (GETP), 9th edition (7)<br>• Chapter 7 |

HFS

## G. Prescribe and implement exercise programs for participants with controlled cardiovascular, pulmonary, and metabolic diseases and other clinical populations. (cont.)

| Knowledge or Skill Statement | Explanation/Examples | Resources |
|---|---|---|
| **Skill** in modifying the exercise prescription and/or exercise choice for individuals with cardiac disease, arthritis, diabetes mellitus, dyslipidemia, hypertension, metabolic syndrome, musculoskeletal injuries, overweight and obesity, osteoporosis, peripheral artery disease, and pulmonary disease | • To make appropriate modifications, the HFS needs to be fully aware of FITT-VP principles because they apply to apparently healthy individuals.<br>• To make appropriate modifications, one needs to fully comprehend the physiology and pathophysiology of these conditions. | *ACSM's Guidelines for Exercise Testing and Prescription* (GETP), 9th edition (7)<br>• Chapter 10 |
| **Skill** in identifying improper exercise techniques and modifying exercise programs for participants with low back, neck, shoulder, elbow, wrist, hip, knee, and/or ankle pain | • To make appropriate modifications, one needs to fully comprehend the physiology and pathophysiology of these conditions.<br>• If warranted, consult with appropriate professional (*i.e.*, AT and/or PT). | *ACSM's Resource Manual for Guidelines for Exercise Testing and Prescription*, 7th edition (8)<br>• Chapters 37 and 42 |

## H. Prescribe and implement exercise programs for healthy special populations (*i.e.*, older adults, youth, pregnant women).

| Knowledge or Skill Statement | Explanation/Examples | Resources |
|---|---|---|
| **Knowledge** of normal maturational changes from childhood to old age and their effects on the skeletal muscle, bone, reaction time, coordination, posture, heat and cold tolerance, maximal oxygen consumption, strength, flexibility, body composition, resting and maximal heart rate, and resting and maximal blood pressure | • Knowledge of related exercise physiology is critical.<br>• This information is fairly extensive and should be covered thoroughly. | *ACSM's Guidelines for Exercise Testing and Prescription* (GETP), 9th edition (7)<br>• Chapter 8<br>*ACSM's Exercise Management for Persons with Chronic Diseases and Disabilities*, 3rd edition (2)<br>• Chapter 5 |
| **Knowledge** of techniques for the modification of cardiovascular, flexibility, and resistance exercises based on age, functional capacity, and physical condition | • To make appropriate modifications, the health fitness specialist (HFS) needs to be fully aware of FITT-VP principles because they apply to apparently healthy individuals.<br>• To make appropriate modifications, the HFS needs to fully comprehend the anatomical and physiological differences between apparently healthy and healthy special populations. | *ACSM's Guidelines for Exercise Testing and Prescription* (GETP), 9th edition (7)<br>• Chapter 8 |
| **Knowledge** of techniques for the development of exercise prescriptions for children, adolescents, and older adults regarding strength, functional capacity, and motor skills | • To make appropriate exercise prescription, the HFS needs to fully comprehend the anatomical and physiological differences between these populations. | *ACSM's Guidelines for Exercise Testing and Prescription* (GETP), 9th edition (7)<br>• Chapter 8 |
| **Knowledge** of the unique adaptations to exercise training in children, adolescents, and older participants regarding strength, functional capacity, and motor skills | • Extensive prior knowledge of related exercise physiology is critical.<br>• This information is fairly extensive and should be covered thoroughly. | *ACSM's Guidelines for Exercise Testing and Prescription* (GETP), 9th edition (7)<br>• Chapter 8<br>*ACSM's Exercise Management for Persons with Chronic Diseases and Disabilities*, 3rd edition (2)<br>• Chapter 5 |

HFS

## H.  Prescribe and implement exercise programs for healthy special populations (*i.e.,* older adults, youth, pregnant women). (cont.)

| Knowledge or Skill Statement | Explanation/Examples | Resources |
|---|---|---|
| **Knowledge** of the benefits and precautions associated with exercise training across the lifespan | • The risk of a cardiovascular event during exercise is very low in apparently healthy individuals.<br>• The risk of a cardiovascular event during exercise is directly related to the intensity of the exercise and the severity of diagnosed or undiagnosed occlusion cardiovascular disease (CVD). | *ACSM's Guidelines for Exercise Testing and Prescription* (GETP), 9th edition (7)<br>• Chapter 1 |
| **Knowledge** of the recommended frequency, intensity, time, and type (FITT) framework for the development of cardiorespiratory fitness, muscular fitness, and flexibility in apparently healthy children and adolescents | • To make appropriate modifications, the HFS needs to be fully aware of FITT-VP principles because they apply to apparently healthy populations.<br>• Children are not miniature adults and therefore, exercise prescription should be modified accordingly. | *ACSM's Resource Manual for Guidelines for Exercise Testing and Prescription*, 7th edition (8)<br>• Chapter 36<br>*ACSM's Guidelines for Exercise Testing and Prescription* (GETP), 9th edition (7)<br>• Chapter 8 |
| **Knowledge** of the effects of the aging process on the musculoskeletal and cardiovascular structures and functions during rest, exercise, and recovery | • Be aware of the effects of the aging process as well as the effects of physical activity or sedentary lifestyle on the musculoskeletal and cardiovascular structures. | *Physiology of Exercise and Healthy Aging* (26)<br>• Chapters 1 and 2 |
| **Knowledge** of the recommended FITT framework necessary for the development of cardiorespiratory fitness, muscular fitness, balance, and flexibility in apparently healthy older adults | • Be aware of any aging-related conditions that may affect exercise prescription. | *ACSM's Resource Manual for Guidelines for Exercise Testing and Prescription*, 7th edition (8)<br>• Chapter 36<br>*ACSM's Guidelines for Exercise Testing and Prescription* (GETP), 9th edition (7)<br>• Chapter 8 |
| **Knowledge** of common orthopedic and cardiovascular exercise considerations for older adults | • When prescribing exercise to older adults, one needs to be aware of all existing mental, physical, and medical conditions and respond accordingly. | *ACSM's Resource Manual for Guidelines for Exercise Testing and Prescription*, 7th edition (8)<br>• Chapter 36 |
| **Knowledge** of the relationship between regular physical activity and the successful performance of activities of daily living (ADL) for older adults | • The physical fitness components that may improve with regular physical activity are muscular strength and endurance, cardiovascular endurance, balance, and flexibility. | *ACSM's Resource Manual for Guidelines for Exercise Testing and Prescription*, 7th edition (8)<br>• Chapter 36 |
| **Knowledge** of the recommended frequency, intensity, type, and duration of physical activity necessary for the development of cardiorespiratory fitness, muscular fitness, and flexibility in apparently healthy pregnant women | • To make appropriate modifications, the HFS needs to be fully aware of FITT-VP principles because they apply to apparently healthy individuals.<br>• Prior to prescribing exercise in this population, the HFS needs to be aware of the physiological responses to exercise, contraindications for exercising, and other special considerations because they relate to this population. | *ACSM's Resource Manual for Guidelines for Exercise Testing and Prescription*, 7th edition (8)<br>• Chapter 36<br>*ACSM's Guidelines for Exercise Testing and Prescription* (GETP), 9th edition (7)<br>• Chapter 8 |

HFS

## H. Prescribe and implement exercise programs for healthy special populations (*i.e.*, older adults, youth, pregnant women). (cont.)

| Knowledge or Skill Statement | Explanation/Examples | Resources |
|---|---|---|
| **Skill** in teaching and demonstrating appropriate exercises for healthy populations with special considerations | • The HFS must be aware of the anatomical and physiological differences between these populations.<br>• The HFS must modify the exercise accordingly.<br>• Lead by example! | *ACSM's Resource Manual for Guidelines for Exercise Testing and Prescription*, 7th edition (8)<br>• Chapter 36<br>*ACSM's Guidelines for Exercise Testing and Prescription* (GETP), 9th edition (7)<br>• Chapter 8 |
| **Skill** in modifying exercises based on age, physical condition, and current health status | • To make appropriate modifications, the HFS needs to fully comprehend the physiological differences between apparently healthy populations and healthy populations with special considerations. | *ACSM's Resource Manual for Guidelines for Exercise Testing and Prescription*, 7th edition (8)<br>• Chapter 36<br>*ACSM's Guidelines for Exercise Testing and Prescription* (GETP), 9th edition (7)<br>• Chapter 8 |

## I. Modify exercise prescriptions based on environmental conditions.

| Knowledge or Skill Statement | Explanation/Examples | Resources |
|---|---|---|
| **Knowledge** of the effects of a hot, cold, or high-altitude environment on the physiologic response to exercise | • This information is fairly extensive and should be covered thoroughly.<br>• This information could be found in any reputable exercise physiology textbook. | *ACSM's Guideline for Exercise Testing and Prescription* (GETP), 9th edition (7)<br>• Chapter 8<br>*Exercise Physiology: Integrating Theory and Application* (19)<br>• Chapter 10 |
| **Knowledge** of special precautions and program modifications for exercise in a hot, cold, or high-altitude environment | • By knowing the physiology as it relates to these conditions, one may develop and implement some prevention strategies. | *ACSM's Guidelines for Exercise Testing and Prescription* (GETP), 9th edition (7)<br>• Chapter 8<br>*Exercise Physiology: Integrating Theory and Application* (19)<br>• Chapter 10 |
| **Knowledge** of the role of acclimatization when exercising in a hot or high-altitude environment | • By knowing the physiology as it relates to these conditions, one may develop an individualized exercise prescription using acclimatization protocols to achieve optimal physical and cognitive (in altitude) performances. | *ACSM's Guidelines for Exercise Testing and Prescription* (GETP), 9th edition (7)<br>• Chapter 8<br>*Exercise Physiology: Integrating Theory and Application* (19)<br>• Chapter 10 |
| **Knowledge** of appropriate fluid intake during exercise in a hot, humid environments as well as cold, and high-altitude | • Be aware of techniques to assess hydration (*i.e.*, urine color and osmolality).<br>• Be aware of hydration needs prior to, during, and after exercise. | *Exercise Physiology: Integrating Theory and Application* (19)<br>• Chapter 9 |

# DOMAIN III: EXERCISE COUNSELING AND BEHAVIORAL STRATEGIES

## A. Optimize adoption and adherence to exercise programs and other healthy behaviors by applying effective communication techniques.

| Knowledge or Skill Statement | Explanation/Examples | Resources |
|---|---|---|
| **Knowledge** of the effective and timely uses of communication modes (*e.g.*, e-mail, telephone, Web site, newsletters) | • The use of the mode of communication may be related to factors such as age, gender, ethnicity, locality, and other subjective preferences. | *ACSM's Resource Manual for Guidelines for Exercise Testing and Prescription*, 7th edition (8)<br>• Chapter 47 |
| **Knowledge** of verbal and nonverbal behaviors that communicate positive reinforcement and encouragement (*e.g.*, eye contact, targeted praise, empathy) | • Because the behavioral aspect needs to be addressed early in the intervention, it is critical that positive reinforcement and encouragement are communicated to your client. | *ACSM's Resource Manual for Guidelines for Exercise Testing and Prescription*, 7th edition (8)<br>• Chapter 46 |
| **Knowledge** of group leadership techniques for working with participants of all ages | • The information and the tools that are being used to motivate and educate participants need to be adjusted to fit the group population. | *ACSM's Resource Manual for Guidelines for Exercise Testing and Prescription*, 7th edition (8)<br>• Chapter 34 |
| **Knowledge** of active listening techniques | • Consider more advanced consoling skills.<br>• Consider both listening and making reflective statements. | *ACSM's Resource Manual for Guidelines for Exercise Testing and Prescription*, 7th edition (8)<br>• Chapter 46 |
| **Knowledge** of learning modes (auditory, visual, kinesthetic) | • Using different modes to enhance task completion. | *The Kinesthetic Classroom Teaching and Learning through Movement* (20)<br>• Chapter 1 |
| **Knowledge** of types of feedback (*e.g.*, evaluative, supportive, descriptive) | • Feedback is vital to behavior modification in an environment that supports a client-centered approach. | *ACSM's Resource Manual for Guidelines for Exercise Testing and Prescription*, 7th edition (8)<br>• Chapters 45 and 46 |
| **Skill** in using active listening techniques | • Consider more advanced consoling skills.<br>• The ability to listen, analyze, and communicate is critical. | *ACSM's Resource Manual for Guidelines for Exercise Testing and Prescription*, 7th edition (8)<br>• Chapter 46 |
| **Skill** in applying teaching and training techniques to optimize participant training sessions | • Extensive knowledge of related behavioral strategies to enhance physical activity participation is critical.<br>• Program should be client centered. | *ACSM's Resource Manual for Guidelines for Exercise Testing and Prescription*, 7th edition (8)<br>• Chapter 45 |
| **Skill** in using feedback to optimize participant training sessions | • Must be familiar with motivational and behavior modification techniques such as client-centered approach and active listening<br>• Must be familiar with basic motivational and behavior modification terms such empathy and rapport | *ACSM's Resource Manual for Guidelines for Exercise Testing and Prescription*, 7th edition (8)<br>• Chapters 45 and 46 |
| **Skill** in applying verbal and nonverbal communications with diverse participant populations | • Vary the mode of communication based on age, gender, ethnicity, locality, and other subjective preferences. | *ACSM's Resource Manual for Guidelines for Exercise Testing and Prescription*, 7th edition (8)<br>• Chapter 47 |

HFS

## B. Optimize adoption of and adherence to exercise programs and other healthy behaviors by applying effective behavioral and motivational strategies.

| Knowledge or Skill Statement | Explanation/Examples | Resources |
|---|---|---|
| **Knowledge** of behavior change models and theories (*e.g.*, health belief model, theory of planned behavior, socioecological model, transtheoretical model, social cognitive theory, cognitive evaluation theory) | • This information is fairly extensive and should be covered thoroughly.<br>• These behavior change models and theories play a key role in the overall process of moving from sedentary to physically active lifestyle. | *ACSM's Resource Manual for Guidelines for Exercise Testing and Prescription*, 7th edition (8)<br>• Chapter 44 |
| **Knowledge** of the basic principles involved in motivational interviewing | • Have a client-centered approach.<br>• May involve various counseling skills | *ACSM's Resource Manual for Guidelines for Exercise Testing and Prescription*, 7th edition (8)<br>• Chapter 46 |
| **Knowledge** of intervention strategies and stress management techniques | • The intervention strategy that may be used should depend on the individual stage of change. | *ACSM's Resource Manual for Guidelines for Exercise Testing and Prescription*, 7th edition (8)<br>• Chapter 44 |
| **Knowledge** of the stages of motivational readiness (*e.g.*, transtheoretical model) | • Be aware of the following: precontemplation, contemplation, preparation, action, and maintenance. | *ACSM's Resource Manual for Guidelines for Exercise Testing and Prescription*, 7th edition (8)<br>• Chapters 43 and 45 |
| **Knowledge** of behavioral strategies for enhancing exercise and health behavior change (*e.g.*, reinforcement; specific, measurable, attainable, realistic and relevant, and time-bound [SMART] goal setting; social support) | • This information is fairly extensive and should be covered thoroughly.<br>• Using sound and effective behavioral strategies are key for enhancing exercise and health behavior change. | *ACSM's Resource Manual for Guidelines for Exercise Testing and Prescription*, 7th edition (8)<br>• Chapter 45 |
| **Knowledge** of behavior modification terminology including but not limited to self-esteem, self-efficacy, antecedents, cues to action, behavioral beliefs, behavioral intentions, and reinforcing factors | • Understanding these concepts play a major role in the overall process of behavior modification and moving from sedentary to physically active lifestyle. | *Behavior Modification: What It Is And How to Do It*, 9th edition (21)<br>• Part II |
| **Knowledge** of behavioral strategies (*e.g.*, exercise, diet, behavioral modification strategies) for weight management | • A successful weight loss program is a lengthy and ongoing process that should include exercise, diet, and behavior modification. | *ACSM's Resource Manual for Guidelines for Exercise Testing and Prescription*, 7th edition (8)<br>• Chapter 35 |
| **Knowledge** of the role that affect, mood, and emotion play in exercise adherence | • Many factors affect exercise adherence (*i.e.*, personal, behavioral). | *ACSM's Resource Manual for Guidelines for Exercise Testing and Prescription*, 7th edition (8)<br>• Chapter 45 |
| **Knowledge** of common barriers to exercise initiation and compliance (*e.g.*, time management, injury, fear, lack of knowledge, weather) | • Recognizing and overcoming barriers to exercise is a vital step in the development of viable behavior change program. | *ACSM's Resource Manual for Guidelines for Exercise Testing and Prescription*, 7th edition (8)<br>• Chapter 45 |
| **Knowledge** of techniques that facilitate motivation (*e.g.*, goal setting, incentive programs, achievement recognition, social support) | • Many aspects are involved in facilitating motivation.<br>• The form of motivation could be described as either extrinsic or intrinsic. | *ACSM's Resource Manual for Guidelines for Exercise Testing and Prescription*, 7th edition (8)<br>• Chapter 45 |

HFS

| B. Optimize adoption of and adherence to exercise programs and other healthy behaviors by applying effective behavioral and motivational strategies. (cont.) |||
|---|---|---|
| **Knowledge or Skill Statement** | **Explanation/Examples** | **Resources** |
| **Knowledge** of the role extrinsic and intrinsic motivation plays in the adoption and maintenance of behavior change | • Program-based incentive is an example of a form of extrinsic motivation.<br>• A personal reward for behavior is an example of a form of intrinsic motivation. | *ACSM's Resource Manual for Guidelines for Exercise Testing and Prescription*, 7th edition (8)<br>• Chapter 45 |
| **Knowledge** of relapse prevention strategies and plans of action | • Relapse in exercising is usually due to an inevitable event (illness or injury, professional engagements, etc.).<br>• Relapse prevention may involve developing a restart plan, the use of reinforcement or rewards system, etc. | *ACSM's Resource Manual for Guidelines for Exercise Testing and Prescription*, 7th edition (8)<br>• Chapter 45 |
| **Knowledge** of applying health coaching principles and lifestyle management techniques related to behavior change | • This topic is fairly extensive and may include strategies to enhance physical activity participation, diet modification, stress reduction techniques, etc. | *ACSM's Resource Manual for Guidelines for Exercise Testing and Prescription*, 7th edition (8)<br>• Chapters 44 and 45 |
| **Knowledge** of strategies that increase nonstructured physical activity levels (*e.g.*, stair walking, parking farther away, bike to work) | • May involve making a conscious decision to become more active<br>• Related to behavior change | *ACSM's Resource Manual for Guidelines for Exercise Testing and Prescription*, 7th edition (8)<br>• Chapters 36 and 45 |
| **Skill** in explaining the purpose and value of understanding perceived exertion | • A valuable secondary tool to monitor exercise tolerance<br>• Scale must be explained prior to the commencement of the test. | *ACSM's Guidelines for Exercise Testing and Prescription* (GETP), 9th edition (2)<br>• Chapter 4<br>• Table 4.7 |
| **Skill** in using imagery as a motivational tool | • The use of images for reinforcing and promoting physical activity | *ACSM's Resource Manual for Guidelines for Exercise Testing and Prescription*, 7th edition (8)<br>• Chapter 45 |
| **Skill** in evaluating behavioral readiness to optimize exercise adherence | • Use tools such as the self-motivation assessment scale and physical activity stages of change. | *ACSM's Resources for the Health Fitness Specialist* (6)<br>• Chapters 10 and 11 |
| **Skill** in applying the theories related to behavior change to diverse populations | • This theoretical knowledge is fairly extensive and should be covered thoroughly.<br>• Consider decision-making theory, social cognitive theory, etc. | *ACSM's Resource Manual for Guidelines for Exercise Testing and Prescription*, 7th edition (8)<br>• Chapter 44 |
| **Skill** in developing intervention strategies to increase self-efficacy and self-confidence | • Applied to different health behavior change theories<br>• Skill to recognize the degree of self-efficacy and self-confidence | *ACSM's Resource Manual for Guidelines for Exercise Testing and Prescription*, 7th edition (8)<br>• Chapter 44 |
| **Skill** in developing reward systems that support and maintain program adherence | • The information is fairly extensive because it applies to different aspects of behavioral strategies to enhance physical activity participation. | *ACSM's Resource Manual for Guidelines for Exercise Testing and Prescription*, 7th edition (8)<br>• Chapters 44 and 45 |
| **Skill** in setting effective behavioral goals | • Goal setting should be realistic, target-specific behaviors, measurable, and time frame specific (long term vs. short term). | *ACSM's Resource Manual for Guidelines for Exercise Testing and Prescription*, 7th edition (8)<br>• Chapters 44–46 |

## C. Provide educational resources to support clients in the adoption and maintenance of healthy lifestyle behaviors.

| Knowledge or Skill Statement | Explanation/Examples | Resources |
|---|---|---|
| **Knowledge** of the relationship between physical inactivity and common chronic diseases (*e.g.*, atherosclerosis, Type 2 diabetes, obesity, dyslipidemia, arthritis, low back pain, hypertension) | • There is an inverse relationship between physical activity and the severity and the number of common chronic diseases.<br>• Dose response related | *ACSM's Guidelines for Exercise Testing and Prescription* (GETP), 9th edition (7)<br>• Chapter 1 |
| **Knowledge** of the dynamic interrelationship between fitness level, body composition, stress, and overall health | • The benefits of regular physical activity may include but not limited to improvement in cardiovascular and respiratory functions, reduction in coronary artery disease (CAD) risk factors, and decreased in overall morbidity and mortality. | *ACSM's Guidelines for Exercise Testing and Prescription* (GETP), 9th edition (7)<br>• Chapter 1<br>• Box 1.2 |
| **Knowledge** of modifications necessary to promote healthy lifestyle behaviors for diverse populations | • To make appropriate modifications, the health fitness specialist (HFS) needs to be fully aware of FITT-VP principles because they apply to apparently healthy populations.<br>• To make appropriate modifications, the HFS needs to fully comprehend the physiology and pathophysiology of common chronic diseases conditions.<br>• To make appropriate modifications, the HFS needs to fully comprehend the anatomical and physiological differences between apparently healthy and healthy special populations. | *ACSM's Guidelines for Exercise Testing and Prescription* (GETP), 9th edition (7)<br>• Chapters 7–10 |
| **Knowledge** of stress management techniques and relaxation techniques (*e.g.*, progressive relaxation, guided imagery, massage therapy) | • Each of these techniques may be useful for stress reduction and may be used individually or in conjunction with one another. | *The Relaxation & Stress Reduction Workbook* (11)<br>• Chapters 4–7 |
| **Knowledge** of the activities of daily living (ADL) and how they relate to overall health | • ADL may be affected negatively by many chronic conditions and may be affected positively by endurance and strength-based exercises. | *ACSM's Resource Manual for Guidelines for Exercise Testing and Prescription*, 7th edition (8)<br>• Chapter 31 |
| **Knowledge** of accessing and disseminating scientifically based, relevant health, exercise, nutrition, and wellness-related resources and information | • Be aware of the concept and importance of research.<br>• Have the ability to "translate" scientific literature to practical use. | *Exercise Physiology: Integrating Theory and Application* (19)<br>• Chapter 1 |
| **Knowledge** of specific, age-appropriate leadership techniques and educational methods to increase client engagement | • The selection of an appropriate program to increase client engagement should be individualized and client centered. | *ACSM's Resource Manual for Guidelines for Exercise Testing and Prescription*, 7th edition (8)<br>• Chapter 45 |
| **Knowledge** of community-based exercise programs that provide social support and structured activities (*e.g.*, walking clubs, intramural sports, golf leagues, cycling clubs) | • These programs could be supported and organized by schools, work sites, religious institutions, etc. | *ACSM's Resource Manual for Guidelines for Exercise Testing and Prescription*, 7th edition (8)<br>• Chapter 48 |

HFS

## C. Provide educational resources to support clients in the adoption and maintenance of healthy lifestyle behaviors. (cont.)

| Knowledge or Skill Statement | Explanation/Examples | Resources |
|---|---|---|
| **Skill** in accessing and delivering health, exercise, and wellness-related information | • The HFS must be able to make use of technology to locate, assess, and use relevant health-related information. | *Exercise Physiology: Integrating Theory and Application* (19)<br>• Chapter 1 |
| **Skill** in educating clients about benefits and risks of exercise and the risks of sedentary behavior | • The HFS must have the skill to access, disseminate, and simplify scientifically based, health-related information.<br>• Be able to explain complex information in layman's terms. | *Exercise Physiology: Integrating Theory and Application* (19)<br>• Chapter 1 |

## D. Provide support within the scope of practice of a health fitness specialist (HFS) and refer to other health professionals as indicated.

| Knowledge or Skill Statement | Explanation/Examples | Resources |
|---|---|---|
| **Knowledge** of the side effects of common over-the-counter and prescription drugs that may impact a client's ability to exercise | • Be aware of the effects of these medications on heart rate (HR), blood pressure (BP), electrocardiogram (ECG), and exercise capacity. | *ACSM's Guidelines for Exercise Testing and Prescription* (GETP), 9th edition (7)<br>• Appendix A |
| **Knowledge** of signs and symptoms of mental health states (*e.g.*, anxiety, depression, eating disorders) that may necessitate referral to a medical or mental health professional | • Affect wide range of populations.<br>• Proper treatment will allow a substantial improvement in psychological functioning and quality of life. | *ACSM's Resource Manual for Guidelines for Exercise Testing and Prescription*, 7th edition (8)<br>• Chapters 9 and 17 |
| **Knowledge** of symptoms and causal factors of test anxiety (*i.e.*, performance, appraisal threat during exercise testing) and how they may affect physiological responses to testing | • Exercise has a positive effect on symptoms of anxiety.<br>• Consider the relationship between anxiety and exercise adherence. | *ACSM's Resource Manual for Guidelines for Exercise Testing and Prescription*, 7th edition (8)<br>• Chapter 17 |
| **Knowledge** of client needs and learning styles that may impact exercise sessions and exercise testing procedures | • A client-centered approach should be adopted for all aspects that are related to exercise.<br>• Exercise prescription should be individualized. | *ACSM's Resource Manual for Guidelines for Exercise Testing and Prescription*, 7th edition (8)<br>• Chapter 34 |
| **Knowledge** of conflict resolution techniques that facilitate communication among exercise cohorts | • Be aware of conflict resolution techniques that may be used to resolve a conflict, argument, or disagreement. | "Conflict Resolution Skills" (25) |
| **Skill** in communicating the need for medical, nutritional, or mental health intervention | • One should be able to evaluate and assess physical activity, nutritional, and psychological statuses and provide and communicate appropriate and sound responses. | *ACSM's Resource Manual for Guidelines for Exercise Testing and Prescription*, 7th edition (8)<br>• Chapters 15, 17, and 20 |

HFS

# DOMAIN IV: LEGAL/PROFESSIONAL

| A. Create and disseminate risk management guidelines for a health/fitness facility, department, or organization to reduce member, employee, and business risk. | | |
|---|---|---|
| **Knowledge or Skill Statement** | **Explanation/Examples** | **Resources** |
| **Knowledge** of employee criminal background checks, child abuse clearances, and drug and alcohol screenings | • Laws may vary between states. | "Performing Pre-Employment Background Checks" (31) |
| **Knowledge** of employment verification requirements mandated by state and federal laws | • Laws may vary between states. | "Performing Pre-Employment Background Checks" (31) |
| **Knowledge** of safe handling and disposal of body fluids and employee safety (Occupational Safety and Health Administration [OSHA] guidelines) | • Applies to occupational exposure to blood/body fluids or other potentially infectious materials | *ACSM's Resource Manual for Guidelines for Exercise Testing and Prescription*, 7th edition (8)<br>• Chapter 19<br>OSHA Standards (29 CFR) 1910.1030(d)(4)(iii)(C) (24) |
| **Knowledge** of insurance coverage common to the health/fitness industry including general liability, professional liability, workers' compensation, property, and business interruption | • Be aware of insurance reimbursement and the role of Medicaid and Medicare.<br>• Be aware of the following topics: malpractice, negligence, and standards of practice. | *ACSM's Resource Manual for Guidelines for Exercise Testing and Prescription*, 7th edition (8)<br>• Chapters 10 and 19 |
| **Knowledge** of sexual harassment policies and procedures | • Must understand the federal law prohibiting sexual harassment in the workplace.<br>• Most states have some additional laws that relates to sexual harassment and discrimination. | "Title VII of the Civil Rights Act of 1964" (30) |
| **Knowledge** of interviewing techniques | • Avoid questions that may violate discrimination laws (what is your sexual orientation, religion, etc.). | "Title VII of the Civil Rights Act of 1964" (30) |
| **Knowledge** of basic precautions taken in an exercise setting to ensure participant safety | • Safety is always first.<br>• Proper screening and emergency policy standards are paramount. | *ACSM's Guidelines for Exercise Testing and Prescription* (GETP), 9th edition (7)<br>• Tables 2.1–2.4<br>• Figures 2.1–2.4<br>*ACSM's Health/Fitness Facility Standards and Guidelines*, 4th edition (3)<br>• Chapter 3<br>• Table 3.1 |
| **Knowledge** of preactivity screening, medical release, and waiver of liability for normal and at-risk participants | • This information is fairly extensive and should be covered thoroughly. | *ACSM's Guidelines for Exercise Testing and Prescription* (GETP), 9th edition (7)<br>• Chapter 2 |
| **Knowledge** of emergency response systems and procedures employee assistance program | • The procedures should be clearly stated, reviewed regularly, and known to all employees. | *ACSM's Health/Fitness Facility Standards and Guidelines*, 4th edition (3)<br>• Chapter 3 |

## A. Create and disseminate risk management guidelines for a health/fitness facility, department, or organization to reduce member, employee, and business risk. (cont.)

| Knowledge or Skill Statement | Explanation/Examples | Resources |
|---|---|---|
| **Knowledge** of the use of signage | • Be aware of the differences between cautionary signage, danger signage, and warning signage. | *ACSM's Health/Fitness Facility Standards and Guidelines,* 4th edition (3)<br>• Chapter 8 |
| **Knowledge** of preventive maintenance schedules and audits | • Be aware of the differences between daily, weekly, and monthly care. | *ACSM's Health/Fitness Facility Standards and Guidelines,* 4th edition (3)<br>• Chapter 7<br>• Tables 7.3 and 7.4 |
| **Knowledge** of techniques and methods of evaluating the condition of exercise equipment to reduce the potential risk of injury | • Be aware of the differences between daily, weekly, and monthly care. | *ACSM's Health/Fitness Facility Standards and Guidelines,* 4th edition (3)<br>• Chapter 7<br>• Tables 7.3 and 7.4 |
| **Knowledge** of the legal implications of documented safety procedures, the use of incident documents, and ongoing safety training documentation for the purpose of safety and risk management | • Be aware of tort and contract principles because they relate to physical activity legal issues.<br>• Regardless of severity, every incident (injury) should be documented. | *ACSM's Resource Manual for Guidelines for Exercise Testing and Prescription,* 7th edition (8)<br>• Chapter 10<br>*ACSM's Health/Fitness Facility Standards and Guidelines,* 4th edition (3)<br>• Chapter 3 |
| **Knowledge** of documentation procedures for cardiopulmonary resuscitation (CPR) and automated external defibrillator (AED) certification for employees. | • CPR and AED certification is critical and required for health fitness specialist (HFS). | *ACSM's Health/Fitness Facility Standards and Guidelines,* 4th edition (3)<br>• Chapter 3 |
| **Knowledge** of AED guidelines for implementation | • AED plays a major role in the resuscitative process in ventricular fibrillation related cardiac arrest.<br>• In some states, a legislation was passed that requires health/fitness facilities to carry AED.<br>• The procedures should be reviewed regularly and known to all AED certified employees. | *ACSM's Health/Fitness Facility Standards and Guidelines,* 4th edition (3)<br>• Chapter 3 |
| **Knowledge** of the components of the American College of Sports Medicine (ACSM) Code of Ethics and the ACSM Certified HFS scope of practice | • The ACSM Code of Ethics has five components.<br>• In recent years, the scope of practice was adjusted and based on the Job Task Analysis (JTA). | *ACSM's Guidelines for Exercise Testing and Prescription* (GETP), 9th edition (7)<br>• Appendix D<br>ACSM's Code of Ethics (5) |
| **Skill** in developing and disseminating a policy and procedures manual | • Chapter 1 provides a good introduction to what a policies and procedures manual should include.<br>• This information is fairly extensive and should be covered thoroughly. | *ACSM's Health/Fitness Facility Standards and Guidelines,* 4th edition (3)<br>• Chapters 1–8 |
| **Skill** in developing and implementing confidentiality policies | • Because personnel in health/fitness facilities are exposed to confidential health-related information, HIPAA regulations should be used as a guide when developing such a policy. | Health Insurance Portability and Accountability Act of 1996 (HIPAA) (28) |

HFS

## A.  Create and disseminate risk management guidelines for a health/fitness facility, department, or organization to reduce member, employee, and business risk. (cont.)

| Knowledge or Skill Statement | Explanation/Examples | Resources |
|---|---|---|
| **Skill** in maintenance of a safe exercise environment (*e.g.*, equipment operation, proper sanitation, safety and maintenance of exercise areas, and overall facility maintenance) | • Follow the recommended daily, weekly, and/or monthly equipment and facility cleaning and maintenance. | *ACSM's Health/Fitness Facility Standards and Guidelines,* 4th edition (3)<br>• Chapter 5<br>• Tables 5.4–5.6<br>• Chapter 7<br>• Tables 7.3 and 7.4 |
| **Skill** in the organization, communication, and human resource management required to implement risk management policies and procedures. | • Be aware of both standards and guidelines for risk management and emergency policies. | *ACSM's Health/Fitness Facility Standards and Guidelines,* 4th edition (3)<br>• Chapter 3 |
| **Skill** in training employees to identify high-risk situations | • Employees should have the appropriate education, certification, and experience to identify high-risk situations.<br>• Employees should be familiar with emergency response protocols. | *ACSM's Health/Fitness Facility Standards and Guidelines,* 4th edition (3)<br>• Chapter 4 |

## B.  Create an effective injury prevention program and ensure that emergency policies and procedures are in place.

| Knowledge or Skill Statement | Explanation/Examples | Resources |
|---|---|---|
| **Knowledge** of emergency procedures (*i.e.*, telephone procedures, written emergency procedures, personnel responsibilities) in a health and fitness setting | • Staff should be familiar with and have access to all written emergency guidelines and procedures.<br>• Emergency plan should be current and documented. | *ACSM's Resource Manual for Guidelines for Exercise Testing and Prescription,* 7th edition (8)<br>• Chapter 19 |
| **Knowledge** of basic first aid procedures for exercise-related injuries, such as bleeding, strains/sprains, fractures, and exercise intolerance (dizziness, syncope, heat and cold injuries) | • This information is fairly extensive and the health fitness specialist (HFS) should have the knowledge to appropriately recognize and treat the emergency. | *ACSM's Resource Manual for Guidelines for Exercise Testing and Prescription,* 7th edition (8)<br>• Chapter 19<br>• Tables 19.2–19.4 |
| **Knowledge** of the HFS responsibilities and limitations and the legal implications of carrying out emergency procedures | • To protect participants/clients and to minimize the risk of legal ramifications, the HFS must be familiar with each facility's policies and procedures (place of employment). | *ACSM's Certified Health Fitness Specialist Scope of Practice* (1)<br>*ACSM's Resource Manual for Guidelines for Exercise Testing and Prescription,* 7th edition (8)<br>• Chapter 10 |
| **Knowledge** of safety plans, emergency procedures, and first aid techniques needed during fitness evaluations, exercise testing, and exercise training | • Be aware of the facility's policies and procedures.<br>• Be aware of different medical conditions/emergencies and the proper acute and emergency (if applicable) response. | *ACSM's Resource Manual for Guidelines for Exercise Testing and Prescription,* 7th edition (8)<br>• Chapter 10 |

## B. Create an effective injury prevention program and ensure that emergency policies and procedures are in place. (cont.)

| Knowledge or Skill Statement | Explanation/Examples | Resources |
|---|---|---|
| **Knowledge** of potential musculoskeletal injuries (*e.g.,* contusions, sprains, strains, fractures), cardiovascular/pulmonary complications (*e.g.,* tachycardia, bradycardia, hypotension/hypertension, dyspnea) and metabolic abnormalities (*e.g.,* fainting/syncope, hypoglycemia/hyperglycemia, hypothermia/hyperthermia) | • The knowledge of these conditions is fairly extensive.<br>• Be aware of the conditions, signs, and symptoms as well as acute responses. | *ACSM's Resource Manual for Guidelines for Exercise Testing and Prescription,* 7th edition (8)<br>• Chapter 19<br>• Table 19.2 |
| **Knowledge** of the initial management and first aid techniques associated with open wounds, musculoskeletal injuries, cardiovascular/pulmonary complications, and metabolic disorders | • The HFS should recognize and be able to provide acute care for each of these conditions. | *ACSM's Resource Manual for Guidelines for Exercise Testing and Prescription,* 7th edition (8)<br>• Chapter 19<br>• Tables 19.2–19.4 |
| **Knowledge** of emergency documentation and appropriate document use | • Regardless of severity, every incident (injury) should be documented. | *ACSM's Health/Fitness Facility Standards and Guidelines,* 4th edition (3)<br>• Chapter 3 |
| **Skill** in applying basic first aid procedures for exercise-related injuries, such as bleeding, strains/sprains, fractures, and exercise intolerance (dizziness, syncope, heat and cold injuries) | • The HFS should recognize (have the knowledge) and be able to provide acute care (be skillful) to each of these conditions. | *ACSM's Resource Manual for Guidelines for Exercise Testing and Prescription,* 7th edition (8)<br>• Chapter 19<br>• Tables 19.2–19.4 |
| **Skill** in applying basic life support, first aid, cardiopulmonary resuscitation (CPR), and automated external defibrillator (AED) techniques | • The HFS must have a current adult CPR/AED certification with a practical skills component. | *ACSM's Health/Fitness Facility Standards and Guidelines,* 4th edition (3)<br>• Chapter 4 |
| **Skill** in designing an evacuation plan | • The plan should be developed as part of the exercise program safety and emergencies procedures. | *ACSM's Resource Manual for Guidelines for Exercise Testing and Prescription,* 7th edition (8)<br>• Chapter 19<br>*ACSM's Health/Fitness Facility Standards and Guidelines,* 4th edition (3)<br>• Appendix J |
| **Skill** in demonstrating emergency procedures during exercise testing and/or training | • The HFS must be familiar with each facility's emergency policies and procedures.<br>• The HFS must have a current adult CPR/AED certification with a practical skills component. | *ACSM's Resource Manual for Guidelines for Exercise Testing and Prescription,* 7th edition (8)<br>• Chapter 19<br>*ACSM's Health/Fitness Facility Standards and Guidelines,* 4th edition (3)<br>• Chapter 4 |

HFS

# DOMAIN V: MANAGEMENT

## A. Manage human resources in accordance with leadership, organization, and management techniques.

| Knowledge or Skill Statement | Explanation/Examples | Resources |
|---|---|---|
| **Knowledge** of industry benchmark compensation and employee benefit guidelines | • The information that is presented by the BLS regarding compensation may vary from year to year.<br>• Employee benefits will vary widely from one employer to another. | Bureau of Labor Statistics (BLS) (10) |
| **Knowledge** of federal, state, and local laws pertaining to staff qualifications and credentialing requirements | • Staff qualifications and credentialing requirements will vary from state to state. | *ACSM's Health/Fitness Facility Standards and Guidelines*, 4th edition (3)<br>• Chapter 4<br>• Tables 4.2–4.5. |
| **Knowledge** of techniques for tracking and evaluating member retention | • Consider using focus groups, surveys, in-depth interviews, and feedback systems. | *ACSM's Resource Manual for Guidelines for Exercise Testing and Prescription*, 7th edition (8)<br>• Chapter 48 |
| **Skill** in applying policies, practices, and guidelines to efficiently hire, train, supervise, schedule, and evaluate employees | • Be very familiar with the facility policies and procedures.<br>• Be very familiar with federal, state, and local laws pertaining to staff qualifications and credentialing requirements. | *ACSM's Health/Fitness Facility Standards and Guidelines*, 4th edition (3)<br>• Chapter 4<br>• Tables 4.2–4.5. |
| **Skill** in applying conflict resolution techniques | • Negotiate and mediate in the interpersonal level (between employees and/or members) in order to resolve a conflict, argument, or disagreement. | "Conflict Resolution Skills" (25) |

## B. Manage fiscal resources in accordance with leadership, organization, and management techniques.

| Knowledge or Skill Statement | Explanation/Examples | Resources |
|---|---|---|
| **Knowledge** of fiduciary roles and responsibilities inherent in managing an exercise and health promotion program | • Be aware of Employee Retirement Income Security Act (ERISA). | "Meeting Your Fiduciary Responsibilities" (29) |
| **Knowledge** of principles of financial planning and goal setting, institutional budgeting processes, forecasting, and allocation of resources | • This information is fairly extensive and requires understanding of the basic principles, rules, and regulations of business administration. | "Understanding the Basics" (32) |
| **Knowledge** of basic software systems that facilitate accounting (*e.g.*, Excel) | • This spreadsheet application is being updated periodically.<br>• There are other basic software systems that may assist facility accounting such as Quicken. | Excel 2010 (22) |
| **Knowledge** of industry benchmarks for budgeting and finance | • This information is fairly extensive and requires understanding of the basic principles, rules, and regulations of business administration. | "Understanding the Basics" (32) |

## B.  Manage fiscal resources in accordance with leadership, organization, and management techniques. (cont.)

| Knowledge or Skill Statement | Explanation/Examples | Resources |
|---|---|---|
| **Knowledge** of basic sales techniques that promote health, fitness, and wellness services | • Be aware of common techniques such as cold calling, drop box leads, etc. | *ACSM's Resource Manual for Guidelines for Exercise Testing and Prescription*, 7th edition (8)<br>• Chapter 48 |
| **Skill** in efficiently managing financial resources and performing related tasks (*e.g.*, planning, budgeting, resource allocation, revenue generation) | • Be very familiar with finance and accounting management because it relates to business administration.<br>• Be very familiar with federal, state, and local laws pertaining to business administration. | "Understanding the Basics" (32) |
| **Skill** in administering fitness- and wellness-related programs within established budgetary guidelines | • Be very familiar with the rules and regulations of business administration. | "Understanding the Basics" (32) |

## C.  Establish policies and procedures for the management of health/fitness facilities based on accepted safety and legal guidelines, standards, and regulations.

| Knowledge or Skill Statement | Explanation/Examples | Resources |
|---|---|---|
| **Knowledge** of accepted guidelines, standards, and regulations used to establish policies and procedures for the management of health/fitness facilities | • Chapter 1 provides a good introduction to what a policy and procedures manual should include.<br>• This information is fairly extensive and should be covered thoroughly. | *ACSM's Health/Fitness Facility Standards and Guidelines*, 4th edition (3)<br>• Chapters 1–8 |
| **Knowledge** of facility design and operation principles | • This information is fairly extensive and should be covered thoroughly.<br>• Be aware of the differences between fitness only and multipurpose facilities in respect to design and overall operations. | *ACSM's Health/Fitness Facility Standards and Guidelines*, 4th edition (3)<br>• Chapters 5 and 16 |
| **Knowledge** of facility and equipment maintenance guidelines | • Be aware of the differences between daily, weekly, and monthly equipment maintenance. | *ACSM's Health/Fitness Facility Standards and Guidelines*, 4th edition (3)<br>• Chapter 5<br>• Tables 5.4–5.6<br>• Chapter 7<br>• Tables 7.3 and 7.4 |
| **Knowledge** of documentation techniques for health/fitness facility management | • Facilities should have written policies and procedures.<br>• Be aware that policies and procedures will vary from state to state. | *ACSM's Health/Fitness Facility Standards and Guidelines*, 4th edition (3)<br>• Chapter 5 |
| **Knowledge** of federal, state, and local laws as they relate to health/fitness facility management | • Check federal, state, and local laws because facility management rules and regulation will vary from state to state. | *ACSM's Health/Fitness Facility Standards and Guidelines*, 4th edition (3)<br>• Chapter 5 |

HFS

## D.   Develop and execute a marketing plan to promote programs, services, and facilities.

| Knowledge or Skill Statement | Explanation/Examples | Resources |
|---|---|---|
| **Knowledge** of lead generation techniques | • Use membership referral, lead boxes, cold calling, etc. | *ACSM's Resources for the Health Fitness Specialist* (6)<br>• Chapters 15 and 17 |
| **Knowledge** of the four *P*'s of marketing: product, price, placement, and promotion | • Marketing plays a major role in the viability of health/fitness facilities.<br>• The management team should consider an array of marketing tools to promote the facility and fitness-related programs. | *ACSM's Resources for the Health Fitness Specialist* (6)<br>• Chapters 15 and 17 |
| **Knowledge** of public relations, community awareness, and sponsorship and their relationship to branding initiatives | • Use tools such as developing alliances with Home Owners Association's HOA's and realtors, initiate community involvement, etc. | *ACSM's Resources for the Health Fitness Specialist* (6)<br>• Chapters 15 and 17 |
| **Knowledge** of advertising techniques | • Consider scatter gun approach, sharp shooter method, promotional massages, etc. | *ACSM's Resources for the Health Fitness Specialist* (6)<br>• Chapters 15 and 17 |
| **Knowledge** of target market (internal) assessment techniques | • Assess internal factors that may provide advantages or disadvantages in meeting the needs of the target market (clients).<br>• Consider market trends, conduct regular evaluations, etc. | *ACSM's Resources for the Health Fitness Specialist* (6)<br>• Chapters 15 and 17 |
| **Knowledge** of target market (external) assessment techniques | • Assess external factors such as offering by competitors, the state of the economy, etc. | *ACSM's Resources for the Health Fitness Specialist* (6)<br>• Chapters 15 and 17 |
| **Skill** in applying marketing techniques that promote client retention | • Use tools such as focus groups, surveys, in-depth interviews, and feedback systems. | *ACSM's Resources for the Health Fitness Specialist* (6)<br>• Chapters 15 and 17 |
| **Skill** in applying marketing techniques that attract new clients | • Must be very familiar with marketing techniques such as lead boxes, direct mail, cold calling, etc. | *ACSM's Resources for the Health Fitness Specialist* (6)<br>• Chapters 15 and 17 |
| **Skill** in designing and writing promotional materials | • Must be very familiar with developing materials that will positively and aggressively market the facility | *ACSM's Resources for the Health Fitness Specialist* (6)<br>• Chapters 15 and 17 |
| **Skill** in collaborating with community and governmental agencies and organizations | • Must be very familiar with strategic alliance strategies | *ACSM's Resources for the Health Fitness Specialist* (6)<br>• Chapters 15 and 17 |
| **Skill** in providing customer service | • Pivotal factor in health/fitness facilities<br>• Some ways to improve customer service relate to providing superior service, maintain exercise equipment, etc. | *ACSM's Resources for the Health Fitness Specialist* (6)<br>• Chapters 15 and 17 |

HFS

## E. Use effective communication techniques to develop professional relationships with other allied health professionals (*e.g.,* nutritionists, physical therapists, physicians, nurses).

| Knowledge or Skill Statement | Explanation/Examples | Resources |
|---|---|---|
| **Knowledge** of communication styles and techniques | • In addition to face-to-face communications (meetings, conferences, etc.), it is common today to use a wide range of electronic communications such as e-mails, tweets, etc. | *ACSM's Resources for the Health Fitness Specialist* (6) <br> • Chapters 15 and 17 |
| **Knowledge** of networking techniques | • Meet and maintain a relationship with other allied health professionals (conferences, webinars, etc.). <br> • Maintain communications (keep in touch). <br> • Consider developing strategic alliances. | *ACSM's Resources for the Health Fitness Specialist* (6) <br> • Chapters 15 and 17 |
| **Skill** in planning meetings | • Requires experience in advertising, the use of other promotional materials, direct mail, etc. | *ACSM's Resources for the Health Fitness Specialist* (6) <br> • Chapters 15 and 17 |

# REFERENCES

## ACSM REFERENCES:

1. American College of Sports Medicine. ACSM's certified health fitness specialist scope of practice. *American College of Sports Medicine* [Internet]. [cited 2011 Sep 22]. Available from: http://www.acsm.org/AM/Template.cfm?Section=HealthFitness_Instructor1&Template=/CM/ContentDisplay.cfm&ContentID=10829#HFI_Scope_of_Practice 2011

2. American College of Sports Medicine. *ACSM's Exercise Management for Persons with Chronic Diseases and Disabilities.* 3rd ed. Champaign (IL): Human Kinetics; 2009. 440 p.

3. American College of Sports Medicine. *ACSM's Health/Fitness Facility Standards and Guidelines.* 4th ed. Champaign (IL): Human Kinetics; 2012. 203 p.

4. American College of Sports Medicine. *ACSM's Health-Related Physical Fitness Assessment Manual.* 4th ed. Philadelphia (PA): Lippincott Williams & Wilkins; 2013. 172 p.

5. American College of Sports Medicine. Code of ethics of American College of Sports Medicine. *American College of Sports Medicine* [Internet]. [cited 2011 Sep 22]. Available from: http://www.acsm.org/Content/NavigationMenu/MemberServices/MemberResources/CodeofEthics/Code_of_Ethics.htm

6. Liguori G, editor. *ACSM's Resources for the Health Fitness Specialist.* Baltimore (MD): Lippincott Williams & Wilkins; 2014.

7. Pescatello LS, senior editor. *ACSM's Guidelines for Exercise Testing and Prescription.* 9th ed. Baltimore (MD): Lippincott Williams & Wilkins; 2014.

8. Swain DP, senior editor. *ACSM's Resource Manual for Guidelines for Exercise Testing and Prescription.* 7th ed. Baltimore (MD): Lippincott Williams & Wilkins; 2014.

## NON-ACSM REFERENCES:

9. Armiger P, Martyn MA. *Stretching for Functional Flexibility.* Philadelphia (PA): Lippincott Williams & Wilkins; 2010. 263 p.

10. Bureau of Labor Statistics. Occupational outlook handbook, 2010–2011 edition, fitness workers. *United States Department of Labor* [Internet]. [cited 2011 Sep 22]. Available from: http://www.bls.gov/oco/ocos296.htm

11. Davis M, Eshelman ER, McKay M. *The Relaxation & Stress Reduction Workbook.* 6th ed. Oakland (CA): New Harbinger Publications; 2008. 371 p.

12. Ehrman JK. *Clinical Exercise Physiology.* 2nd ed. Champaign (IL): Human Kinetics; 2009. 691 p.

13. Fleck SJ, Kraemer WJ. *Designing Resistance Training Programs.* 3rd ed. Champaign (IL): Human Kinetics; 2004. 377 p.

14. Garber CE, Blissmer B, Deschenes MR, et al. American College of Sports Medicine position stand. Quantity and quality of exercise for developing and maintaining cardiorespiratory, musculoskeletal, and neuromotor fitness in apparently healthy adults: guidance for prescribing exercise. *Med Sci Sports Exerc.* 2011;43(7):1334–59.

15. Goldenberg L, Twist P. *Strength Ball Training.* 2nd ed. Champaign (IL): Human Kinetics; 2007. 285 p.

16. Hall SJ. *Basic Biomechanics.* 6th ed. Boston (MA): WCB/McGraw-Hill; 2011. 577 p.

17. Heyward VH. *Advanced Fitness Assessment and Exercise Prescription.* 4th ed. Champaign (IL): Human Kinetics; 2002. 369 p.

18. Higgins M. *Therapeutic Exercise: From Theory to Practice.* Philadelphia (PA): F. A. Davis Company; 2011. 807 p.

19. Kraemer WJ, Fleck SJ, Deschenes MR. *Exercise Physiology: Integrated Theory and Application.* Philadelphia (PA): Lippincott Williams & Wilkins; 2011. 488 p.

20. Lengel T, Kuczala M. *The Kinesthetic Classroom : Teaching and Learning through Movement.* Thousand Oaks (CA): Corwin Press; 2010. 156 p.

21. Martin G, Pear J. *Behavior Modification: What It Is and How to Do It.* 9th ed. Boston (CA): Pearson Education/Allyn & Bacon; 2011. 462 p.

22. Microsoft Corporation. Excel 2010. *Microsoft Corporation* [Internet]. [cited 2011 Sep 26]. Available from: http://office.microsoft.com/en-us/excel/

23. Newton H. *Explosive Lifting for Sports—Enhanced Edition.* Champaign (IL): Human Kinetics; 2006. 191 p.

HFS

24. Occupational Safety & Health Administration. Occupational safety and health standards: toxic and hazardous substances (standard number 1910.1030). *United States Department Labor* [Internet]. [cited 2011 Sep 22]. Available from: http://www.osha.gov/pls/oshaweb/owadisp.show_document?p_table=standards&p_id=10051

25. Segal J, Smith M. Conflict resolution skills. *Helpguide* [Internet]. [cited 2011 Sep 22]. Available from: http://helpguide.org/mental/eq8_conflict_resolution.htm

26. Taylor AW, Johnson MJ. *Physiology of Exercise and Healthy Aging.* Champaign (IL): Human Kinetics; 2008. 274 p.

27. U.S. Department of Agriculture. USDA center for nutrition policy and promotion. *United States Department of Agriculture* [Internet]. [cited 2011 Sep 26]. Available from: http://www.choosemyplate.gov/index.html

28. U.S. Department of Health & Human Services. Summary of the HIPAA privacy rule. *U.S. Department of Health & Human Services* [Internet]. [cited 2011 Sep 22]. Available from: http://www.hhs.gov/ocr/privacy/hipaa/understanding/summary/privacysummary.pdf

29. U.S. Department of Labor. Meeting your fiduciary responsibilities. *United States Department of Labor* [Internet]. [cited 2011 Sep 26]. Available from: http://www.dol.gov/ebsa/publications/fiduciaryresponsibility.html

30. U.S. Equal Employment Opportunity Commission. Title VII of the Civil Rights Act of 1964. *U.S. Equal Employment Opportunity Commission* [Internet]. [cited 2011 Sep 22]. Available from: http://www.eeoc.gov/laws/statutes/titlevii.cfm

31. U.S. Small Business Administration. Performing pre-employment background check. *U.S. Small Business Administration* [Internet]. [cited 2011 Sep 22]. Available from: http://www.sba.gov/content/performing-pre-employment-background-Checks

32. U.S. Small Business Administration. Understanding the basics. *U.S. Small Business Administration* [Internet]. [cited 2011 Sep 22]. Available from: http://www.sba.gov/category/navigation-structure/starting-managing-business/starting-business/preparing-your-finances/understanding-basics

HFS

*Note: HFS certification candidates should also review the practice examination found in Part 1, ACSM Certified Personal Trainer (CPT).*

DIRECTIONS: Each of the numbered items or incomplete statements in this section is followed by answers or by completions of the statement. Select the ONE lettered answer or completion that is BEST in each case.

1. Which of the following medications is designed to modify blood cholesterol levels?
   A) Nitrates
   B) β–Blockers
   C) Antihyperlipidemics
   D) Aspirin

2. Which of the following represents more than 90% of the fat stored in the body and is composed of a glycerol molecule connected to three fatty acids?
   A) Phospholipids
   B) Cholesterol
   C) Triglycerides
   D) Free fatty acids

3. Limited flexibility of which of the following muscle groups increases the risk of low back pain?
   A) Quadriceps
   B) Hamstrings
   C) Hip flexors
   D) Biceps femoris

4. Which of the following terms represents an imaginary horizontal plane passing through the midsection of the body and dividing it into upper and lower portions?
   A) Sagittal
   B) Frontal
   C) Transverse
   D) Superior

5. Which of the following blood pressure (BP) readings would characterize hypertension in the adult?
   A) 100/60 mm Hg
   B) 110/70 mm Hg
   C) 120/80 mm Hg
   D) 140/90 mm Hg

6. For every one metabolic equivalent (MET) increase in exercise intensity during submaximal exercise, systolic blood pressure (SBP) (mm Hg) should increase _____.
   A) Approximately 10 mm Hg
   B) 15–20 mm Hg
   C) 25–30 mm Hg
   D) 30–35 mm Hg

7. Which of the following would not terminate a maximal or submaximal exercise test in a low-risk adult?
   A) Subject requests to stop
   B) Shortness of breath
   C) A slight decrease in diastolic pressure
   D) Failure of heart rate (HR) to increase with increased intensity

8. If a 150-lb man exercised for 30 min on a Monark cycle ergometer at an intensity of 27.5 mL $\cdot$ kg$^{-1}$ $\cdot$ min$^{-1}$, what would his caloric expenditure be for the entire 30-min session?
   A) 280.50 kcal
   B) 137.50 kcal
   C) 9.35 kcal
   D) 5.50 kcal

9. To promote weight loss, cardiovascular endurance exercise should be performed for _____.
   A) At least 30 min on 3 or more days per week (moderate intensity)
   B) At least 50–60 min $\cdot$ d$^{-1}$ totaling 300 min $\cdot$ wk$^{-1}$ (moderate intensity)
   C) At least 20–25 min on 3 or more days per week (vigorous intensity)
   D) At least 10 min on most days of the week (vigorous intensity)

10. For adults with arthritis, which of the following apply?
    A) Progression in duration of activity should be emphasized over increased intensity.
    B) Physical activity should be completed at the same time every day.
    C) Avoid all joint movement during periods of acute flares and inflammation.
    D) All of the above.

11. Uncoordinated gait, headache, dizziness, vomiting, and elevated body temperature are signs and symptoms of _____.
    A) Acute exposure to the cold
    B) Hypothermia
    C) Heat exhaustion and heat stroke
    D) Acute altitude sickness

12. What is a subject's work rate in watts if he pedals on a Monark cycle ergometer at 50 revolutions per minute (RPM) at a resistance of 2.0 kp? Assume that 1 revolution of the cycle ergometer flywheel is 6 m long.
    A) 10 W
    B) 50 W
    C) 100 W
    D) 200 W

13. Regular exercise will result in what chronic adaptation in cardiac output ($\dot{Q}$) during exercise at the same workload?
    A) Increase
    B) Decrease
    C) No change
    D) Increase during dynamic exercise only

14. Which of the following conditions is characterized by a decrease in bone mass and density, producing bone porosity and fragility?
    A) Osteoarthritis
    B) Osteomyelitis
    C) Epiphyseal osteomyelitis
    D) Osteoporosis

15. When using the original Borg scale (6–20) for the general public, moderate intensity should be maintained between _____.
    A) 8 and 12
    B) 12 and 16
    C) 17 and 18
    D) 19 and 20

16. Rotation of the anterior surface of a bone toward the midline of the body is called _____.
    A) Medial rotation
    B) Lateral rotation
    C) Supination
    D) Pronation

17. $\dot{Q}$ can be calculated by multiplying _____.
    A) HR and stroke volume
    B) Stroke volume and the difference between the oxygen-carrying capacity of the arterial blood and venous blood
    C) Oxygen consumption and HR
    D) HR and blood volume

18. A source of intimal injury thought to initiate the process of atherogenesis is _____.
    A) Dyslipidemia
    B) Hypertension
    C) Turbulence of blood flow within the vessel
    D) All of the above

19. At what level is high-density lipoprotein (HDL) considered a risk factor in the development of cardiovascular disease?
    A) $<200$ mg $\cdot$ dL$^{-1}$
    B) $<110$ mg $\cdot$ dL$^{-1}$
    C) $<60$ mg $\cdot$ dL$^{-1}$
    D) $<40$ mg $\cdot$ dL$^{-1}$

20. What could be an alternative to the contraindicated, high-risk plough exercise?
    A) Squats to 90 degrees
    B) Flexion with rotation
    C) Double knee to chest
    D) Lateral neck stretches

21. Which of the following is NOT true regarding the psychological benefits of regular exercise in the elderly?
    A) Self-concept
    B) Life satisfaction
    C) Stimulate appetite
    D) Self-efficacy

22. To determine program effectiveness, psychological theories provide a conceptual framework for assessment and _____.
    A) Management of programs or interventions
    B) Application of cognitive-behavioral or motivational principles
    C) Measurement
    D) All of the above

23. As a result of regular exercise training, which of the following is NOT affected during maximal exercise?
    A) $\dot{Q}$
    B) Stroke volume
    C) Maximal heart rate (HR$_{max}$)
    D) None of the above

24. When exercise training children, _____.
    A) Exercise programs should increase physical fitness in the short term and strength and stamina in the long term.
    B) Strength training should be avoided for safety reasons.
    C) Increasing the rate of training intensity more than approximately 10% per week increases the likelihood of overuse injuries of bone.
    D) Children with exercise-induced asthma are often unable to lead active lives.

25. Which of the following risk factors for the development of coronary artery disease (CAD) has the greatest likelihood of being influenced by regular exercise?
    A) Smoking
    B) Cholesterol
    C) Type 1 diabetes
    D) Hypertension

26. At minimum, professionals performing fitness assessments on others should possess which combination of the following?
    A) Cardiopulmonary resuscitation (CPR) and American College of Sports Medicine (ACSM) Health Fitness Specialist (HFS)
    B) Advanced cardiac life support and ACSM Exercise Specialist
    C) Advanced cardiac life support and ACSM Registered Clinical Exercise Physiologist
    D) Only physicians can perform fitness assessments

27. Which of the following components of the exercise prescription work inversely with each other?
    A) Intensity and duration
    B) Mode and intensity
    C) Mode and duration
    D) Mode and frequency

28. Which statement is true regarding physical activity for children?
    A) Children should participate in several bouts of physical activity lasting 15 min or more each day.
    B) Children should perform 30 min of moderate-intensity and 30 min of vigorous-intensity physical activity on most days of the week.
    C) Children should focus on just one or two modes of physical activity so as to develop exceptional skills in those areas.
    D) Children need to have several periods of 2 h or more of inactivity during the day in order to have adequate rest.

29. Which statement is true regarding resistance training in children?
    A) We now know that it is appropriate and effective to use maximal (one repetition maximum [1-RM]) resistance training with children.
    B) The child should perform 8–15 repetitions (reps) per exercise.
    C) In terms of progression, focus mainly on the amount of resistance for the child.
    D) If a child cannot perform a minimum of 8 reps with good form, the resistance is too heavy and should be reduced.

30. Which mode would be inappropriate for most elderly (older) individuals?
    A) Walking as part of a social group
    B) Aquatic (water) exercise in a group setting
    C) Plyometrics as part of a health club class
    D) Stationary cycling for those with poor balance
    E) A, B, and D

31. How many reps should an elderly individual perform on each resistance exercise?
    A) 8–10 reps
    B) 12–15 reps
    C) 6–8 reps
    D) 4 reps

32. Which would NOT be a special consideration for exercise prescription in individuals with arthritis?
    A) Water exercise may help alleviate pain and stiffness.
    B) Vigorous, highly repetitive exercise should be encouraged in order to strengthen connective tissues at the joint.
    C) People with arthritis may be anemic due to regular use of nonsteroidal anti-inflammatory drugs (NSAIDs) causing gastrointestinal bleeding.
    D) For those with rheumatoid arthritis, morning exercise should be avoided due to significant morning stiffness.

33. In the term "arthritis," the prefix "arth" stands for _____, whereas the suffix "itis" stands for _____.
    A) Paste, inflammation
    B) Diseased, inflammation
    C) Joint, inflammation
    D) Joint, condition of

34. Which resistance exercise would strengthen both the biceps and latissimus dorsi muscles?
    A) Chin-ups
    B) Dead lifts
    C) Back extensions
    D) Upright rows

35. What at-home, single exercise using one's own body weight as resistance could be performed to strengthen the chest and triceps?
    A) Chin-ups
    B) Crunches
    C) Pec deck flyes
    D) Push-ups

36. At 6-MET intensity, an individual who has a 10-MET maximal capacity fitness level would be at an intensity classification of what?
    A) Light
    B) Moderate
    C) Hard
    D) Very hard

37. Which activity/activities below is/are considered as activities of daily living (ADL)?
    A) Reading and writing
    B) Lifting medium-weight items
    C) Transferring (walking)
    D) Speaking

38. When working with an individual with diabetes, what should you have on hand at all times?
    A) Sugar
    B) NutraSweet (artificial sweetener)
    C) Nitroglycerin
    D) Insulin

39. What exercises should be avoided after the first trimester for a pregnant woman?
    A) Upright exercises such as walking stairs
    B) Supine position exercises
    C) Prone position exercises
    D) Sitting exercises such as cycling

40. When periodizing training for a marathon runner (26.2 miles) who is doing a long run each Sunday, which is appropriate? Each Sunday run should _____.
    A) Be the same distance at about 20–22 miles.
    B) Gradually increase in distance weekly with a slightly lower distance Sunday every fourth week or so.
    C) Gradually increase in distance every week by about 10%.
    D) Rapidly increase distance weekly then avoid all long runs the last 2 mo.

41. In prevention of osteoporosis, it is important to regularly perform what kind of exercise?
    A) High-intensity
    B) Aquatic
    C) Low-intensity
    D) Weight-bearing

42. Both the Karvonen (heart rate reserve) and the straight $HR_{max}$ formulas of calculating target heart rate (THR) begin subtracting variables from a set number. What is this first number used in both formulas?
    A) Estimated maximal HR
    B) Maximal SBP
    C) Body Weight
    D) Gender

43. Which grouping lists the three training principles that you need to consider when prescribing exercise for individuals?
    A) Overload, intensity, progression
    B) Frequency, intensity, duration
    C) Specificity, overload, redundancy
    D) Overload, specificity, progression

44. If you want your client to exercise at 55%–70% of her maximum HR in today's workout and she is 24 yr old and does not know her observed maximum HR, what HR should be using today?
    A) 97–123 bpm
    B) 108–137 bpm
    C) 110–140 bpm
    D) 121–154 bpm

45. Which of the following types of muscle stretching can cause residual muscle soreness, is time consuming, and typically requires a partner?
    A) Static
    B) Ballistic
    C) Proprioceptive neuromuscular facilitation (PNF)
    D) All of the above

46. From rest to maximal exercise, the SBP should _____ progressively with an increasing workload.
    A) Increase
    B) Decrease
    C) Stay the same
    D) Decrease with isometric or increase with isotonic contractions

47. Most sedentary people who begin an exercise program are likely to stop within _____.
    A) 1–2 d
    B) 3–6 wk
    C) 1 mo
    D) 3–6 mo

48. Reasons for fitness testing of the older adult include _____.
    A) Evaluation of progress
    B) Exercise prescription
    C) Motivation
    D) All of the above

49. What is the energy cost of running at 6.5 mph up a grade of 5%?
    A) 8.2 MET
    B) 10.2 MET
    C) 13.2 MET
    D) 15.2 MET

50. Feeling good about being able to perform an activity or skill, such as finally being able to run a mile or to increase the speed of walking a mile, is an example of an _____.
    A) Extrinsic reward
    B) Intrinsic reward
    C) External stimulus
    D) Internal stimulus

51. What muscles does a "standing leg curl" exercise strengthen?
    A) Gluteal and quadriceps
    B) Hamstrings and calves
    C) Hamstrings only
    D) Calves only

52. What is the maneuver called where an individual holds his or her breath during a resistance training exercise in hopes of temporarily enhancing his or her strength?
    A) Karvonen
    B) Diaphragmatic
    C) Valsalva
    D) Anginal

53. If you prescribe that your client stretch his hamstrings, which flexibility exercise would NOT accomplish this?
    A) Modified hurdler stretch
    B) Forward wall push stretch
    C) Straddle stretch
    D) Cross-legged standing toe touch

54. In the *New Dietary Guidelines for Americans 2005*, it is recommend that for the general population to sustain weight loss in adulthood that they participate in at least _____ min of daily moderate-intensity physical activity while not exceeding caloric intake requirements.
    A) 20–40
    B) 30–60
    C) 60–90
    D) 90–120

55. If planning a 60-min walk (as opposed to some dynamic/ballistic activity like gymnastics tumbling), when is the most important time to stretch in relation to the walk?
    A) Before you warm-up
    B) After you warm-up
    C) Immediately after the completion of the 60-min walk
    D) After the cool-down

56. During exercise performed at high altitudes, HR will be _____ at the same rating of perceived exertion (RPE) observed at sea level.
    A) Lower
    B) Higher
    C) The same

57. An important safety consideration for exercise equipment in a fitness center includes _____.
    A) Flexibility of equipment to allow for different body sizes
    B) Size of equipment to accommodate small and large clients
    C) Affordability of equipment to allow for changing out equipment periodically
    D) Mobility of equipment to allow for easy rearrangement

58. The ACSM recommendation for intensity, duration, and frequency of cardiorespiratory exercise for apparently healthy individuals includes _____.
    A) Intensity of 60%–90% $HR_{max}$, duration of 20–60 min, and frequency of 3–5 d a week
    B) Intensity of 85%–90% $HR_{max}$, duration of 30 min, and frequency of 3 d a week
    C) Intensity of 50%–70% $HR_{max}$, duration of 15–45 min, and frequency of 5 d a week
    D) Intensity of 60%–90% $HR_{max}$ reserve, duration of 20–60 min, and frequency of 7 d a week

59. A method of strength and power training that involves an eccentric loading of muscles and tendons followed immediately by an explosive concentric contraction is called _____.
    A) Plyometrics
    B) Periodization
    C) Supersets
    D) Isotonic reversals

60. Which of the following personnel is responsible for program design as well as implementation of that program?
    A) Administrative assistant
    B) Exercise specialist
    C) Manager or director
    D) HFS

61. What is the purpose of agreements, releases, and consent forms?
    A) To inform the client of participation risks, as well as the rights of the client and the facility.
    B) To inform the client what he or she can and cannot do in the facility.
    C) To define the relationship between the facility operator and the HFS.
    D) To detail the rights and responsibilities of the club owner to reject an application by a prospective client.

62. After 30 yr of age, skeletal muscle strength begins to decline, primarily because of which of the following?
    A) A gain in fat tissue
    B) A gain in lean tissue
    C) A loss of muscle mass caused by a loss of muscle fibers
    D) Myogenic precursor cell inhibition

63. The Health Belief Model assumes that people will engage in a behavior, such as exercise, when _____.
    A) There is a perceived threat of disease.
    B) External motivation is provided.
    C) Optimal environmental conditions are met.
    D) Internal motivation outweighs external circumstances.

HFS

64. The informed consent document _____.
    A) Is a legal document
    B) Provides immunity from prosecution
    C) Provides an explanation of the test to the client
    D) Legally protects the rights of the client

65. A measure of muscular endurance is _____.
    A) 1-RM
    B) Three-repetition maximum
    C) Number of curl-ups in 1 min
    D) Number of curl-ups in 3 min

66. If a client exercises too much without rest days or develops a minor injury and does not allow time for the injury to heal, what can occur?
    A) An overuse injury
    B) Shin splints
    C) Sleep deprivation
    D) Decreased physical conditioning

67. The ACSM recommends that exercise intensity be prescribed within what percentage of $HR_{max}$ range?
    A) 40% and 60%
    B) 50% and 80%
    C) 60% and 90%
    D) 70% and 100%

68. The ACSM recommends how many reps of each exercise for muscular strength and endurance?
    A) 5–6
    B) 8–12
    C) 12–20
    D) More than 20

69. For higher intensity activities, _____.
    A) The benefit outweighs any potential risk.
    B) The risk of orthopedic and cardiovascular complications is increased.
    C) The risk of orthopedic and cardiovascular complications is minimal.
    D) There is no increased risk of orthopedic and cardiovascular complications.

70. What is the recommended rep range when resistance training adults for general muscular fitness?
    A) 1–5
    B) 6–10
    C) 8–12
    D) 15–20

71. Which of the following is an example of how to progressively overload the muscular system via resistance training?
    A) Increase amount of resistance lifted.
    B) Perform more sets per muscle group.
    C) Increase days per week the muscle groups are trained.
    D) All of the above are examples of progressive overload.

72. Which of the following resistance training exercises is an example of a multijoint exercise?
    A) Bicep curls
    B) Leg curls
    C) Leg press
    D) Calf raises

73. Which of the following is the recommended rest interval between sets of resistance training exercise?
    A) 30 s
    B) 1–2 min
    C) 2–3 min
    D) 3–4 min

74. For novice trainees, how many sets of each resistance training exercise are needed to improve muscular fitness?
    A) 1
    B) 2
    C) 3
    D) 4

75. Exercise adherence is increased when _____.
    A) There is social and health care provider support for the individual.
    B) A regular schedule of exercise is established.
    C) Muscle soreness and injury are minimal.
    D) Individualized, attainable goals, and objectives are identified.
    E) All of the above.

76. Which of the following are changes seen as a result of regular, chronic exercise?
    A) Decreased HR at rest
    B) Increased stroke volume at rest
    C) No change in $\dot{Q}$ at rest
    D) All of the above

77. While assessing the behavioral changes associated with an exercise program, which of the following would be categorized under the cognitive process of the Transtheoretical Model?
    A) Stimulus control
    B) Reinforcement management
    C) Self-reevaluation
    D) Self-liberation

78. Fitness assessment is an important aspect of the training program because it provides information for which of the following?
    A) Developing the exercise prescription
    B) Evaluating proper nutritional choices
    C) Diagnosing musculoskeletal injury
    D) Developing appropriate billing categories

HFS

79. Following an acute musculoskeletal injury, the appropriate action calls for stabilization of the area and incorporating the RICE treatment method. RICE is the acronym for which of the following?
    A) Recovery, Ibuprofen, Compression, Education
    B) Rest and Ice, Care for Injury
    C) Rest, Ice, Compression, Elevation
    D) Rotate, Ice, Care, Evaluate

80. A resistance training program that starts with light weights and high reps for the first set and then gradually moves to heavier weights and fewer reps for each successive set would be an example of which of the following training style?
    A) Circuits
    B) Supersets
    C) Split routines
    D) Pyramids

81. For individuals undertaking nonmedically supervised weight loss initiatives to reduce energy intake, the ACSM recommends weight loss of approximately _____.
    A) 1–2 lb · wk$^{-k}$ (0.5–1 kg)
    B) 5–8 lb · wk$^{-1}$ (2.3–4 kg)
    C) 8–10 lb · wk$^{-1}$ (4–4.5 kg)
    D) 10–15 lb · wk$^{-1}$ (4.5–7 kg)

82. A client with scoliosis exhibits which of the following conditions?
    A) A chronic, inflammatory, demyelinating disease
    B) An abnormal curvature of the spine
    C) Softening of the articular cartilage
    D) Inflammation of the growth plate at the tibial tuberosity

83. Which of the following assumes that a person will adopt appropriate health behaviors if he or she feels the consequences are severe and feel personally vulnerable?
    A) Learning theories
    B) Health Belief Model
    C) Transtheoretical Model
    D) Stages of Motivational Readiness

84. Identify the appropriate self-directed evaluation tool used as a quick health screening before beginning any exercise program.
    A) Minnesota Multiphasic Personality Inventory (MMPI)
    B) RPE-Borg scale
    C) Physical Activity Readiness Questionnaire (PAR-Q)
    D) Exercise Electrocardiogram (E-ECG)

85. You have examined your patient's health screening documents and obtained physiologic resting measurements, and you decide to proceed with a single session of fitness assessments. Identify the recommended order of administration.
    A) Flexibility, cardiorespiratory fitness, body composition, and muscular fitness
    B) Flexibility, body composition, muscular fitness, and cardiorespiratory fitness
    C) Body composition, cardiorespiratory fitness, muscular fitness, and flexibility
    D) Body composition, flexibility, cardiorespiratory fitness, and muscular fitness

86. Implementing emergency procedures must include the fitness center's _____.
    A) Management
    B) Staff
    C) Clients
    D) Management and staff

87. Which of the following is a possible medical emergency that a client can experience during an exercise session?
    A) Hypoglycemia
    B) Hypotension
    C) Hyperglycemia
    D) All of the above

88. Which of the following muscle actions occurs when muscle tension increases but the length of the muscle does not change?
    A) Concentric isotonic
    B) Eccentric isotonic
    C) Isokinetic
    D) Isometric

89. Which of the following activities provides the greatest improvement in aerobic fitness for someone who is beginning an exercise program?
    A) Weight training
    B) Downhill snow skiing
    C) Stretching
    D) Walking

90. In commercial settings, clients should be more extensively screened for potential health risks. The information solicited should include which of the following?
    A) Personal medical history
    B) Present medical status
    C) Medication
    D) All of the above

91. Generally, low-fit or sedentary persons may benefit from _____.
    A) Shorter duration, higher intensity, and higher frequency of exercise
    B) Longer duration, higher intensity, and higher frequency of exercise
    C) Shorter duration, lower intensity, and higher frequency of exercise
    D) Shorter duration, higher intensity, and lower frequency of exercise

92. What is the planning tool that addresses the organization's short- and long-term goals; identifies the steps needed to achieve the goals; and gives the time line, priority, and allocation of resources to each goal?
    A) Financial plan
    B) Strategic plan
    C) Risk management plan
    D) Marketing plan

93. When performing multiple fitness assessments in one session, you would begin by taking nonexercise or resting measurements and then test _____.
    A) Flexibility
    B) Cardiorespiratory endurance
    C) Muscular strength
    D) Muscular endurance

94. Which of the following is a contractile protein in skeletal muscle?
    A) Myosin
    B) Fascicle
    C) Myofibril
    D) Muscle fiber

95. Through which valve in the heart does blood flow when moving from the right atrium to the right ventricle (RV)?
    A) Bicuspid valve
    B) Tricuspid valve
    C) Pulmonic valve
    D) Aortic valve

96. Which of the following will increase stability?
    A) Lowering the center of gravity.
    B) Raising the center of gravity.
    C) Decreasing the base of support.
    D) Moving the center of gravity farther from the edge of the base of support.

97. During aerobic exercise, which of the following responses would NOT be considered normal?
    A) Increased SBP
    B) Increased pulse pressure
    C) Increased mean arterial pressure
    D) Increased diastolic blood pressure (DBP)

98. An exercise program for elderly persons generally should emphasize increased _____.
    A) Frequency
    B) Intensity
    C) Duration
    D) Intensity and frequency

99. The loss of elasticity (or "hardening") of the arteries is known as _____.
    A) Atherosclerosis
    B) Arteriosclerosis
    C) Atheroma
    D) Adventitia

100. Which of the following is a FALSE statement regarding an informed consent?
    A) The informed consent is not a legal document.
    B) The informed consent does not provide legal immunity to a facility or individual in the event of injury to an individual.
    C) Negligence, improper test administration, inadequate personnel qualifications, and insufficient safety procedures are all items that are expressly covered by the informed consent.
    D) The consent form does not relieve the facility or individual of the responsibility to do everything possible to ensure the safety of the individual.

# HFS EXAMINATION ANSWERS AND EXPLANATIONS

**1—C.** Antihyperlipidemics

Nitrates and nitroglycerine are antianginals (used to reduce chest pain associated with angina pectoris). β-Blockers are antihypertensives (used to reduce BP by inhibiting the action of adrenergic neurotransmitters at the β-receptor, thereby promoting peripheral vasodilation). β-Blockers also are designed to reduce BP by inhibiting the action of adrenergic neurotransmitters at the β-receptors, thereby decreasing $\dot{Q}$. Antihyperlipidemics control blood lipids, especially cholesterol and low-density lipoprotein (LDL). Aspirin is used to control for blood platelet stickiness.

**2—C.** Triglycerides

Dietary fats include triglycerides, sterols (*e.g.*, cholesterol), and phospholipids. Triglycerides represent more than 90% of the fat stored in the body. A *triglyceride* is a glycerol molecule connected to three fatty acid molecules. The fatty acids are identified by the amount of "saturation" or the number of single or double bonds that link the carbon atoms. Saturated fatty acids only have single bonds. Monounsaturated fatty acids have one double bond, and polyunsaturated fatty acids have two or more double bonds.

**3—B.** Hamstrings

An adequate range of motion or joint mobility is requisite for optimal musculoskeletal health. Specifically, limited flexibility of the low back and hamstring regions may relate to an increased risk for development of chronic low back pain and disability. Activities that will enhance or maintain musculoskeletal flexibility should be included as a part of a comprehensive preventive or rehabilitative exercise program.

**4—C.** Transverse

The body has three cardinal planes, and each individual plane is perpendicular to the other two. Movement occurs along these planes. The sagittal plane divides the body into right and left parts, and the midsagittal plane is represented by an imaginary vertical plane passing through the midline of the body, dividing it into right and left halves. The frontal plane is represented by an imaginary vertical plane passing through the body, dividing it into front and back halves. The transverse plane represents an imaginary horizontal plane passing through the midsection of the body and dividing it into upper and lower portions.

**5—D.** 140/90 mm Hg

To be classified as hypertensive, the SBP must equal or exceed 140 mm Hg or the diastolic pressure must equal or exceed 90 mm Hg as measured on two separate occasions, preferably days apart. An elevation of either the systolic or diastolic pressure is classified as hypertension.

**6—A.** Approximately 10 mm Hg

During dynamic exercise, SBP will increase in a direct proportion to exercise intensity. The increase in SBP is due to the increase in $\dot{Q}$, which helps to facilitate increase in blood flow to the exercising muscles. The increase in SBP is expected to rise 5–10 mm Hg per MET of effort. By definition, 1 MET being roughly equivalent to the energy expended during rest.

**7—C.** A slight decrease in diastolic pressure

During dynamic exercise, DBP may not change much or even decrease slightly because it represents the pressure in heart during diastole (rest).

**8—A.** 280.5 kcal

The steps are as follows:
a. Convert 150 lb to 68 kg (divide by 2.2)
b. If he exercises at a volume of oxygen consumed per unit time ($\dot{V}O_2$) of 27.5 mL · kg$^{-1}$ · min$^{-1}$ (relative) and he weighs 68 kg, that is equal to a $\dot{V}O_2$ of 1.87 L · min$^{-1}$ (absolute).
c. With an absolute $\dot{V}O_2$ of 1.87 L · min$^{-1}$, you can multiply that by 30 min of exercise and by 5 kcal · min$^{-1}$ (conversion of L · min$^{-1}$ to kcal · min$^{-1}$) that equals to 280.5 kcal total for the exercise session.

**9—B.** At least 50–60 min · d$^{-1}$ totaling 300 min · wk$^{-1}$ (moderate intensity)

According to ACSM guidelines, in order to promote weight loss through the use of cardiovascular endurance exercise, one needs to exercise 30–60 min · d$^{-1}$, 5 d · wk$^{-1}$ (150–300 total minutes per week).

**10—D.** All of the above

Because adults with arthritis are usually at a lower level of fitness, an increase in duration first will allow for a more graduate adaptation to the exercise program and minimize the risk for muscle soreness, discomfort, and injury. Further, the risk for muscle soreness, discomfort, and injury may also be reduced when the exercise is done at the same time of the day and avoided during periods of acute flares and inflammation.

**11—C.** Heat exhaustion and heat stroke
Heat exhaustion and heat stroke are serious conditions that result from a combination of the metabolic heat generated from exercise accompanied by dehydration and electrolyte loss from sweating. Signs and symptoms include uncoordinated gait, headache, dizziness, vomiting, and elevated body temperature. If these conditions are present, exercise must be stopped. Attempts to rehydrate, perhaps intravenously, should be attempted, and the body must be cooled by any means possible. The person should be placed in the supine position, with the feet elevated.

**12—A.** 10 W
This question does not require the use of a metabolic formula because it is asking for the subject's work rate. The steps to answering this question are as follows: Write down the known values and convert those values to the appropriate units — 5 RPM × 6 m = 30 m · $min^{-1}$ (each revolution on a Monark cycle ergometer = 6 m); 2.0 kp = 2.0 kg. Write down the formula for work rate: Work rate = force × distance/time. Substitute the known values for the variable name: Work rate = 2.0 kg × 30 m · $min^{-1}$; Work rate = 60 kg · m · $min^{-1}$. The question asks for watts, so divide the work rate (kg · m · $min^{-1}$) by 6.

$$W = kg \cdot m \cdot min^{-1}/6$$
$$= 600 \ kg \cdot m \cdot min^{-1}/6$$
$$= 10$$

**13—C.** No change
$\dot{Q}$ does not change significantly, primarily because the person is performing the same amount of work and, thus, responds with the same $\dot{Q}$. It should be noted, however, that the same $\dot{Q}$ is now being generated with a lower HR and higher stroke volume compared with when the person was untrained.

**14—D.** Osteoporosis
Every population that has been studied exhibits a decline in bone mass with aging. Therefore, bone loss is considered by most clinicians to be an inevitable consequence of aging. *Osteoporosis* refers to a condition that is characterized by a decrease in bone mass and density, producing bone porosity and fragility, and it refers to the clinical condition of low bone mass and the accompanying increase in

susceptibility to fracture from minor trauma. The age at which bone loss begins and the rate at which it occurs vary greatly between males and females. Risk factors for age-related bone loss and development of clinical osteoporosis include being a white or Asian female, being thin-boned or petite, having a low peak bone mass at maturity, having a family history of osteoporosis, premature or surgically induced menopause, alcohol abuse and/or cigarette smoking, sedentary lifestyle, and inadequate dietary calcium intake.

**15—B.** 12 and 16
Although some learning is required on the part of the participant, the RPE should be considered an adjunct to HR measures. The RPE can be used as a reliable barometer of exercise intensity. The RPE is particularly useful when participants are incapable of monitoring their pulse accurately or when medications such as β-blockers alter the HR response to exercise. The ACSM recommends an exercise intensity that will elicit an RPE within a range of 12–16 on the original Borg scale of 6–20.

**16—A.** Medial rotation
*Rotation* is the turning of a bone around its own longitudinal axis or around another bone. Rotation of the anterior surface of the bone toward the midline of the body is *medial rotation*, whereas rotation of the same bone away from the midline is *lateral rotation*. *Supination* is a specialized rotation of the forearm that results in the palm of the hand being turned forward (anteriorly). *Pronation* (the opposite of supination) is the rotation of the forearm that results in the palm of the hand being directed backward (posteriorly).

**17—A.** HR and stroke volume
$\dot{Q}$ is calculated by multiplying HR and stroke volume. During dynamic exercise, $\dot{Q}$ increases with increasing exercise intensity. Stroke volume increases only until approximately 40%–50% of $\dot{V}O_{2max}$. Above this point, increases in $\dot{Q}$ are accounted for only by an increase in HR. During static exercise, $\dot{Q}$ may fall as a result of a drop in venous return. When the contraction is released, a rapid increase in $\dot{Q}$ occurs as the venous return increases.

**18—D.** All of the above
Initial causes of CAD are thought to be an irritation of, or an injury to, the tunica intima (the innermost of the three layers in the wall) of the blood vessel. Sources of this initial injury are thought to be caused by dyslipidemia

(elevated total blood cholesterol), hypertension (chronic high BP, either an elevation of SBP or DBP measured on two different days), immune responses, smoking, tumultuous and nonlaminar blood flow in the lumen of the coronary artery (turbulence), vasoconstrictor substances (chemicals that cause the smooth muscle cells in the walls of the vessel to contract, resulting in a reduction in the diameter of the lumen), and viral infections.

**19—C.** $<60$ mg $\cdot$ dL$^{-1}$
Risk factors that contribute to the development of CAD include age (men, $>45$ yr; women, $>55$ yr), a family history of myocardial infarction or sudden death (male first-degree relatives $<55$ yr and female first-degree relatives $<65$ yr), cigarette smoking, hypertension (arterial BP $>140/90$ mm Hg measured on two separate occasions), hypercholesterolemia (total cholesterol $>200$ mg $\cdot$ dL$^{-1}$ or 5.2 mmol $\cdot$ L$^{-1}$, or HDL $<35$ mg $\cdot$ dL$^{-1}$ or 0.9 mmol $\cdot$ L$^{-1}$), diabetes mellitus in individuals older than 30 yr or in individuals who have had Type 1 diabetes more than 15 yr or Type 2 diabetes in individuals older than 35 yr. Other risk factors contribute to the development of CAD but are not primary risk factors.

**20—C.** Double knee to chest
Double knee-to-chest stretches are a safe alternative to the plough. Squats to 90 degrees and lateral neck stretches are considered safe alternative exercises to full squats and full neck rolls, respectively. Flexion with rotation is considered a contraindicated high-risk exercise and is not recommended. An alternative to the flexion with rotation is supine curl-ups with flexion followed by rotation.

**21—C.** Stimulate appetite
Older people who exercise regularly report greater life satisfaction (older people who exercise regularly have a more positive attitude toward their work and generally are in better health than sedentary persons), greater happiness (strong correlations have been reported between the activity level of older adults and self-reported happiness), higher self-efficacy (older persons taking part in exercise programs commonly report that they can do everyday tasks more easily than before they began exercising), improved self-concept and self-esteem (older adults improve their score on self-concept questionnaires following participation in an exercise program), and reduced psychological stress (exercise is effective in reducing psychological stress without unwanted side effects).

**22—B.** Application of cognitive-behavioral or motivational principles
Psychological theories are the foundations for effective use of strategies and techniques of effective counseling and motivational skill-building for exercise adoption and maintenance. Theories provide a conceptual framework for development, rather than management, of programs or interventions. Psychological theories facilitate evaluation of program effectiveness, not just measurement of outcomes. Within the field of behavioral change, a theory is a set of assumptions that accounts for the relationships between certain variables and the behavior of interest.

**23—C.** Maximal heart rate (HR$_{max}$)
HR$_{max}$ does not change significantly with exercise training, although it declines with age. Maximal stroke volume increases after training as a result of an increase in contractility or in the size of the heart. Because HR$_{max}$ is unchanged and maximal stroke volume increases, maximal Q̇ must increase.

**24—C.** Increasing the rate of training intensity more than approximately 10% per week increases the likelihood of overuse injuries of bone. Increasing the rate of progression of training more than approximately 10% per week is a risk factor for overuse injuries of bone. Exercise programs for children and adolescents should increase physical fitness in the short term and lead to adoption of a physically active lifestyle in the long term. Strength training in youth carries no greater risk of injury than comparable strength training programs in adults if proper instruction, exercise prescription, and supervision are provided. Children who have exercise-induced asthma often are physically unfit because of restriction of activity imposed by the child, parents, or physicians.

**25—D.** Hypertension
Regular exercise will decrease SBP and DBP. Exercise has no effect on age and family history of heart disease and no direct effect on cigarette smoking, although some individuals may choose to quit smoking after beginning to exercise. Regular endurance exercise does increase HDL, but it has limited influence on total cholesterol. Exercise has no direct effect on Type 1 diabetes, but it can promote weight loss and improve glucose tolerance for those with Type 2 diabetes.

**26—A.** CPR and ACSM HFS
At minimum, professionals performing fitness assessments on others should possess CPR and ACSM HFS certification.

**27—A.** Intensity and duration
Intensity and duration of exercise must be considered together and are inversely related. Similar improvements in aerobic fitness may be realized if a person exercises at a low intensity for a longer duration or at a higher intensity for less time.

**28—A.** Children should participate in several bouts of physical activity lasting 15 min or more each day.
Activity that is intermittent in nature is preferred for children over continuous exercise because this is the type of activity they naturally self-select. Active play versus exercise should be emphasized. Although children should attempt to accumulate 60 or more minutes of physical activity daily, it should not be continuous. Children should not focus on just one or two modes. Exposing them to a wide variety of physical activities is suggested to enhance adherence. Finally, children should not have prolonged periods during the day that are sedentary because this may promote negative health consequences.

**29—D.** If a child cannot perform a minimum of 8 reps with good form, the resistance is too heavy and should be reduced.
Maximal (1-RM) resistance training should not be performed with children because it may promote injury as well as it may discourage young children. Children should perform 8–15 reps per exercise and increased only when the child can perform the desired number of reps with good form. Do not focus on the amount of resistance, instead focus on participation and proper technique.

**30—C.** Plyometrics as part of a health club class
Plyometrics does not work well for most older individuals due to joint issues as well as decreased flexibility and balance problems. There would be a high risk of acute musculoskeletal injury. Walking, water exercise, and stationary cycling are all preferred modes for the elderly due to their low impact and ease. It is ideal to have elderly individuals exercise socially in a place that is accessible, convenient, and enjoyable to enhance adherence.

**31—C.** 6–8 reps
Research supports that one set is all that is necessary to adequately strengthen in the elderly population. Muscular endurance is more important in this population than strength or power so a higher number of reps is performed.

**32—B.** Vigorous, highly repetitive exercise should be encouraged in order to strengthen connective tissues at the joint.
Repetitive motion should be avoided because it could cause increased inflammation at the affected joints. Warm water exercise should be encouraged because it can promote physical activity with less pain. Mornings should be avoided due to stiffness, and finally, expect that people who regularly medicate with NSAIDs may develop anemia because of continuous blood loss via abdominal bleeding.

**33—C.** Joint, inflammation
"Arth" means joint indicating where the "itis" (inflammation) is taking place. The prefix "arth" is not to be confused with the prefix "athero," which is Greek for gruel or paste.

**34—A.** Chin-ups
Chin-ups strengthen the lats, rhomboids, and biceps. Dead lifts do strengthen the lats but do not strengthen the biceps. Back extensions primarily strengthen the lower back, the glutes, and hamstrings. Finally, an upright row does strengthen the biceps, deltoids, and trapezius but not the lats.

**35—D.** Push-ups
Push-ups work both the chest and triceps. Chin-ups strengthen the lats, rhomboids, and biceps, not the chest or triceps. Crunches strengthen the abdominals and hip flexors, whereas pec deck flyes primarily strengthen the chest.

**36—B.** Moderate
A person with a 10-MET maximal capacity fitness level would have the following classifications of intensity: very light <2.8 MET, light = 2.8–4.5 MET, moderate = 4.6–6.3 MET, hard = 6.4–8.6 MET, and very hard = ≥ 8.7 MET.

**37—C.** Transferring (walking)
Walking is the only one of these four that is considered an ADL. The six ADL are eating, bathing, dressing, toileting, transferring (walking), and continence. Although it is great to be able to lift a medium weight, speak, read, and write, it is not necessary for ADL.

**38—A.** Sugar

You'd want to have sugar available in the case that the individual develops hypoglycemia. The sugar will allow individuals with diabetes to feel back to normal soon. Insulin should never be given to a client who is having a diabetic emergency unless it is absolutely 100% known that he or she forgot to take his or her insulin. Giving an extra dose of insulin could seriously damage the individual or cause death. Nitroglycerin is only given in the event of angina (chest pain). NutraSweet is not a real sugar so it will do no good.

**39—B.** Supine position exercises

Exercises in the supine (lying on your back) position could cause mild obstruction of venous return, which decreases $\dot{Q}$, and may cause BP to drop dangerously low. Exercise in the prone position may be uncomfortable if not contraindicated. Walking is a good exercise for most pregnant women with no other special conditions. Sitting exercises such as riding a bicycle are fine to do provided that the comfort level is adequate.

**40—B.** Gradually increase in distance weekly with a slight lower distance Sunday every fourth week or so.

The runner could become overtrained if he or she just built up to a longer distance each week without a down week built in periodically, even if done gradually. Doing the same distance weekly will not allow the runner to reach the race distance, therefore never allowing them to prepare for the actual race mileage. Periodization must be done gradually. If increased too rapidly, the runner may become injured or overtrained.

**41—D.** Weight bearing

Regularly participating in weight-bearing exercises such as walking or running is important to keep bone mineral density high in order to decrease risk of developing osteoporosis. Water exercise is not considered weight bearing because of the buoyancy effect of the water. Intensity, whether it is high or low is not relevant in this case. What matters is if the exercise involves supporting the weight.

**42—A.** Estimated maximal HR

The number that you subtract from originally is the estimated maximum HR. With each year of life (age), we estimate that we lose one beat in terms of our $HR_{max}$. (*i.e.*, 220-age). It has nothing to do with SBP, weight, or gender.

**43—D.** Overload, specificity, progression

The three training principles are overload, specificity, and progression. Redundancy does not have anything to do with it. Although frequency, intensity, and duration are important items to consider with exercise programming, they are not considered training principles. *Overload* is pushing the body beyond what it is used to, *specificity* is being careful to choose exercises that closely relate to the outcome goal, and *progression* has to do with developing a systematic method of improving.

**44—B.** 108–137 bpm

You begin by subtracting her age of 24 yr from 200. So $220 - 24 = 196$ bpm, which is her estimated $HR_{max}$ at her current age. Then multiply both 0.55 and 0.70 to 196 bpm to get your answers: $0.55 \times 196 = 108$ bpm and $0.70 \times 196 = 137$ bpm. Answer letter A is incorrect because it subtracted her age from 200 instead of 220. Answer letter C is incorrect because it used 200 with no age adjustment, and answer letter D is incorrect because it used 220 with no age adjustment, which gave too high of a value.

**45—C.** PNF

PNF is a stretching technique that combines the use of isometric contractions with passive static stretching. This stretching technique involves the use of a partner and a few cycles and, therefore, is more time consuming that the other stretching techniques (static and dynamic).

**46—A.** Increase

SBP is an indicator of $\dot{Q}$ (the amount of blood pumped out of the heart in 1 min) in a healthy vascular system. $\dot{Q}$ normally increases as workload increases, because the peripheral and central stimuli that control $\dot{Q}$ normally increase with an increase in workload. Thus, SBP should increase with an increase in workload. Failure of the SBP to increase as workload increases indicates that $\dot{Q}$ is not increasing, which, in turn, indicates an abnormal response to increasing workload. Additionally, an abnormally elevated SBP response to aerobic exercise indicates an unhealthy vascular system.

**47—D.** 3–6 mo

Most sedentary people are not motivated to initiate exercise programs and, if exercise is initiated, they are likely to stop within 3–6 mo. In general, participants in earlier stages benefit most from cognitive strategies,

HFS

such as listening to lectures and reading books without the expectation of actually engaging in exercise, whereas individuals in later stages depend more on behavioral techniques, such as reminders to exercise and developing social support to help them establish a regular exercise habit and be able to maintain it.

**48—D.** All of the above

Fitness testing is conducted in older adults for the same reasons as in younger adults, including exercise prescription, evaluation of progress, motivation, and education.

**49—C.** 13.2 MET

The steps are as follows:

a. Write out the running equation (accurate for speeds in excess of 5 mph):

$\dot{V}O_2$ (mL $\cdot$ kg$^{-1}$ $\cdot$ min$^{-1}$) = Horizontal + Vertical + Resting
$\dot{V}O_2$ (mL $\cdot$ kg$^{-1}$ $\cdot$ min$^{-1}$) = (Speed $\times$ 0.2) + (Speed $\times$ Grade $\times$ 0.9) + 3.5

b. Convert speed (6.5 mph) to meters per minute:

$6.5 \times 26.8 = 174.2$ m $\cdot$ min$^{-1}$

c. Solve for the unknown:

$\dot{V}O_2$ (mL $\cdot$ kg$^{-1}$ $\cdot$ min$^{-1}$) = (174.2 $\times$ 0.2) + (174.2 $\times$ 0.05 $\times$ 0.9) + 3.5 $\cdot$ $\dot{V}O_2$ (mL $\cdot$ kg$^{-1}$ $\cdot$ min$^{-1}$) = 46.18 mL $\cdot$ kg$^{-1}$ $\cdot$ min$^{-1}$

d. Convert 46.18 mL $\cdot$ kg$^{-1}$ $\cdot$ min$^{-1}$ to MET:

1 MET = 3.5 mL $\cdot$ kg$^{-1}$ $\cdot$ min$^{-1}$
$46.18 \div 3.5 = 13.2$ MET

**50—B.** Intrinsic reward

*Reinforcement* is the positive or negative consequence for performing or not performing a behavior. *Positive consequences* are rewards that motivate behavior. This can include both intrinsic and extrinsic rewards. *Intrinsic rewards* are the benefits gained because of the rewarding nature of the activity. *Extrinsic* or external rewards are the positive outcomes received from others, which may include encouragement and praise or material reinforcements such as T-shirts and money.

**51—B.** Hamstrings and calves

The hamstrings and calves are the prime movers of a standing leg curl. It takes both, not just one or the other. The quadriceps would be an antagonist muscle group and the glutes are not involved in this motion.

**52—C.** Valsalva

The Valsalva maneuver is quite dangerous, especially to an individual that may already have hypertension. With a closed glottis, intrathoracic pressure is increased, which if it gets high enough could cause an aneurysm to rupture causing a stroke. Karvonen is the researcher who developed the THR zone formula. *Diaphragmatic* is a type of deep-breathing exercise used to manage stress. *Angina* means chest pain, which is unrelated.

**53—B.** Forward wall push stretch

The standing wall push stretch would stretch primarily the calf region. Modified hurdler (with knee angled in instead of out) would probably be the safest stretch; however, the straddle stretch would work effectively too provided there is no bouncing and no pushing past the point of tension into pain. The cross-legged standing toe touch would stretch the hamstrings; however, it is very important not to bounce in order to avoid muscle strains. There are certainly more effective, safer hamstring stretches than this last one.

**54—C.** 60–90

They recommend 60–90 min moderate-intensity activity daily to *sustain* the weight loss. To help *manage* body weight and *prevent* weight gain in adulthood, they recommend 60 min, and to reduce the risk of chronic disease in adulthood, they recommend engaging in at least 30 min daily.

**55—D.** After the cool-down

If not warming up for a ballistic, dynamic, or explosive power activity but instead warming up for a steady activity like cycling, walking, running, swimming, etc., the prestretch is not crucial. Instead, the poststretch following the cool-down is the best time to gain flexibility as the muscles are very warm, flexible, and pliable. It would however be crucial to prestretch following a warm-up for explosive activities.

**56—B.** Higher

HR at high altitude will be higher than at sea level for the same perceived exertion because of the decreased supply of oxygen available. In terms of endurance competition, it would be wise to properly acclimate to the race altitude prior to the race. Dehydration is often an issue at high altitudes, which are also generally dryer so make sure to adequately hydrate before, during, and after training.

**57—A.** Flexibility of equipment to allow for different body sizes.

Creating a safe environment in which to exercise is a primary responsibility of any fitness facility. In developing and operating facilities and equipment for use by exercisers, the managers and staff are obligated to meet a standard of care for exerciser safety. The equipment to be used not only includes testing, cardiovascular, strength, and flexibility pieces but also rehabilitation, pool, locker room, and emergency equipment. You must evaluate several criteria when selecting equipment. These criteria include correct anatomic positioning, ability to adjust to different body sizes, quality of design and materials, durability, repair records, and then price.

**58—A.** Intensity of 60%–90% $HR_{max}$, duration of 20–60 min, and frequency of 3–5 d a week.

The ability to take in and to use oxygen depends on the health and integrity of the heart, lungs, and circulatory systems. Efficiency of the aerobic metabolic pathways also is necessary to optimize cardiorespiratory fitness. The degree of improvement that may be expected in cardiorespiratory fitness relates directly to the frequency, intensity, duration, and mode or type of exercise. Maximal oxygen uptake may improve between 5% and 30% with training. The exercise prescription can be altered for different populations to achieve the same results. However, for an apparently healthy person, the ACSM recommends an intensity of 60%–90% $HR_{max}$, duration of 20–60 min, and frequency of 3–5 d a week.

**59—A.** Plyometrics

*Plyometrics* is a method of strength and power training that involves an eccentric loading of muscles and tendons followed immediately by an explosive concentric contraction. This stretch-shortening cycle may allow an enhanced generation of force during the concentric (shortening) phase. Most well-controlled studies have shown no significant difference in power improvement when comparing plyometrics with high-intensity strength training. The explosive nature of this type of activity may increase the risk for musculoskeletal injury. Plyometrics should not be considered a practical resistance exercise alternative for health/fitness applications but may be appropriate for select athletic or performance needs.

**60—C.** Manager or director

The characteristics of a good manager or director include designing programs and monitoring the implementation of programs. He or she also guides the staff or clients through the program. He or she is a good communicator who also purchases equipment and supplies. A good manager monitors the safety of the program or facility and surveys clients and staff to assess the success and value of the program.

**61—A.** To inform the client of participation risks, as well as the rights of the client and the facility.

Agreements, releases, and consents are documents that clearly describe what the client is participating in, the risks involved, and the rights of the client and the facility. If signed by the client, he or she is accepting some of the responsibility and risk by participating in this program. All fitness facilities are strongly encouraged to have program or service agreements and informed consents drafted by a lawyer for their protection.

**62—C.** A loss of muscle mass caused by a loss of muscle fibers

After 30 yr of age, skeletal muscle strength begins to decline. However, the loss of strength is not linear, with most of the decline occurring after 50 yr of age. By 80 yr of age, strength loss usually is in the range of 30%–40%. The loss of strength with aging results primarily from a loss of muscle mass, which, in turn, is caused by both the loss of muscle fibers and the atrophy of the remaining fibers.

**63—A.** There is a perceived threat of disease.

The Health Belief Model assumes that people will engage in a behavior (*e.g.*, exercise) when there exist a perceived threat of disease and a belief of susceptibility to disease, and the threat of disease is severe. This model also incorporates cues to action as critical to adopting and maintaining behavior. The concept of self-efficacy (confidence) is also added to this model. Motivation and environmental considerations are not a part of the Health Belief Model.

**64—C.** Provides an explanation of the test to the client.

Informed consent is not a legal document. It does not provide legal immunity to a facility or individual in the event of injury to a client nor does it legally protect the rights of the client. It simply provides evidence that the client was made aware of the purposes, procedures, and risks associated with the test or exercise program. The consent form does not relieve the facility or individual of the responsibility to do everything possible to ensure the safety of the client. Negligence, improper test administration, inadequate personnel qualifications, and insufficient safety procedures all are items that are not expressly covered by informed consent. Because of the limitations associated with informed consent documents, legal counsel should be sought during the development of the document.

**65—C.** Number of curl-ups in 1 min
Three common assessments for muscular endurance include the bench press, for upper body endurance (a weight is lifted in cadence with a metronome or other timing device; the total number of lifts performed correctly and in time with the cadence); the push-up, for upper body endurance (the client assumes a standardized beginning position with the body held rigid and supported by the hands and toes for men and the hands and knees for women; the body is lowered to the floor, then pushed back up to the starting position; the score is the total number of properly performed push-ups completed without a pause by the client, with no time limit); and the curl-up (crunch), for abdominal muscular endurance (the client begins in the bent-knee sit-up with knees at 90 degrees, the arms at the side, palms facing down with middle fingers touching masking tape. A second piece of tape is placed 10 cm apart. OR set a metronome to 50 bpm and the client performs slow, controlled curl-ups to lift the shoulder blades off the mat with the trunk making a 30-degree angle, in time with the metronome at a rate of 25 per minute done for 1 min. OR the client performs as many curl-ups as possible in 1 min).

**66—A.** An overuse injury
Overuse injuries become more common when people participate in more cardiovascular exercise by increasing time, duration, or intensity too quickly. A client exercises too much without time for rest and recovery or develops a minor injury and does not reduce or change that exercise allowing the injury to heal.

**67—C.** 60% and 90%
Several methods are available to define exercise intensity objectively. The ACSM recommends that exercise intensity be prescribed within a range of 64%–70% and 94% of $HR_{max}$ or between 40%–50% and 85% of oxygen uptake reserve ($\dot{V}O_{2max}R$). Lower intensities will elicit a favorable response in individuals with very low fitness levels. Because of the variability in estimating $HR_{max}$ from age, it is recommended

that, whenever possible, an actual $HR_{max}$ from a graded exercise test be used. Factors to consider when determining appropriate exercise intensity include age, fitness level, medications, overall health status, and individual goals.

**68—B.** 8–12
The ACSM recommends that one set of 8–12 reps of each exercise should be performed to volitional fatigue for healthy individuals. Choose a range of reps between 3 and 20 (*i.e.*, 3–5, 8–10, 10–15) that can be performed at a moderate-repetition duration (~3 s concentric, ~3 s eccentric) based on age, fitness level, assessment, and ability. The ACSM recommends exercising each muscle group two to three nonconsecutive days per week.

**69—B.** The risk of orthopedic and cardiovascular complications is increased.
The risk of orthopedic and, perhaps, cardiovascular complications can be increased with high-intensity activity. Factors to consider when determining exercise intensity include the individual's level of fitness, presence of medications that may influence exercise performance, risk of cardiovascular or orthopedic injury, and individual preference for exercise and individual program objectives.

**70—C.** 8–12
Eight to twelve (8–12) reps represent a relatively low intensity of 67%–80% of 1-RM. This low intensity allows the development of muscular endurance and reduces the risk of musculoskeletal related injuries.

**71—D.** All of the above are examples of progressive overload.
By definition, *progressive overload* is a principle of training that states that the stress on the musculoskeletal system needs to progressively increase in order to keep producing greater force. This could be achieved by increasing the intensity (resistance), the number of rep or sets, and/or the number of exercise session per week.

**72—C.** Leg press
The leg press is considered a multijoint exercise because the movement occurs around the hip, knee, and ankle joints. The rest of the exercises are considered a single joint movement.

**73—C.** 2–3 min
Generally, the length of the rest periods depends on the type of exercise performed. During resistance training, 2–3 min rest

interval between sets allows the exercising muscles sufficient to recover, which may allow optimal performance during subsequent sets.

**74—A.** 1
The baseline weight training fitness level of a novice trainee is quite minimal. Therefore, and in the beginning of the training program, one set per exercise should be sufficient enough to stress the musculoskeletal system and improve muscular fitness.

**75—E.** All of the above.
Different factors affect exercise adherence. Some are situational in nature such as social support and time commitment, whereas others are personal (individualized). In order for a trainee to "stick" to an exercise routine, many of these factors must be met.

**76—D.** All of the above.
The effects of regular (chronic) exercise can be classified or grouped into those that occur at rest, during moderate (or submaximal) exercise, and during maximal effort work. For example, you can measure an untrained individual's resting heart rate ($HR_{rest}$), train the person for several weeks or months, and then measure $HR_{rest}$ again to see what change has occurred. $HR_{rest}$ declines with regular exercise, probably because of a combination of decreased sympathetic tone, increased parasympathetic tone, and decreased intrinsic firing rate of the sinoatrial node. Stroke volume increases at rest as a result of increased time for ventricular filling and an increased myocardial contractility. Little or no change occurs in $\dot{Q}$ at rest, because the decline in HR is compensated for by the increase in stroke volume.

**77—C.** Self-reevaluation
Key components of the Transtheoretical Model are the processes of behavioral change. These processes include five cognitive processes (consciousness raising, dramatic relief, environmental reevaluation, self-reevaluation, and social liberation) and five behavioral processes (counterconditioning, helping relationships, reinforcement management, self-liberation, and stimulus control).

**78—A.** Developing the exercise prescription.
The purpose of the fitness assessment is to develop a proper exercise prescription (the data collected through appropriate fitness assessments assist the health fitness specialist in developing safe, effective programs of exercise based on the individual client's current fitness status), to evaluate the rate of progress (baseline and follow-up testing indicate progression toward fitness goals), and to motivate (fitness assessments provide information needed to develop reasonable, attainable goals). Progress toward or attainment of a goal is a strong motivator for continued participation in an exercise program.

**79—C.** Rest, Ice, Compression, Elevation
Basic principles of care for musculoskeletal injuries include the objectives for care of exercise-related injuries, which are to decrease pain, reduce swelling, and prevent further injury. These objectives can be met in most cases by following "RICE" guidelines. RICE stands for Rest, Ice, Compression, and Elevation. Rest will prevent further injury and ensure that the healing process will begin. Ice is used to reduce swelling, bleeding, inflammation, and pain. Compression also helps to reduce swelling and bleeding. Compression is achieved by the use of elastic wraps or tape. Elevation helps to decrease the blood flow and excessive pressure to the injured area.

**80—D.** Pyramids
Various systems of resistance training exist that differ in their combinations of sets, reps, and resistance applied, all in an effort to overload the muscle. Circuit weight training uses a series of exercises performed in succession with minimal rest between exercises. Various health benefits as well as modest improvements in aerobic capacity have been demonstrated as a result of circuit weight training. *Supersets* refer to consecutive sets for antagonistic muscle groups with no rest between sets or multiple exercises for a specific muscle group with little or no rest. Split routines entail exercising different body parts on different days or during different sessions. Pyramids are performed either in ascending (increasing the resistance within a set of reps or from one set to the next) or descending (decreasing the resistance within a set of reps or from one set to the next) fashion.

**81—A.** 1–2 lb · wk$^{-1}$ (0.5–1.0 kg)
The goal of the exercise component of a weight reduction program should be to maximize caloric expenditure. Frequency, intensity, and duration must be manipulated in conjunction with a dietary regimen in an attempt to create a caloric deficit of 500–1,000 cal · d$^{-1}$. The recommended maximal rate for weight loss is 1–2 lb · wk$^{-1}$.

**82—B.** An abnormal curvature of the spine
*Scoliosis* is a lateral deviation in the alignment of the vertebrae. *Kyphosis* is a posterior thoracic curvature. *Lordosis* is an anterior lumbar curvature. A chronic, inflammatory, demyelinating disease describes *multiple sclerosis*. Softening of the articular cartilage describes *chondrosis*. Inflammation of the growth plate at the tibial tuberosity is a condition known as *Osgood-Schlatter disease*.

**83—B.** Health Belief Model
The Health Belief Model is a theoretical framework to help explain and predict interventions to increase physical activity. The model originated in the 1950s based on work by Rosenstock. Learning theories assume that an overall complex behavior arises from many small simple behaviors. By reinforcing partial behaviors and modifying cues in the environment, it is possible to shape the desired behavior.

**84—C.** PAR-Q
The PAR-Q is a screening tool for self-directed exercise programming. The MMPI is a psychological scale. The RPE-Borg scale is used to measure or to rate perceived exertion during exercise or during an exercise test. The E-ECG would involve continuous electrical heart monitoring during exercise stress test used in a clinical setting when deemed appropriate by a physician.

**85—C.** Body composition, cardiorespiratory fitness, muscular fitness, and flexibility
To get the best and most accurate information, the following order of testing is recommended: resting measurements (*e.g.*, HR, BP, blood analysis), body composition, cardiorespiratory fitness, muscular fitness, and flexibility. Some methods of body composition assessment are sensitive to hydration status and some tests of cardiorespiratory and muscular fitness may affect hydration, so it is inappropriate to administer those before the body composition assessment. Assessing cardiorespiratory fitness often uses measures of HR. Some tests of muscular fitness and flexibility affect HR, so they are inappropriate to administer before cardiorespiratory fitness testing, because the elevated HR from those assessments may, in turn, affect the cardiorespiratory fitness testing results.

**86—D.** Management and staff
When an emergency or injury occurs, safe and effective management of the situation will assure the best care for the individual.

Implementing emergency procedures is an important part of the training of the staff. In-services, safety plans, and emergency procedures should be a part of the staff training. In addition, all exercise staff should be CPR certified and knowledgeable of first aid. Therefore, the fitness center management and staff all are included in the implementation of an emergency plan.

**87—D.** All of the above
Possible medical emergencies during exercise include heat exhaustion or heat stroke, fainting, hypoglycemia, hyperglycemia, simple or compound fractures, bronchospasm, hypotension or shock, seizures, bleeding, and other cardiac symptoms.

**88—D.** Isometric
*Isometric muscle action*, also known as static muscle action, occurs when muscle tension increases with no overt muscular or limb movement; the length of the muscle does not change. These actions occur when with an attempt to push or pull against an immovable object. Measures of static strength are specific to both the muscle group and joint angle being tested; therefore, these tests' usefulness to generalize overall muscular strength is limited.

**89—D.** Walking
Large muscle group activity performed in rhythmic fashion over prolonged periods facilitates the greatest improvements in aerobic fitness. Walking, running, cycling, swimming, stair climbing, aerobic dance, rowing, and cross-country skiing are examples of these types of activities. Weight training should not be considered an appropriate activity for enhancing aerobic fitness but should be part of in a comprehensive exercise program to improve muscular strength and muscular endurance. The mode(s) of activity should be selected based on the principle of specificity — that is, with attention to the desired outcomes — and to maintain the participation and enjoyment of the individual.

**90—D.** All of the above
Different types of health screenings are used for various purposes. In commercial settings, clients should be screened more extensively for potential health risks. At minimum, a personal medical history should be taken. In addition, present medical status should be examined and questions asked regarding the use of medications (both prescription and over-the-counter).

**91—C.** Shorter duration, lower intensity, and higher frequency of exercise

The number of times per day or per week that a person exercises is interrelated with both the intensity and the duration of activity. Generally, sedentary persons or those with poor fitness may benefit from multiple short-duration, low-intensity exercise sessions per day. Individual goals, preferences, limitations, and time constraints also will determine frequency and the relationship between duration, frequency, and intensity.

**92—B.** Strategic plan

The strategic plan addresses strategic decisions of the organization in defining short- and long-term goals and serves as the overarching planning tool. Health and fitness programs, financial plans, risk management efforts, and marketing plans only address subsegments within the overall strategic plan.

**93—A.** Flexibility

When choosing the correct sequence of testing, one needs to consider the energy systems that being involved during the exercise and time for complete recovery. Nonfatiguing tests (height, weight, flexibility, etc.) should be performed first followed by tests that stress the phosphagen system (shorter recovery) followed by tests that stress the other energy systems.

**94—A.** Myosin

The skeletal muscle consists of bundles of muscle fibers called *muscle fascicles*, or *fasciculi*. Each fasciculus contains muscle cells. Within the muscle cells are cylinders called *myofibrils*, which are responsible for the contraction of the muscle fiber. The myofibrils have this ability because they contain myofilaments, which are the contractile proteins, actin and myosin. *Actin* is a thin filament that is twisted into a strand. *Myosin* is a thick filament that has a tail and a head. During activation of the muscle, actin and myosin interact, causing cross bridging between the two filaments. The myosin pulls the actin, which shortens the muscle and causes tension development.

**95—B.** Tricuspid valve

Blood from the peripheral anatomy flows to the heart through the superior and inferior venae cavae into the right atrium. From the right atrium, the blood passes through the tricuspid valve to the RV, then out through the pulmonary semilunar valve to the pulmonary arteries, and then to the lungs to be oxygenated.

The tricuspid valve is so named because of the three cusps, or flaps, of which it is made. The bicuspid valve is a similar valve, having only two cusps; it is found between the left atrium and left ventricle (LV). Blood leaving the LV will pass through the aortic semilunar valve to the ascending aorta and then out to the systemic circulation.

**96—A.** Lowering the center of gravity

Lowering the center of gravity will increase stability. Stability would also be increased by increasing the size of the base of support, by moving the center of gravity closer to the center of the base of support, or both.

**97—D.** Increased DBP

Because of the vasodilation associated with exercise-induced stimulation of the sympathetic nervous system, diastolic pressure remains unchanged, or even slightly decreased, during exercise.

**98—A.** Frequency

Increased frequency of exercise is generally recommended for older adults to optimize cardiovascular as well as balance and flexibility adaptations. The recommended duration of exercise depends on the intensity of the activity; higher-intensity activity should be conducted over a shorter period of time.

**99—B.** Arteriosclerosis

*Arteriosclerosis*, also called hardening of the arteries, is a loss of arterial elasticity and is associated with aging. Atherosclerosis is a form of arteriosclerosis characterized by an accumulation of obstructive lesions within the arterial wall. The *adventitia*, the outermost layer of the artery wall, provides the media and intima with oxygen and other nutrients.

**100—C.** Negligence, improper test administration, inadequate personnel qualifications, and insufficient safety procedures are all items that are expressly covered by the informed consent.

Negligence, improper test administration, inadequate personnel qualifications, and insufficient safety procedures are all items that are expressly NOT covered by the informed consent. The informed consent is also not a legal document; it does not provide legal immunity to a facility or individual in the event of injury to a person and it does not relieve the facility or individual of the responsibility to do everything possible to ensure the safety of an individual.

## HFS EXAMINATION QUESTIONS BY DOMAIN

Use the following table as a guide to assist you in your studying process. It is important to note that some questions can be classified as testing multiple domains by the knowledge, skills, and abilities (KSAs).

| Domain Number | I | II | III | IV | V |
|---|---|---|---|---|---|
| Domain Name | Health and Fitness Assessment | Exercise Prescription, Implementation (and Ongoing Support) | Exercise Counseling and Behavioral Strategies | Legal/ Professional | Management |
| Percentage of Questions from Domain | 30% | 30% | 15% | 10% | 15% |
| Question Numbers | 1, 2, 5, 6, 7, 18, 19, 46, 78, 84, 85, 93 | 3, 4, 8, 9, 10, 12, 13, 14, 15, 16, 17, 20, 23, 24, 25, 27, 47, 48, 49, 58, 59, 62, 67, 68, 69, 70, 76, 80, 81, 82, 87, 88, 89, 94, 95, 96, 97, 98, 99 | 11, 21, 28, 29, 30, 31, 32, 33, 34, 35, 36, 37, 38, 39, 40, 41, 42, 43, 44, 45, 50, 51, 52, 53, 54, 55, 56, 63, 66, 71, 72, 73, 74, 75, 77, 83, 91 | 26, 64, 100 | 22, 57, 60, 61, 65, 79, 86, 90, 92 |

# ACSM Certified Clinical Exercise Specialist (CES)

PAUL SORACE, MS, ACSM-RCEP, *Associate Editor*

*Note: CES certification candidates should also review the case studies found in Part 1, ACSM Certified Personal Trainer (CPT) and Part 2, ACSM Certified Health Fitness Specialist (HFS).*

## DOMAIN I: PATIENT/CLIENT ASSESSMENT

**CASE STUDY CES.I**

Author: **Trent A. Hargens, PhD**
Author's Certifications: **ACSM-CES**

You are an exercise physiologist at a hospital-based wellness facility. A client, Drew, recently joins your facility. Drew is a 47-yr-old male. He currently weighs 315 lb and is 5 ft 11 in tall. His waist circumference is currently 127 cm. Due to his waist girth and weight, body composition estimation was not possible via skinfolds. He currently does no regular physical activity. At his initial consultation with you, you measured his resting heart rate ($HR_{rest}$) at 58 bpm, and his resting blood pressure (BP) was 138/72 mm Hg. At his most recent doctor visit, his fasting blood measures were the following: total cholesterol = 192 mg $\cdot$ dL$^{-1}$, high-density lipoprotein cholesterol (HDL-C) = 41 mg $\cdot$ dL$^{-1}$, low-density lipoprotein (LDL) = 117 mg $\cdot$ dL$^{-1}$, triglycerides = 169 mg $\cdot$ dL$^{-1}$, and glucose = 137 mg $\cdot$ dL$^{-1}$. On his health history questionnaire, he states that he has previously been diagnosed with high cholesterol, high BP, and diabetes mellitus. He is currently on several medications including Lipitor (statin for cholesterol), atenolol ($\beta$-blocker for BP), and metformin (biguanide for glucose control). He reports that his father previously was diagnosed with diabetes in his 40s and had a nonfatal heart attack at age 52 yr. He also reports that no symptoms suggestive of ischemia.

During your initial consultation with Drew, he discussed his desire to improve his overall health and to try to prevent a premature myocardial infarction (MI). He realizes that he is not in good health and not physically active. He wishes to make the necessary changes to lose weight, to improve his risk factor profile, and hopefully not go down the same path as his father.

## MULTIPLE-CHOICE QUESTIONS FOR CASE STUDY CES.I

1. According to the most recent edition of the *American College of Sports Medicine's* (ACSM's) *Guidelines for Exercise Testing and Prescription* (GETP), what is recommended prior to his beginning exercise at a moderate-to-vigorous intensity in your facility?
   A) Signed informed consent form only
   B) Signed informed consent form and medical clearance from physician
   C) Signed informed consent form, medical clearance from physician, and graded exercise test (GXT)
   D) Signed informed consent form, medical clearance from physician, and GXT with physician supervision

2. Atenolol, one of the medications that Drew is currently taking, has which effect that needs to be considered?
   A) Increases his exercise tolerance
   B) Decreases his exercise heart rate (HR)
   C) Increases his $HR_{rest}$
   D) Increases his exercise breathing rate

3. Drew states during his initial consultation that he does not feel that his glucose reading of 137 mg · dL⁻¹ does not reflect his usual level of glucose control and that he usually "does better." What follow-up test would you recommend that would BEST determine Drew's level of glucose control?
   A) Another fasted blood glucose test
   B) An oral glucose tolerance test
   C) A glycolated hemoglobin (HbA1C) test
   D) No follow-up test is needed

4. Given what Drew has relayed to you in your initial consultation with him, what stage of change is Drew currently at?
   A) Precontemplation
   B) Contemplation
   C) Preparation
   D) Action

5. Given Drew's extensive cardiovascular risk profile and diagnosed metabolic disease, what potential cardiovascular complication possibility exists with his performing physical activity?
   A) Silent ischemia
   B) Hypoglycemia
   C) Ketoacidosis
   D) Peripheral neuropathy

## DISCUSSION QUESTION FOR CASE STUDY CES.I

1. What do you believe to be Drew's major health concern and should Drew's main goal be as he begins his lifestyle program?

# DOMAIN II: EXERCISE PRESCRIPTION

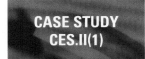
**CASE STUDY CES.II(1)**

Author: **Donald M. Cummings, PhD**
Author's Certifications: **ACSM-CES**

You are a clinical exercise physiologist in a cardiopulmonary rehabilitation department at a medical facility. A new patient, Greg, a 55-yr-old male, has been referred by his physician to participate in a 12-wk exercise rehabilitation program due to a recent episode of chest pain and a positive GXT result. Subsequent Lexiscan nuclear test confirms a 75% occlusion of the right coronary artery (RCA) and an 80% occlusion of the circumflex artery (CXA). A brief synopsis of Greg's medical history, fasting blood laboratory report, and recent GXT results is provided as follows.

### Medical History

Greg is a 55-yr-old male who has a height of 5 ft 9 in and weighs 178 lb (26.3 kg · m⁻² body mass index [BMI]). He reports a family history of his father having high BP and dying of a heart attack at the age of 58 yr. His mother is still living with an unremarkable medical history. He has two younger siblings, brother and sister, with the brother currently being treated for high BP as the only sibling reportable medical history. Greg reports never smoking. He states that his exercise consists of hiking with his dog for 30–45 min, 2–3 d · wk⁻¹. He currently is being treated for hypertension and hyperlipidemia. He has been prescribed an angiotensin-converting enzyme (ACE) inhibitor (enalapril 10 mg OD), a diuretic (spironolactone 50 mg bid), a hydroxymethylglutaryl coenzyme A (HMG CoA) reductase inhibitor (atorvastatin 20 mg OD), and a nitrate (nitroglycerin lingual spray 0.4 mg prn). Greg denies any other significant medical history prior to the current episode of chest pain. He reports that while he was working in the yard (landscaping), he developed substernal chest pressure that lasted for 20 min, associated with a feeling of shortness of breath (SOB) (dyspnea) and profuse sweating (diaphoresis). After resting for 15 min in a chair, Greg reports that the symptoms subsided. He was referred for blood analysis and a GXT.

Blood Laboratory Analysis (Fasting):

| | |
|---|---|
| Glucose | 94 mg · dL$^{-1}$ |
| Urea nitrogen | 12 mg · dL$^{-1}$ |
| Creatinine | 1.0 mg · dL$^{-1}$ |
| Sodium | 142 mmol · L$^{-1}$ |
| Potassium | 4.2 mmol · L$^{-1}$ |
| Chloride | 105 mmol · L$^{-1}$ |
| Carbon dioxide | 28 mmol · L$^{-1}$ |
| Calcium | 8.8 mg · dL$^{-1}$ |
| Cholesterol | 171 mg · dL$^{-1}$ |
| Triglycerides | 77 mg · dL$^{-1}$ |
| HDL cholesterol | 46 mg · dL$^{-1}$ |
| Total protein | 6.9 g · dL$^{-1}$ |
| Albumin | 3.7 g · dL$^{-1}$ |
| Aspartate aminotransferase (AST) | 36 U · L$^{-1}$ |
| Alanine aminotransferase (ALT) | 42 U · L$^{-1}$ |
| Alkaline phosphatase (ALKP) | 98 U · L$^{-1}$ |
| Total bilirubin | 0 .6 mg · dL$^{-1}$ |
| Unconjugated bilirubin | 0.7 mg · dL$^{-1}$ |
| Direct bilirubin | 0 mg · dL$^{-1}$ |
| LDL | 99 mg · dL$^{-1}$ |
| Very low-density lipoprotein (VLDL) | 15 mg · dL$^{-1}$ |
| Cholesterol/HDL | 3.71 mg · dL$^{-1}$ |

| GXT Results: | Name: | | Greg | |
|---|---|---|---|---|
| | Age: | | 55 yr | |
| | HR$_{rest}$ | | 76 bpm | |
| | Resting electrocardiogram (ECG) | | Normal sinus rhythm (NSR) | |
| | Resting BP | | | |
| | Supine | | 142/88 mm Hg | |
| | Standing | | 140/88 mm Hg | |

| Time | Speed | Grade | HR (bpm) | BP (mm Hg) | Rating of Perceived Exertion (RPE) | Metabolic Equivalent (MET) | Symptoms (scales all out of 4) | ECG |
|---|---|---|---|---|---|---|---|---|
| 1 | 1.7 | 10 | 94 | | | | | Sinus rhythm |
| 2 | 1.7 | 10 | 102 | | | | | Sinus rhythm |
| 3 | 1.7 | 10 | 110 | 168/88 | 10 | 4.7 | | Sinus rhythm |
| 4 | 2.5 | 12 | 115 | | | | | Sinus rhythm |
| 5 | 2.5 | 12 | 125 | | | | | Sinus rhythm, 1 premature ventricular contraction (PVC) |
| 6 | 2.5 | 12 | 134 | 186/84 | 14 | 7.0 | 1+ Chest pain | 1.0 mm horizontal ST depression |
| 7 | 3.4 | 14 | 144 | | | | 2+ Chest pain, 1+ SOB | 1.0 mm horizontal ST depression, 1 PVC |

CES

| Time | Speed | Grade | HR (bpm) | BP (mm Hg) | Rating of Perceived Exertion (RPE) | Metabolic Equivalent (MET) | Symptoms (scales all out of 4) | ECG |
|------|-------|-------|----------|------------|------|------|---------|-----|
| 8 | 3.4 | 14 | 150 | | | | 2+ Chest pain, 1+ SOB | 1.5 mm horizontal ST depression |
| 9 | 3.4 | 14 | 158 | 194/84 | 18 | 10.1 | 3+ Chest pain, 2+ SOB | 2.0 mm horizontal ST depression, 1 PVC |
| 10 | Recovery | Supine | 154 | 186/86 | | | 2+ Chest pain, 1+ SOB | 2.0 mm horizontal ST depression |
| 11 | Recovery | Supine | 136 | 180/84 | | | 1+ Chest pain | 1.0 mm horizontal ST depression, 1 PVC |
| 12 | Recovery | Supine | 125 | 176/84 | | | Chest pain Resolved | Sinus rhythm |
| 13 | Recovery | Supine | 94 | | | | | Sinus rhythm |
| 14 | Recovery | Supine | 84 | 156/88 | | | | Sinus rhythm |

## MULTIPLE-CHOICE QUESTIONS FOR CASE STUDY CES.II(1)

1. According to the most recent edition of the *ACSM's GETP* and based on Greg's GXT results, the approximate maximum "safe" exercise MET level he should exercise would be
   A) 5 MET
   B) 6 MET
   C) 7 MET
   D) 8 MET
   E) 9 MET

2. According to the most recent edition of the *ACSM's GETP* and based on Greg's GXT results, a good index of exercise intensity would be an exercise HR no greater than
   A) 110 bpm
   B) <124 bpm
   C) 134 bpm
   D) 144 bpm
   E) 150 bpm

3. According to the most recent edition of the *ACSM's GETP*, which classes of medications prescribed to Greg may have adverse side effects during exercise?
   A) Antihypertensive medications
   B) Antilipidemic medications
   C) Antiangina medications
   D) All of Greg's medication classes may have acute adverse side effects during exercise.
   E) Only Greg's antihypertensive and antiangina medications may have acute adverse side effects during exercise.

4. According to the most recent edition of the *ACSM's GETP*, which classes of medications prescribed to Greg may have an effect on his HR during exercise?
   A) Antihypertensive medications
   B) Antilipidemic medications
   C) Antiangina medications
   D) All of Greg's medication classes may have an effect on his HR during exercise.
   E) None of Greg's medication classes may have an effect on his HR during exercise.

5. The use of ACSM's metabolic calculations for the treadmill would suggest which of the following as a maximal safe workload for exercise training?
   A) 2.0 mph and 15.0% grade
   B) 3.0 mph and 6.5% grade
   C) 4.0 mph and 8.0% grade
   D) 5.0 mph and 5.5% grade
   E) Cannot be determined from the data given

6. The use of ACSM's metabolic calculations for the cycle ergometer would suggest which of the following as a maximal safe workload for exercise training?
   A) 375 kgm · min$^{-1}$
   B) 450 kgm · min$^{-1}$
   C) 535 kgm · min$^{-1}$
   D) 630 kgm · min$^{-1}$
   E) Cannot be determined from the data given

CES

7. According to the most recent edition of the *ACSM's GETP*, a resistance program may be initiated for Greg at which of the following repetition maximum (RM)?
   A) one repetition maximum (1-RM)
   B) 6–8 RM
   C) 8–12 RM
   D) 12–15 RM
   E) Any of the above levels of RM would be appropriate for Greg.

8. According to the most recent edition of the *ACSM's GETP*, a resistance program of 12–15 RM represents approximately which percent range of 1-RM for the upper body?
   A) 10%–20%
   B) 30%–40%
   C) 50%–60%
   D) 70%–80%

9. According to the most recent edition of the *ACSM's GETP*, if you DID NOT have the GXT results for Greg, which of the following initial exercise MET levels would be appropriately safe?
   A) 1 MET
   B) 2–4 MET
   C) 5–7 MET
   D) 8–10 MET
   E) Patients with heart disease cannot exercise without a preexercise GXT.

10. Based on the maximum MET level as determined in Question 1, at what approximate percent of reserve volume of oxygen consumed per unit of time ($\dot{V}O_2R$) is Greg working?
    A) 45%
    B) 55%
    C) 65%
    D) 75%
    E) 85%

## DISCUSSION QUESTIONS FOR CASE STUDY CES.II(1)

1. If Greg followed the exercise program that you developed for 6 mo and does not change his diet, what kind of changes would you tell him that he may expect in his blood chemistries?

2. How could you use the rate pressure product as a tool to use for the progression of Greg's exercise program?

**CASE STUDY CES.II(2)**

Author: **James H. Ross, MS**
Author's Certifications: **ACSM-RCEP, ACSM-CES**

You are a clinical exercise specialist at a health/fitness facility. You have a new client joining your facility. He is a 55-yr-old male who currently weighs 193 lb and is 66 in. in height. Body composition by skinfolds was estimated at 32% body fat and waist circumference was 42 in. He is a current smoker (smokes one pack a day). HR_rest was 76 bpm and resting BP 132/88 mm Hg. Fasting blood values were measured 2 wk ago as the following: total cholesterol = 227 mg · dL$^{-1}$, HDL-C = 33 mg · dL$^{-1}$, triglycerides = 156 mg · dL$^{-1}$, and glucose = 126 mg · dL$^{-1}$. He has been walking the dog for the last 4 wk each day but reports no other exercise. He reports no symptoms of exercise intolerance except SOB when walking up hills. His brother died of a fatal heart attack at age 60 yr. Currently, he is taking a diuretic (hydrochlorothiazide [HCTZ]) to control his BP. He has recently joined your health/fitness facility to increase his fitness level and manage his weight, cholesterol, and BP.

Your client recently had a Bruce maximal exercise test ordered by his physician (due to SOB concerns). The physician interpreted the test as equivocal because he did not reach 85% of predicted maximal heart rate (HR_max). The test interpretation also indicated ~0.5–1 mm of ST depression in the lateral leads at peak exercise but no clinical signs of ischemia. His HR_max and BP were 130 bpm and 168/94 mm Hg, respectively. His maximal oxygen consumption was estimated to be 6.6 MET. His physician ordered a pulmonary function test with the following results: forced expiratory volume in one second (FEV$_{1.0}$)(L) = 2.6 and his forced vital capacity (FVC)(L) = 3.4. Based on these results, his physician has given approval for your client to start an exercise program.

Upon receiving the results, you set up a meeting with your client to help in the development of an appropriate exercise prescription.

# MULTIPLE-CHOICE QUESTIONS FOR CASE STUDY CES.II(2)

1. According to the most recent edition of the *ACSM's GETP*, when prescribing exercise, the optimal intensity of exercise for aerobic fitness benefits would be set at
   A) 20%–30% of one's maximal oxygen uptake reserve
   B) 50%–85% of one's maximal oxygen uptake reserve
   C) 85%–95% of one's maximal oxygen uptake reserve
   D) 100% of one's maximal oxygen uptake reserve

2. According to the most recent edition of the *ACSM's GETP*, the recommended frequency of exercise to achieve health benefits would be
   A) 1–2 d $\cdot$ wk$^{-1}$
   B) 3–5 d $\cdot$ wk$^{-1}$
   C) 5–6 d $\cdot$ wk$^{-1}$
   D) Daily

3. What risk stratification would you assign for your client?
   A) Low risk
   B) Moderate risk
   C) High risk

4. Given his health information provided, your client likely has
   A) Metabolic syndrome
   B) Heart disease
   C) Diabetes
   D) Apparently healthy

5. An appropriate target heart rate (THR) for your client would be
   A) 107–127 bpm
   B) 149–162 bpm

C) 97–108 bpm
D) 103–122 bpm

6. The use of ACSM's metabolic calculations for the treadmill would suggest which of the following workloads as appropriate for an initial workload for exercise training?
   A) 5.0 mph and 4% grade
   B) 1.5 mph and 2% grade
   C) 3.0 mph and 2% grade
   D) Cannot be determined from the data given

7. Your client is about 131 lb of lean body mass and would need to lose about 30 lb of fat to attain a weight of 163 lb at 20% body fat. Approximately how many calories would he need to lose to achieve a 30-lb loss and how many minutes of exercise might it take to do? (Use calculations from Question 6.)
   A) 105,000 cal; 12,235 min
   B) 10,500 cal; 1,223 min
   C) 105,000 cal; 16,632 min
   D) Cannot be determined from the data given

8. Muscle strengthening and flexibility exercises should include >_____ d $\cdot$ wk$^{-1}$ at a _____ intensity.
   A) 5; moderate
   B) 7; light
   C) 2; moderate
   D) 3–5; vigorous

# DISCUSSION QUESTIONS FOR CASE STUDY CES.II(2)

1. What questions will you ask your client prior to developing his exercise prescription?

2. What do you believe to be his major health concern and what exercise/physical activity program might you suggest he follow to manage that health concern?

**CASE STUDY CES.II(3)**

Author: **James H. Ross, MS**
Author's Certifications: **ACSM-RCEP, ACSM-CES**

You are a clinical exercise specialist in a cardiac rehabilitation program. A new patient referred to your program is a 45-yr-old male, who currently weighs 223 lb and is 68 in. in height. He quitted 6 mo ago after smoking 23 yr of two packs a day. His HR$_{rest}$ and BP were measured at 62 bpm and 142/78 mm Hg, respectively, and his waist circumference was 46 in. Fasting blood values were recently measured as the following: total cholesterol = 197 mg $\cdot$ dL$^{-1}$, HDL-C = 40 mg $\cdot$ dL$^{-1}$, triglycerides = 156 mg $\cdot$ dL$^{-1}$, LDL = 125 mg $\cdot$ dL$^{-1}$, and glucose = 106 mg $\cdot$ dL$^{-1}$. He admits that he has not been exercising but has played golf once each week prior to his hospitalization for a lateral wall MI (heart attack) and had two stents implanted (1-Left Anterior Descending [1-LAD]; 1-circumflex) 6 wk ago. His ejection fraction (EF) was estimated to be 54% during a stress echo. He reports that his father died of a heart attack at age 42 yr. He is currently taking atenolol to lower his BP and Lipitor for high cholesterol. During the consultation, he stated that he wants to work out on his own but agreed to come to Cardiac Rehabilitation Program (CRP) because of his physician's insistence.

The patient was administered a physician-supervised Bruce exercise test 1 wk ago. The supervising physician concluded that the test was uninterpretable because the presence of a left bundle-branch block (LBBB). The test was terminated because of leg fatigue and dyspnea. No clinical signs of ischemia were noted during the exercise test. His $HR_{max}$ and BP were 115 bpm and 208/86 mm Hg, respectively. His maximal oxygen consumption was estimated using the ACSM's walking metabolic calculations at 10 MET.

## MULTIPLE-CHOICE QUESTIONS FOR CASE STUDY CES.II(3)

1. What primary goal will you recommend for your patient while at cardiac rehabilitation?
   A) Weight reduction
   B) Lowering fasting blood glucose
   C) Lowering lipids
   D) Maintenance of smoking cessation

2. What mode of exercise will you suggest for your patient?
   A) Walking track
   B) Exercise bike
   C) Treadmill
   D) The one your patient most enjoys

3. What risk stratification is appropriate for your patient with heart disease?
   A) Lowest risk
   B) Moderate risk
   C) Highest risk

4. How would you classify your patient's disease risk given his BMI and waist circumference?
   A) Normal
   B) Increased risk
   C) High risk
   D) Very high risk

5. An appropriate THR for your client would be
   A) 62–82 bpm
   B) 70–95 bpm
   C) 83–104 bpm
   D) 80–100 bpm

6. The use of ACSM's metabolic calculations for the cycle ergometer would suggest which of the following workload as appropriate for an initial workload for exercise training?
   A) 150 W
   B) 75 W
   C) 25 W
   D) Cannot be determined from the data given

7. After a few weeks of exercise, you suggest extra exercise sessions above the 3 d · $wk^{-1}$ cardiac rehabilitation schedule. Your patient prefers bike riding but does not have an exercise bike at home. He wants to walk in the neighborhood near his house but doesn't know what pace he should use. Choose a workload that is appropriate for him to work at ~40% of peak volume of oxygen consumed per unit of time ($\dot{V}O_{2peak}$).
   A) 5.0 mph and 4% grade
   B) 1.5 mph and 2% grade
   C) 4.0 mph and 0% grade
   D) Cannot be determined from the data given

## DISCUSSION QUESTIONS FOR CASE STUDY CES.II(3)

1. Do you think that the use of the ACSM's walking formula for determination of MET levels on the Bruce test is appropriate?

2. What adaptations should be made for your patient using a treadmill test to prescribe exercise on a cycle ergometer?

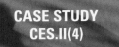

**CASE STUDY CES.II(4)**

Author: **James H. Ross, MS**
Author's Certifications: **ACSM-RCEP, ACSM-CES**

You are the clinical exercise specialist in a pulmonary rehabilitation program. The new patient referred to your program is a 53-yr-old female who currently weighs 153 lb and is 58 in. in height. She recently quit smoking after 30 yr of 1.5 packs a day. She was recently diagnosed with emphysema, and her $HR_{rest}$ and BP were measured at 82 bpm and 128/80 mm Hg, respectively. Her fasting blood lipids were measured last week as the following: total cholesterol = 177 mg $\cdot$ dL$^{-1}$, HDL-C = 50 mg $\cdot$ dL$^{-1}$, triglycerides = 136 mg $\cdot$ dL$^{-1}$, LDL = 112 mg $\cdot$ dL$^{-1}$, and glucose = 100 mg $\cdot$ dL$^{-1}$. She has not participated in regular physical activity for 30 yr but did like to garden and mow her own yard until the last couple years. She recently had pulmonary function tests performed by her pulmonologist with the following results: FVC = 1.35 L $\cdot$ min$^{-1}$, $FEV_{1.0}$ = 0.60 L $\cdot$ min$^{-1}$. Her medications include albuterol and theophylline. During the consultation, she stated that she doesn't exercise because of her dyspnea, which comes on after a couple minutes of exercise.

The patient performed a physician-supervised maximal cycle ergometer test 2 wk ago. She exercised for 2 min, and the test was stopped because of dyspnea. The physician's interpretation was negative for any signs of ischemia. Her $HR_{max}$ and BP were 150 bpm and 182/86 mm Hg, respectively. Her maximal oxygen consumption was estimated using the ACSM's leg ergometer metabolic calculations at 3.11 MET. Oxygen saturation was monitored by pulse oximeter throughout the test and was 86% at maximal exercise. In the last minute of exercise, she stated that she was at 3 on the 4-point dyspnea scale. She did not use supplemental oxygen during the exercise test.

## MULTIPLE-CHOICE QUESTIONS FOR CASE STUDY CES.II(4)

1. What method of prescribing exercise intensity will you use for your patient?
   A) 50%–85% of heart rate reserve (HRR)
   B) 3–4 on a 4-point dyspnea scale
   C) 50%–85% of maximal oxygen consumption
   D) None of the above

2. What mode of exercise will you suggest for your patient?
   A) Walking track
   B) Exercise bike
   C) Treadmill
   D) Arm ergometer

3. According to the Global Initiative for Chronic Obstructive Pulmonary Disease (COPD), how would you classify your patient's disease condition given her pulmonary values?
   A) Mild
   B) Moderate
   C) Severe
   D) Very severe

4. The patient's use of albuterol shortly prior to exercise may impact _____.
   A) Symptoms of heart disease
   B) HR range
   C) Symptoms of dyspnea
   D) B and C

5. Using the ACSM's leg ergometer metabolic equations, what is the work rate at maximal exercise?
   A) 100 W
   B) 75 W
   C) 25 W
   D) Cannot be determined from the data given

6. What muscle groups will you primarily emphasize with your pulmonary patient's resistance training?
   A) Shoulder girdle and inspiratory muscles
   B) Quadriceps, hamstrings, and gluteal muscles
   C) Abdominal and back muscles
   D) Gastrocnemius and soleus muscles

7. What will be your recommendations for exercise frequency for your pulmonary patient?
   A) 2–4 d $\cdot$ wk$^{-1}$
   B) 3–5 d $\cdot$ wk$^{-1}$
   C) 5–7 d $\cdot$ wk$^{-1}$
   D) None of the above

CES

# DISCUSSION QUESTIONS FOR CASE STUDY CES.II(4)

1. What adaptations should be made for your patient using a cycle ergometer test to prescribe exercise for a person walking?

2. Discuss the importance of closely monitoring exercise intensity, dyspnea, and oxygen saturation during exercise bouts.

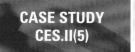

**CASE STUDY CES.II(5)**

Author: **Janet P. Wallace, PhD, FACSM**
Author's Certifications: **ACSM-CES, ACSM-PD**

Exercise prescription is the development of a specific exercise program based on a comprehensive evaluation, whereas exercise programming is basic exercise advice based on a limited evaluation. However, in several cardiac rehabilitation settings, exercise prescriptions are given without a comprehensive evaluation, including exercise testing. This scenario challenges your exercise prescription skills in an exercise programming environment.

# MULTIPLE-CHOICE QUESTIONS FOR CASE STUDY CES.II(5)

1. It is not unusual for patients with heart disease to enter outpatient cardiac rehabilitation without preliminary exercise test. Reasons for this scenario include
   A) Cardiac transplantation
   B) When RPE will be used for exercise prescription
   C) Exercise testing was clinically nonessential because coronary anatomy has been documented.
   D) Stable disease

2. According to the *ACSM's GETP*, the initial MET intensity prescription for a stable asymptomatic 50-yr-old post-MI patient with no prior exercise or pharmacological test available would be
   A) 1–2 MET
   B) 2–3 MET
   C) 2–4 MET
   D) 3–5 MET

3. How would you adjust the MET intensity $R_x$ for this patient (in Question 2) if he answered the following questions on the Duke Activity Status Index (DASI)?
   A) 8–10 MET
   B) 6–8 MET
   C) 4–6 MET
   D) 10–12 MET

| Yes/No | Question | Weight | Score |
|--------|----------|--------|-------|
| yes | Take care of yourself; that is, eat, dress, bathe, or use the toilet? | 2.75 | |
| yes | Walk indoors, such as around your house? | 1.75 | |
| yes | Walk a block or two on level ground? | 2.75 | |
| yes | Climb a flight of stair or walk up a hill? | 5.50 | |
| yes | Run a short distance? | 8.00 | |
| | Do light work around the house like dusting or washing dishes? | 2.70 | |
| | Do moderate work around the house like vacuuming, sweeping floors, or carrying groceries? | 3.50 | |
| yes | Do heavy work around the house like scrubbing floors or lifting or moving heavy furniture? | 8.00 | |
| yes | Do yard work like raking leaves, weeding, or pushing a power mower? | 4.50 | |
| yes | Have sexual relations? | 5.25 | |
| yes | Participate in moderate recreational activities like golf, bowling, dancing, double tennis, or throwing a baseball or football? | 6.00 | |
| | Participate in strenuous sports like swimming, singles tennis, football, basketball, or skiing? | 7.50 | |
| | | Total | |

Adapted with permission from Hlatky MA, Boineau RE, Higginbotham MB et al. A brief self-administered questionnaire to determine functional capacity (the Duke Activity Status Index). *Am J Cardiol.* 1989;64:651–4.

CES

4. How would you confirm that the intensity estimated in Question 3 was safe for this patient?
   A) After a proper warm-up, observe his RPE and HR/BP response during the exercise at the selected MET.
   B) After a proper warm-up, observe his ECG, RPE, and signs/symptoms during the exercise at the selected MET.
   C) After a proper warm-up, monitor his RPE, ECG, HR/BP response, and signs/symptoms during exercise at the selected MET.
   D) After a proper warm-up, monitor his ECG and HR/BP response to the selected MET.

5. How would you give him a THR for activities outside of the outpatient rehabilitation setting?
   A) Estimate his $HR_{max}$ with 220 − age and then use the Karvonen formula to give him a THR between 70%–85% intensity.
   B) 20 beats above $HR_{rest}$
   C) Give him a THR no higher than the HR he has been exercising at in outpatient rehabilitation.
   D) Don't give him a THR without an exercise test, use RPE only.

6. What would be the beginning exercise intensity for a 65-yr-old woman who exhibited 1 mm ST segment depression with +1 angina and hypokinetic lateral ventricular wall with 45% EF during her pharmacologic myocardial perfusion imaging with dipyridamole?
   A) 1–2 MET
   B) 20 beats > $HR_{rest}$
   C) 10 beats < HR at ST segment depression
   D) 2–4 MET

7. What if she had no pharmacologic myocardial perfusion imaging, what beginning exercise intensity would you give her?
   A) 1–2 MET
   B) 15 beats > $HR_{rest}$
   C) 10 beats > $HR_{rest}$
   D) 2–4 MET

8. How would you adjust the initial intensity for the following response on the Veterans Administration Specific Questionnaire (VASQ)?

| MET | Draw one line BELOW the activities you are able to do routinely with minimal or no symptoms, such as SOB, chest discomfort, and fatigue. |
|---|---|
| 1 | Eating, getting dressed, working at a desk |
| 2 | Taking a shower |
|  | Walking down eight steps |
| 3 | Walking slowly on a flat surface for one or two blocks |
|  | ———————————————— |
|  | A moderate amount of work around the house like vacuuming, sweeping the floors, or carrying groceries |

| 4 | Light yard work (i.e., raking leaves, weeding, or pushing a power mower) |
|---|---|
|  | Painting or light carpentry |
| 5 | Walking briskly (i.e., 4 mi in 1 h) |
|  | Social dancing, washing the car |
| 6 | Playing nine holes of golf carrying your own clubs |
|  | Heavy carpentry, mow lawn with push mower |
| 7 | Perform heavy outdoor work (i.e., digging, spading soil) |
|  | Play tennis singles, carry 60 lb |
| 8 | Move heavy furniture |
|  | Jog slowly, climb stairs quickly, carry 20 lb upstairs |
| 9 | Bicycling at a moderate pace, sawing wood, jumping rope slowly |
| 10 | Brisk swimming, bicycle up a hill, walking briskly uphill, jog 6 miles · h$^{-1}$ |
| 11 | Cross-country skiing |
|  | Play basketball full court |
| 12 | Running briskly, continuously on level ground, 8 miles · h$^{-1}$ |
| 13 | Any competitive activity including those which involve intermittent sprinting |
|  | Running competitively, rowing, backpacking |

Adapted with permission from Meyer J, Do D, Herbert W, Ribisl P, Froelicher VF. A nomogram to predict exercise capacity from a Specific Activity Questionnaire and Clinical Data. *Am J Cardiol*. 1994;73:591–6.

   A) 1–2 MET
   B) 2–3 MET
   C) 2–4 MET
   D) 10 beats above standing HR

9. Using the VASQ, her predicted exercise capacity is

Reprinted with permission from Meyer J, Do D, Herbert W, Ribisl P, Froelicher VF. A nomogram to predict exercise capacity from a Specific Activity Questionnaire and Clinical Data. *Am J Cardiol* 1994;73:591–6.

   A) 3 MET
   B) 3.5 MET
   C) 4.0 MET
   D) 4.5 MET

CES

10. She has had a normal response to the exercise program exhibiting no ischemia or symptoms. Her HR and RPE are now lower at the initial work rate. How would you progress her exercise program to increase her physical work capacity?
   A) Keep her RPE at 11–14 but increase her absolute intensity 1–2 MET.
   B) Increase her RPE to 13–15 with an increase of 1–2 MET.
   C) Increase her THR >10 beats · min$^{-1}$ with an increase of 1–2 MET.
   D) Keep her RPE at 11–14 but increase her relative intensity 1–2 MET.

# DOMAIN III: PROGRAM IMPLEMENTATION AND ONGOING SUPPORT

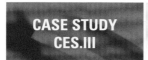

**CASE STUDY CES.III**

Author: **David E. Verrill, MS, FAACVPR**
Author's Certifications: **ACSM-RCEP, ACSM-CES**

You are the clinical exercise physiologist at a local hospital pulmonary rehabilitation program. A new patient, Earl, is a 72-yr-old male just starting the program and you are performing his initial assessment. He arrives from a small town outside the city limits (45–55-min drive). Earl has COPD manifested by a combination of emphysema, chronic bronchitis, and bronchiectasis. He also has a history of blood clots in his lungs, peripheral arterial disease, hyperlipidemia, osteoporosis, and osteoarthritis. He reports increasing fatigue and dyspnea in recent weeks as well as being more depressed. He is on 3 L · min$^{-1}$ of oxygen by nasal cannula in resting (sedentary) conditions, and he increases his oxygen liter flow to 6 L · min$^{-1}$ with exertional activities per physician order. Earl currently weighs 131 lb and is 6 ft tall (BMI = 17.8 kg · m$^{-2}$). You measured his body composition by skinfolds and the value predicted was 8% body fat. He quitted smoking 6 mo ago, but over his lifespan, he smoked 2.5 packs of cigarettes per day for 60 yr. During his initial assessment (while on 3 L · min$^{-1}$ oxygen), the following resting physiological data was assessed and recorded: HR = 109 bpm; BP = 106/56 mm Hg; percent saturation of arterial oxygen (SaO2) = 94%; chest sounds = coarse (but mild) bilateral crackles during inspiration. Earl currently takes prednisone, Advair Diskus (fluticasone and salmeterol), a baby aspirin, Niaspan (intermediate release niacin), Atrovent (ipratropium), Plavix (clopidogrel), and Lexapro (escitalopram). Earl was short of breath when he entered the facility, and his wife stated that he had not been feeling "up to par" over the past few weeks.

You conducted a 6-min walk test (6MWT) test today on Earl immediately after his initial assessment. His highest HR and BP achieved were 136 bpm and 148/78 mm Hg, respectively. His peak SaO2 was 80% on 6 L · min$^{-1}$ of oxygen, and this increased to 92% within 3 min of recovery. He walked 901 ft with one rest break (below average for his age category). He rated his peak level of exertion as 15 on the Borg category scale and his peak dyspnea as 5 on the Borg dyspnea scale. He had moderate-to-marked dyspnea (2–3 on the 0–4 scale) at test termination and mild calf pain in both legs. Other fitness tests you conducted demonstrated an average score for both upper body muscular strength (handgrip dynamometer) and leg endurance (30-s sit-to-stand test).

## MULTIPLE-CHOICE QUESTIONS FOR CASE STUDY CES.III

1. The first action for developing Earl's initial treatment plan (ITP) would be to
   A) Formulate his exercise prescription based upon his 6MWT results.
   B) Call Earl's pulmonologist and discuss his 6MWT results with the medical staff.
   C) Increase his supplemental oxygen flow to 8 L · min$^{-1}$ during his rehabilitation exercise to compensate for his lower exercise SaO2 values seen during the 6MWT.
   D) Develop his individual short- and long-term goals that he wishes to strive for during program participation.

2. The initial exercise prescription for Earl should
   A) Be deferred until Earl's pulmonologist provides follow-up recommendations based upon his initial assessment.
   B) Include recumbent cycling of 15–20 W at 30–40 rpm for 8 min.
   C) Include treadmill walking at 2.8 mph with a 1% incline for 10 min.
   D) Include arm ergometry exercise of 10 W at 20–30 rpm for 8 min.

3. Prednisone is a drug prescribed to
   A) Help provide immediate airway relief in the event of an asthma attack.
   B) Help loosen mucus in the airways for easier removal.
   C) Help shrink the swelling and inflammation of the airways.
   D) Help provide long-term relief of dyspnea through dilation of the airways.

4. Earl has a smoking history of _____ pack per years.
   A) 60
   B) 150
   C) 24
   D) 90

5. Earl has complained recently of fatigue, worsening dyspnea, and some depression. To address these problems, you would
   A) Self-refer Earl to a psychologist or psychiatrist for his depression.
   B) Have Earl perform a GXT to see if he has any cardiac involvement that might be contributing to these issues.
   C) Collect as much information as possible in your initial assessment about these issues and contact his physician with this information.
   D) Ask Earl's pulmonologist to refer him to the pulmonary function testing laboratory to reassess his FVC and $FEV_{1.0}$ values.

6. During your initial assessment, you give Earl surveys to assess his quality of life (QOL), level of dyspnea with activities of daily living (ADL), and depression. One commonly used tool to assess dyspnea with ADL in pulmonary rehabilitation participants is
   A) The University of California at San Diego Shortness of Breath Questionnaire
   B) The Beck Depression-II survey
   C) The Ferrans and Powers' QOL survey (Pulmonary Version)
   D) The Physical Activity Readiness Questionnaire (PAR-Q)

7. Earl's BMI classifies him as _____ by expert panel normative data.
   A) Underweight
   B) Normal weight
   C) Overweight
   D) Obese (class I)

8. Specific components that categorize Earl's ITP would consist of all of the following except
   A) A plan to address his worsening depression.
   B) Vitamin B and D supplementation to help improve his $FEV_{1.0}$ and FVC values.
   C) A diet and exercise plan to increase his body weight and muscle mass.
   D) Pursed-lip breathing training to help him lessen his dyspnea.

9. Assuming Earl completes 12–16 wk of pulmonary rehabilitation participation, which of the following combination of follow-up tests would you perform for outcomes tracking and to provide feedback for his physician?
   A) 6MWT, 30-s sit-to-stand test, grip dynamometer test, dyspnea survey
   B) Submaximal GXT, QOL surveys, depression survey, 30-s sit-to-stand test
   C) 6MWT, Diet Habit Survey (DHS), skinfold assessment, depression survey
   D) Shuttle test, dyspnea survey, QOL survey, skinfold assessment

10. Which of the following statements is true regarding factors to consider for Earl's ITP?
   A) Because Earl quitted smoking 6 mo ago, there is no longer a need to focus on smoking cessation interventions.
   B) Training techniques to improve Earl's upper and lower body strength should take precedence over techniques to improve his 6MWT performance.
   C) Earl's BMI puts him at a significantly lower risk of early mortality.
   D) Bronchiectasis is structural damage to airway cartilage and muscle tissue involving one or more lobes of the lung.

## DISCUSSION QUESTIONS FOR CASE STUDY CES.III

1. List and discuss some short- and long-term goals that Earl should be trying to achieve throughout his pulmonary rehabilitation program.

2. What problems do you foresee Earl having with program participation, compliance, and completion?

3. How would you develop Earl's exercise prescription from the results of his 6MWT?

# DOMAIN IV: LEADERSHIP AND COUNSELING

**CASE STUDY CES.IV**

Author: **Shala E. Davis, PhD, FACSM**
Author's Certifications: **ACSM-ETT, ACSM-CES, ACSM-PD**

Kimberly is a 43-yr-old woman (65 in tall and 159 lb) who is an office manager at a large shipping company. She is divorced and has two school-aged children (8 and 11 yr old). Kimberly has no known cardiovascular, pulmonary, or metabolic disease but considers herself to be highly deconditioned. Kimberly has been diagnosed with fibromyalgia syndrome (FMS). She works 45 h $\cdot$ wk$^{-1}$ and commutes 30 min each way daily. Her medications are limited to over-the-counter sleep aids and nonsteroidal anti-inflammatory drugs (NSAIDs). Kimberly has initiated multiple exercise programs with little success over the past 2 yr and complains of low motivation and depression-like symptoms.

## MULTIPLE-CHOICE QUESTIONS FOR CASE STUDY CES.IV

1. Which of the following are common symptoms of clients diagnosed with FMS?
   A) Sleep disturbances
   B) Undue fatigue
   C) Diffuse soft tissue pain
   D) Depression
   E) None of the above
   F) All of the above

2. FMS symptoms may be increased by which of the following?
   A) Emotional stress
   B) Low-intensity exercise
   C) Poor sleep
   D) A and B
   E) A and C
   F) B and C

3. Which of the following theories related to exercise behavior is based on the principle that the person, behavior, and environment all influence future behavior?
   A) Transtheoretical model
   B) Social cognitive theory
   C) Health behavior model
   D) Self-determination model

4. Which of the following is not a strategy or strategies used to increase self-efficacy?
   A) Experiencing successful completion of tasks
   B) Modeling experiences
   C) Social persuasion
   D) Challenging self with difficult goals

5. Which of the following is not part of the SMART principles of goal setting?
   A) Goals should be realistic.
   B) Goals should have a reasonable time frame.
   C) Goals should be challenging.
   D) Goals should be specific.

## DISCUSSION QUESTIONS FOR CASE STUDY CES.IV

1. Identify three barriers and elaborate on how each barrier impacts exercise compliance for this client.

2. Provide strategies to address the barriers identified.

3. How would you approach goal setting for this client?

CES

# DOMAIN V: LEGAL AND PROFESSIONAL CONSIDERATIONS

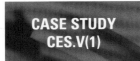

**CASE STUDY CES.V(1)**

Author: **Timothy S. Maynard, MS**
Author's Certifications: **ACSM-PD**

The words *privacy* and *confidentiality* are often used to mean the same thing. However, there is a difference in the meaning of the two words.

- *Privacy* refers to a person's right to be free from interference by another person.
- *Confidentiality* relates to the protection of information.

In the context of medical care, *privacy* means that no one has the right to interfere with a patient who is receiving care in a health care organization. *Confidentiality* in health care settings means that no one can view private health care information without a patient's permission.

The law protects all citizens from unwanted invasion of their privacy. A patient's name or photograph cannot be used without the patient's permission or consent. Using a patient's name or photograph without consent violates the right to privacy and can lead to legal action.

The U.S. Department of Health and Human Services created Standards for Privacy of Individually Identifiable Health Information, or the Privacy Rule, as part of the Health Insurance Portability and Accountability Act (HIPAA) of 1996 (HIPAA is pronounced HIP-ah). This law was passed to protect the use and release of a patient's health information. Organizations that process health information, such as health insurers and medical billers, must obey HIPAA laws. Hospital staff must also obey HIPAA laws.

The HIPAA privacy and confidentiality laws apply to health information that can be shared verbally, in writing, or on a computer. Examples of a patient's health information include the following:

- Names
- Addresses
- Birth dates
- Social security numbers
- Information that is related to a past, present, or future physical or mental condition

HIPAA protects any information that can be used to identify a person. Do not share such information with anyone who is not directly caring for the patient.

According to the HIPAA laws, your organization does not need to ask a patient's permission to use or release health information that is needed

- For treatment,
- To process payments, and
- To carry out general health care operations.

Examples of general health care operations include activities such as tracking and reporting data for quality assurance or use review.

Only share a patient's medical or personal information with other health care workers on a need-to-know basis. This means that you can share health information with those who are directly involved in the care, treatment, or services given to a patient. When sharing information, use the precautions defined by your organization's policies and procedures to ensure a patient's privacy and confidentiality. You must even be careful when telling others about the admission or discharge of a patient.

## TRUE OR FALSE AND MULTIPLE-CHOICE QUESTIONS FOR CASE STUDY CES.V(1)

1. You are assisting with the cardiac rehabilitation department with patient orientation. A woman in work cloths and wearing a hospital badge picks up one of your patients' medical records and begins to read through it.

   True or False: At this point, there is no need to question the woman because it is okay for health care workers employed by your organization to review patient medical records.

2. You are working in a rehabilitation center where you assist with the performance of stress testing on subjects with suspected cardiac diseases. You routinely construct exercise prescriptions for these subjects following the completion of these tests. A visitor stops you in the hallway and begins to ask you questions about the care of a patient, his wife, who has recently completed a stress test in your center. The visitor asks you to tell him the results of the stress test and what other tests have been ordered for his wife because he is afraid that she is dying.

   What should you do?
   A) Show the patient's medical records to her husband.
   B) Give the visitor the number to the stress test and the laboratory departments so that he can call and check on those tests.
   C) Tell the visitor the stress test results and which tests have been ordered for his wife, but do not tell him the results.
   D) Tell the visitor that you are very sorry, but you cannot release any patient-related information without written consent from the patient to do so.

3. True or False: A hospital or health clinic must obtain a patient's permission to release information before it can give information to the state health department about a patient's exposure to tuberculosis (TB).

4. Health care workers who violate privacy and confidentiality laws by selling a patient's personal information to another person or organization are subject to what type of penalties?
   A) Criminal penalties of up to $5,000 and 2 yr in prison
   B) Criminal penalties of up to $5,000 and 6 yr in prison
   C) Criminal penalties of up to $150,000 and 8 yr in prison
   D) Criminal penalties of up to $250,000 and 10 yr in prison

5. You are helping the department secretary for a Rehab and Wellness Center to answer the phone while she has gone to get a cup of coffee. A credit card company calls and is asking about your coworker, Nancy. They claim Nancy is applying for a credit line and they want to verify some information.

   What should you do?
   A) Provide them with the information because Nancy is a coworker.
   B) Do not answer any questions and transfer the call to the human resources department or human resources manager.
   C) Report the credit company to the Better Business Bureau for inappropriate requests for information.
   D) Tell that person that you will call them back when you have more time to talk.

6. You are assigned to help prepare a patient for his first independent exercise session in a new surrounding after completing your hospital-based cardiac rehabilitation program. Your patient is a local politician who is well known to the community and regularly in the news. Your best friend, who also works for your hospital in the radiology department hears about this patient and calls you to ask why the politician was in cardiac rehabilitation.

   What should you do?
   A) Pull the chart to confirm the patient's medical history and diagnosis before sharing it so you may be sure to be accurate.
   B) Speak with the patient and ask him if you may share his medical information with your friend because she is a big fan.
   C) Tell your friend that it would be a violation of the law to discuss the patient's case with her.
   D) Obtain the forms for the patient to sign allowing you to share this medical information with your friend.

7. Who is permitted to view the medical information about a hospital employee who is receiving care in your department?
   A) The employee's manager or supervisor may see the record so they may determine the employee's limitations upon return to work.
   B) The employee's coworkers so they may be aware of the employee's limitation upon return to work.
   C) Only the employees of the hospital who are directly involved with the care of that employee may view the medical records on a need-to-know basis.

**CASE STUDY CES.V(2)**

Author: **Timothy S. Maynard, MS**
Author's Certifications: **ACSM-PD**

The Occupational Safety and Health Administration (OSHA) developed Bloodborne Pathogen Standards for health care workers to decrease their risk of accidental contact with bloodborne pathogens. These standards state that health care organizations must provide workers with information on what bloodborne pathogens are and how to prevent exposure to or contact with them.

An organizational Bloodborne Pathogen Exposure Control Plan should be developed to communicate information to employees about the following:

- Bloodborne pathogens
- Risk of exposure
- How your organization plans to decrease and eliminate exposure to bloodborne pathogens
- Hepatitis B vaccinations
- Postexposure evaluation and follow-up
- Communication of hazards to employees

The exposure control plan should outline your risk of exposure to bloodborne pathogens based on the tasks you perform as an employee.

To find out more about the OSHA's requirements about bloodborne pathogens and an organization's exposure control plan you may see this OSHA Web site: www.osha.gov

## TRUE OR FALSE AND MULTIPLE-CHOICE QUESTIONS FOR CASE STUDY CES.V(2)

1. True or False: The purpose of a health care organization's Bloodborne Pathogen Exposure Control Plan is to reduce an employee's risk of exposure to radiation.

2. True or False: A health care organization should develop a Bloodborne Pathogen Exposure Control Plan after 60% of its employees have been exposed to bloodborne pathogens.

**CASE STUDY CES.V(3)**

Author: **Timothy S. Maynard, MS**
Author's Certifications: **ACSM-PD**

Use standard precautions when providing patient care or while handling items that may be contaminated with blood and body fluids. Standard precautions help prevent the spread of bloodborne pathogens from patient to health care worker and from health care worker to patient. Unless otherwise directed, you should use standard precautions with every patient.

| Standard Precautions | |
|---|---|
| Recommendations from the U.S. Centers for Disease Control and Prevention (CDC) for the use of standard precautions for the care of patients in all health care settings. | |
| **Hand hygiene** | Perform after touching blood, body fluids, secretions, excretions, and contaminated items; after removing gloves; and between patient contacts. |
| **Gloves** | Use when touching blood; body fluids; secretions; excretions; contaminated items; mucous membranes; and skin with cuts, abrasions, or other openings. |
| **Gown** | Use during procedures and patient care activities when contact of clothing or exposed skin with blood, body fluids, secretions, or excretions may occur. |

CES

| Standard Precautions (cont.) | |
|---|---|
| **Mask, eye protection (goggles), face shield** | Use during procedures and patient care activities that are likely to cause splashes or sprays of blood, body fluids, or secretions, especially during suctioning and endotracheal intubation. |
| **Soiled patient care equipment** | Handle in a manner that prevents transfer of microorganisms to others and to the environment; wear gloves if visibly contaminated; and perform hand hygiene. |
| **Environmental control** | Routinely care for, clean, and disinfect environmental surfaces, especially frequently touched surfaces in patient care areas. |
| **Material and laundry** | Handle in a manner that prevents transfer of microorganisms to others and to the environment. |
| **Needles and other sharps** | Do not recap, bend, break, or hand manipulate used needles. If recapping is required, use a one-handed scoop technique only. Use safety features when available. Place used sharps in a puncture-resistant container. |
| **Patient resuscitation** | Use a mouthpiece, resuscitation bag, and other ventilation devices to prevent contact with mouth and oral secretions. |
| **Patient placement** | Make it a priority to place a patient in a single-patient room if the patient is at increased risk for spreading an infection to others, does not maintain appropriate hygiene, or is at increased risk for acquiring infection or developing an adverse outcome following an infection. |
| **Respiratory hygiene and cough etiquette** | Instruct symptomatic persons to cover their mouth and nose when sneezing or coughing, use tissues and dispose of them in a no-touch receptacle, perform hand hygiene after soiling of hands with respiratory secretions, wear a surgical mask if tolerated, or maintain separation greater than 3 ft of space if possible. |

Source: http://www.cdc.gov

## Engineering Controls

Engineering controls are used to reduce workplace exposure to bloodborne pathogens. Examples of engineering controls include the following:

• Sharps disposal containers
• Self-sheathing or retractable needles
• Needleless intravenous (IV) systems

A number of these controls isolate or remove the risk for exposure to bloodborne pathogens using safety mechanisms. When using engineering controls, you should also use personal protective equipment (PPE) to eliminate the risk of exposure to bloodborne pathogens.

For nurses, needlesticks during IV therapy are the most common cause of exposure to blood.

## Communicating Hazards to Employees

Health care organizations must provide information to workers on the risks for exposure to bloodborne pathogens and methods for safe disposal of contaminated waste.

## Labels

OSHA requires that health care organizations educate workers on the disposal of waste that is contaminated with blood and body fluids. As part of meeting this requirement, organizations should tell health care workers when to use warning labels and how to recognize contaminated material. OSHA recommends using warning labels on the following:

• Containers of regulated waste
• Refrigerators and freezers containing blood or other material that may be infected
• Containers used to store, transport, or ship blood or other potentially infected materials

The labels and signs should be fluorescent orange or orange-red, with lettering and symbols in a contrasting color. Red bags or red containers may be substituted for labels.

CES

Your organization also communicates about your risk for exposure to bloodborne pathogens through information and training sessions. Training should address the following:

- Your risk for exposure to bloodborne pathogens
- Methods to reduce and eliminate exposure to bloodborne pathogens
- What you should do if you are exposed to bloodborne pathogens

## What Is an Exposure Incident?

An exposure incident happens when you have direct contact with blood or body fluid through the following:

- Splash or spray to your eyes, mouth, or other mucosal surface
- Needlestick, laceration, or other piercing of the skin by an object contaminated with blood or other body fluids
- Contact with contaminated blood or body fluid that enters a cut, abrasion, or other lesion on your skin
- Your organization's exposure control plan describes specific steps to follow when you are exposed to contaminated substances in the workplace. The exposure control plan should tell you about the free postexposure evaluation and follow-up care provided by your organization. The postexposure evaluation and follow-up are confidential.

| Exposure Incident | What to Do |
|---|---|
| Hands or skin | Immediately wash the area with soap and water. |
| Mucous membranes | Flush the exposed area with water. |
| Any exposure incident | Notify your supervisor of the exposure incident immediately. In some cases, preventive treatment may be necessary and must be started within only a few hours of the exposure. The patient involved in the exposure may require testing. |

Source: http://www.osha.gov

## MULTIPLE-CHOICE QUESTIONS FOR CASE STUDY CES.V(3)

1. Which practice is included in standard precautions?
   A) Using gloves when handling blood or body fluids to prevent exposure to bloodborne pathogens and washing hands between patient contacts
   B) Wearing masks for every patient-related activity
   C) Wearing shoe covers at all times to protect shoes from contamination
   D) Wearing eye protection at all times

2. What type of germ is a bloodborne pathogen?
   A) A germ that is carried in the blood that can cause disease
   B) A germ that everyone is born with
   C) A germ normally found in blood products
   D) A cancer-causing germ

3. Which viruses are bloodborne pathogens?
   A) TB, hepatitis B virus, and hepatitis C virus
   B) Poison ivy, hepatitis B virus, and human immunodeficiency virus (HIV)
   C) Hepatitis B virus, hepatitis C virus, and HIV
   D) Flu virus, hepatitis E virus, and HIV

4. Which situation describes an exposure incident to a potential bloodborne pathogen?
   A) Testing blood glucose from a finger stick on a patient with hepatitis B
   B) Touching the blood of a patient infected with HIV with gloved hands
   C) A splash of blood on intact skin
   D) An accidental needlestick while changing a patient's bed linens

5. Which example of a work practice control decreases the risk of exposure to bloodborne pathogens?
   A) Recapping used needles as soon as possible
   B) Eating your lunch at your work station
   C) Sorting dirty laundry, such as bed linens, in a patient's room
   D) Placing used needles and sharps in a puncture-resistant container

6. According to OSHA, who must give input for decisions about safety devices?
   A) Leaders within the organization who make purchasing decisions
   B) Patients who receive care within the health care organization
   C) Nonmanagerial employees who are responsible for direct patient care
   D) Materials management employees responsible for stocking supplies

7. What information must be included in your health care organization's exposure control plan?
   A) Your risk for exposure to bloodborne pathogens
   B) The needle size for different patient care procedures
   C) The correct steps to take to clean a patient's room
   D) How to draw blood from a patient

8. Which type of precautions must be followed for every patient whom you come in contact with?
   A) Airborne precautions
   B) Standard precautions
   C) Contact precautions
   D) Health care precautions

9. What is the purpose of an exposure control plan?
   A) To decrease the spread of the common cold among health care workers
   B) To decrease the exposure of health care workers to secondhand smoke
   C) To increase the use of contact precautions in health care organizations
   D) To eliminate or decrease health care workers exposure to bloodborne pathogens

10 How are bloodborne pathogens spread from an infected person to a noninfected person?
   A) Rough broken or open skin and mucous membranes
   B) Through contaminated air
   C) Through contact with personal items, such as the telephone
   D) Through contaminated water

## ECG CASE STUDIES

**CES.ECG(1)**

Authors: **Dennis Kerrigan (DK), PhD, and Clinton A. Brawner (CAB), MS, FACSM**
Authors' Certifications: **DK: ACSM-CES; CAB: ACSM-RCEP, ACSM-CES**

A 75-yr-old male patient with a recent history (2 mo ago) of coronary bypass surgery presents to cardiac rehabilitation for his initial visit with the following rhythm. His vitals are as follows: weight = 230 lb, BP = 102/84 mm Hg.

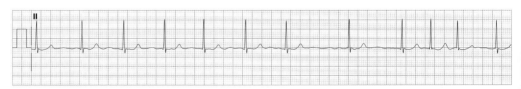

### SHORT-ANSWER QUESTIONS FOR CES.ECG(1)

1) What is the rate? _____

2) Regular or Irregular? _____

3) Interpret the rhythm. _____

CES

## MULTIPLE-CHOICE QUESTIONS FOR CES.ECG(1)

1) Name the medication usually prescribed that prevents a common complication due to this arrhythmia?
   A) Lisinopril
   B) Warfarin
   C) Metoprolol
   D) Simvastatin

2) What effect does this arrhythmia typically have on cardiac output (CO)?
   A) CO is elevated due to the increased contractions in the atria.
   B) The "atrial kick" has negligible effect on CO.

C) CO is reduced.
D) None of the above.

3) How should exercise be prescribed in this patient, assuming he performed a sign- and symptom-limited exercise stress test prior to cardiac rehabilitation?
   A) RPE
   B) An HR 20–30 beats above rest
   C) 50%–85% of HRR
   D) The patient should not exercise with this arrhythmia.

**CES.ECG(2)**

Authors: **Dennis Kerrigan (DK), PhD, and Clinton A. Brawner (CAB), MS, FACSM**
Authors' Certifications: **DK: ACSM-CES; CAB: ACSM-RCEP, ACSM-CES**

A patient with a history of cardiac arrest and MI is walking on the treadmill in cardiac rehabilitation when you observe this rhythm.

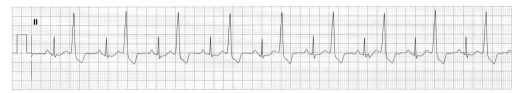

## SHORT-ANSWER QUESTIONS FOR CES.ECG(2)

1) What is the underlying rhythm? _____

2) What is the dysrhythmia? _____

## MULTIPLE-CHOICE QUESTIONS FOR CES.ECG(2)

1. Assuming this patient has a history of this dysrhythmia, what actions should be taken?
   A) Continue to monitor.
   B) Stop the exercise immediately.
   C) Call an emergency code, and grab the automatic defibrillator.
   D) Slow treadmill speed and call physician.

2. What might be some potential causes of this dysrhythmia?
   A) Caffeine
   B) Anxiety/stress
   C) Forgetting to take medications
   D) All of the above

CES

**CES.ECG(3)**

Authors: **Dennis Kerrigan (DK), PhD, and Clinton A. Brawner (CAB), MS, FACSM**
Authors' Certifications: **DK: ACSM-CES; CAB: ACSM-RCEP, ACSM-CES**

A 52-yr-old male without a history of heart disease is scheduled in your laboratory for a standard sign- and symptom-limited exercise stress test with ECG to evaluate a recent episode of angina while performing yard work.

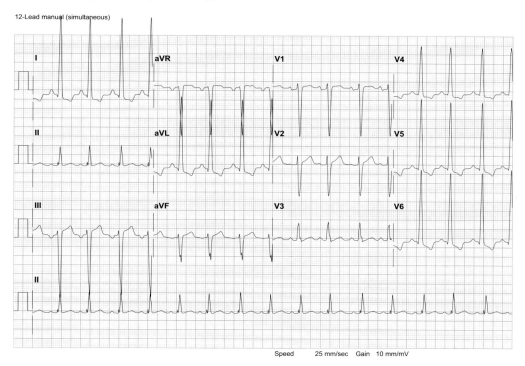

12-Lead manual (simultaneous)

Speed     25 mm/sec    Gain   10 mm/mV

## SHORT-ANSWER QUESTIONS FOR CES.ECG(3)

1) What is the rate? _____

2) Regular or Irregular? _____

3) Interpret the ECG. _____

## TRUE OR FALSE AND MULTIPLE-CHOICE QUESTIONS FOR CES.ECG(3)

1.  Assuming the patient is asymptomatic at rest, what course of action would you follow?
    A)  Proceed with the stress test using a low-level treadmill protocol.
    B)  Send patient directly to emergency department.
    C)  Attempt Valsalva maneuver.
    D)  Contact referring physician to verify the test ordered.

2.  True or False. If the aforementioned patient presented with the observed ECG abnormality AND severe chest pain, this could indicate an acute MI.

CES

**CES.ECG(4)**

Authors: **Dennis Kerrigan (DK), PhD, and Clinton A. Brawner (CAB), MS, FACSM**
Authors' Certifications: **DK: ACSM-CES; CAB: ACSM-RCEP, ACSM-CES**

A 42-yr-old male with hypertension is undergoing a symptom-limited exercise stress test on a treadmill in response to a recent episode of syncope he experienced while running. The following ECG was taken during stage IV of the Bruce protocol.

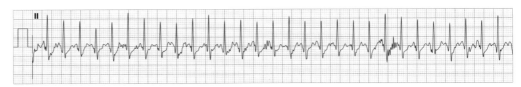

## SHORT-ANSWER QUESTIONS FOR CES.ECG(4)

1) What is the rate? _____

2) Regular or Irregular? _____

3) Interpret the rhythm. _____

## MULTIPLE-CHOICE QUESTIONS FOR CES.ECG(4)

1. If the aforementioned ECG was taken during rest, what might you suspect?
   A) Second-degree atrioventricular (AV) block, type I
   B) Supraventricular tachycardia (SVT)
   C) Ventricular tachycardia
   D) Both A and B

2. Which of the following medications for hypertension is he likely NOT taking
   A) ACE inhibitor
   B) Diuretic
   C) Angiotensin 2 receptor antagonists
   D) β-blocker

3. Based on the ECG alone and information given earlier, should the stress test be stopped?
   A) Yes
   B) No

**CES.ECG(5)**

Authors: **Dennis Kerrigan (DK), PhD, and Clinton A. Brawner (CAB), MS, FACSM**
Authors' Certifications: **DK: ACSM-CES; CAB: ACSM-RCEP, ACSM-CES**

A 53-yr-old female with ischemic cardiomyopathy is performing a symptom-limited exercise stress test in your laboratory. During stage III of the Naughton protocol, you observe for the first time the following on the ECG.

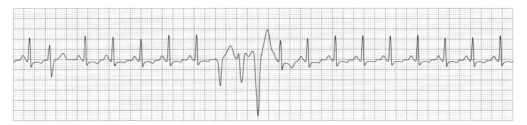

## SHORT-ANSWER QUESTIONS FOR CES.ECG(5)

1) What is the rate? _____

2) Regular or Irregular? _____

3) Interpret the rhythm _____

## MULTIPLE-CHOICE QUESTIONS FOR CES.ECG(5)

1. What course of action should you take?
   A) Stop the test immediately.
   B) Continue with the test.
   C) Take an immediate BP.
   D) Administer a sublingual nitroglycerin.

2. What can be said about the ectopic beats?
   A) They are multifocal.
   B) They are unifocal.
   C) They are junctional beats.
   D) They are both ventricular and supraventricular in nature.

**CES.ECG(6)**

Authors: **Dennis Kerrigan (DK), PhD, and Clinton A. Brawner (CAB), MS, FACSM**
Authors' Certifications: **DK: ACSM-CES; CAB: ACSM-RCEP, ACSM-CES**

A 16-yr-old hockey player has an ECG as part of his preparticipation screening. The following is his resting ECG.

12-Lead manual (simultaneous)

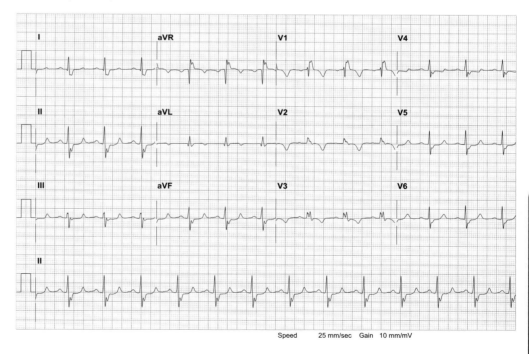

Speed    25 mm/sec    Gain    10 mm/mV

## SHORT-ANSWER QUESTIONS FOR CES.ECG(6)

1) What is the rate? _____

2) Regular or Irregular? _____

3) Interpret the ECG. _____

## MULTIPLE-CHOICE QUESTIONS FOR CES.ECG(6)

1. Based on the ECG, what will likely happen with this athlete?
   A) The athlete will be cleared to participate without any further workup.
   B) The athlete will likely play hockey next year after receiving treatment.
   C) The athlete will no longer be able to participate in sports.
   D) The athlete will likely undergo additional evaluation before returning to play.

**CES.ECG(7)**

Authors: **Dennis Kerrigan (DK), PhD, and Clinton A. Brawner (CAB), MS, FACSM**
Authors' Certifications: **DK: ACSM-CES; CAB: ACSM-RCEP, ACSM-CES**

A 32-yr-old apparently healthy male cyclist is self-referred for a maximal exercise test to assess his $\dot{V}O_{2peak}$ and anaerobic threshold in preparation for an upcoming race. The following is his resting ECG.

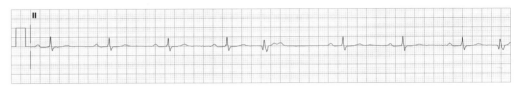

## SHORT-ANSWER QUESTIONS FOR CES.ECG(7)

1) What is the rate? _____

2) Regular or Irregular? _____

3) Interpret the rhythm. _____

## TRUE OR FALSE AND MULTIPLE-CHOICE QUESTIONS FOR CES.ECG(7)

1. True or False. The length of the PR interval is directly responsible for the rate.

2. What are the testing implications of this ECG?
   A) Physician should be notified due to the likelihood of a complete heart block.
   B) Due to the decreased CO, a $\dot{V}O_{2peak}$ will be blunted.
   C) This is a benign finding, which will have no effect on the test.
   D) There is a slight risk for atrial reentry tachycardia.

**CES.ECG(8)**

Authors: **Dennis Kerrigan (DK), PhD, and Clinton A. Brawner (CAB), MS, FACSM**
Authors' Certifications: **DK: ACSM-CES; CAB: ACSM-RCEP, ACSM-CES**

An 84-yr-old female is exercising in cardiac rehabilitation for the first time. While on the recumbent cycle, you see the following on the monitor.

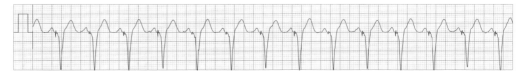

CES

## SHORT-ANSWER QUESTIONS FOR CES.ECG(8)

1) What is the rate? _____

2) Regular or Irregular? _____

3) Interpret the rhythm. _____

## MULTIPLE-CHOICE QUESTIONS FOR CES.ECG(8)

1. Which of the following conditions might be the reason she received a pacemaker?
   A) Sick sinus syndrome
   B) Ventricular tachycardia
   C) Third-degree AV block
   D) Both A and C

2. During her first three visits, she experiences chest pain. As a result, her physician sends her for a symptom-limited exercise stress test with nuclear imaging. Why was the nuclear imaging specified?
   A) She is unable to walk very long on a treadmill.
   B) Her pacemaker would interfere with an echocardiogram.
   C) If present, ischemia would not be undetectable by ECG alone due to the pacemaker depolarization.
   D) All of the above.

---

**CES.ECG(9)**

Authors: **Dennis Kerrigan (DK), PhD, and Clinton A. Brawner (CAB), MS, FACSM**
Authors' Certifications: **DK: ACSM-CES; CAB: ACSM-RCEP, ACSM-CES**

A 64-yr-old male with a history of an MI and stent 15 yr ago is exercising in your phase 3 cardiac rehabilitation program. While on the treadmill, he complains of jaw pain and nausea. You place him in a semisupine position with the upper body slightly elevated and attach an ECG.

12-Lead manual (simultaneous)

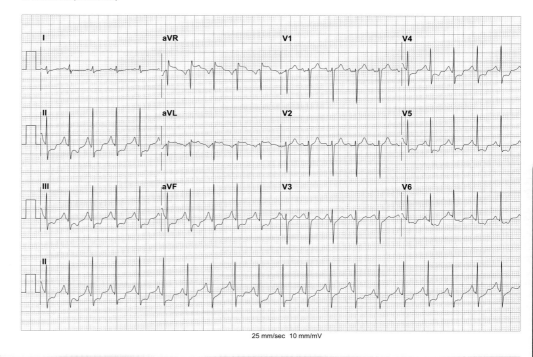

25 mm/sec  10 mm/mV

## SHORT-ANSWER QUESTIONS FOR CES.ECG(9)

1) What is the rate? _____

2) Regular or Irregular? _____

3) Interpret the rhythm. _____

## MULTIPLE-CHOICE QUESTIONS FOR CES.ECG(9)

1. Which of the following medications may improve his jaw pain?
   A) Nitroglycerin
   B) Plavix
   C) Epinephrine
   D) Both A and C

2. Based on the ECG, what regions of the heart are ischemic?
   A) Inferior
   B) Septal
   C) Lateral
   D) Both A and C

### CES.ECG(10)

Authors: **Dennis Kerrigan (DK), PhD, and Clinton A. Brawner (CAB), MS, FACSM**
Authors' Certifications: **DK: ACSM-CES; CAB: ACSM-RCEP, ACSM-CES**

A 58-yr-old female has just completed a low-level exercise test as a predischarge requirement following an ST elevated MI a few days ago. While seated in recovery, you notice a change in the ECG.

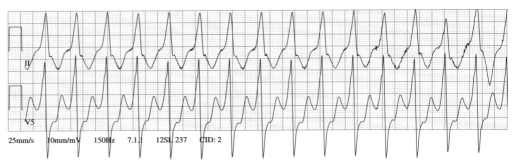

25mm/s    10mm/mV    150Hz    7.1.1    12SL 237    CID: 2

## SHORT-ANSWER QUESTIONS FOR CES.ECG(10)

1) What is the rate? _____

2) Regular or Irregular? _____

3) Interpret the rhythm. _____

## MULTIPLE-CHOICE QUESTIONS FOR CES.ECG(10)

1. What actions should you take?
   A) Check the patient.
   B) Notify the physician.
   C) Prepare the crash cart.
   D) All of the above.

2. Your patient suddenly loses consciousness, what was likely the cause of this?
   A) Low blood glucose
   B) Vasovagal response
   C) Seizure
   D) Low CO

# CES CASE STUDIES ANSWERS AND EXPLANATIONS

## CASE STUDY CES.I

### Multiple-Choice Answers for Case Study CES.I

**1—D.** Signed informed consent form, medical clearance from physician, and GXT with physician supervision

*Resource:* Pescatello LS, senior editor. *ACSM's Guidelines for Exercise Testing and Prescription.* 9th ed. Baltimore (MD): Lippincott Williams and Wilkins; 2014.

**2—B.** Decreases his exercise HR

*Resource:* Pescatello LS, senior editor. *ACSM's Guidelines for Exercise Testing and Prescription.* 9th ed. Baltimore (MD): Lippincott Williams and Wilkins; 2014.

**3—C.** An HbA1C test

*Resource:* Colberg SR, et al. Exercise and Type 2 Diabetes: The American College of Sports Medicine and the American Diabetes Association: Joint Position Statement Diabetes Care. 2010;33:e147–e167.

**4—C.** Preparation

*Resource:* Pescatello LS, senior editor. *ACSM's Guidelines for Exercise Testing and Prescription.*
9th ed. Baltimore (MD): Lippincott Williams and Wilkins; 2014.

**5—A.** Silent ischemia

*Resource:* Pescatello LS, senior editor. *ACSM's Guidelines for Exercise Testing and Prescription.* 9th ed. Baltimore (MD): Lippincott Williams and Wilkins; 2014.

### Discussion Question Answer for Case Study CES.I

1. Drew's main concern at this juncture is his likely diabetes related to his excess body fat. Drew's main goal should be to increase his physical activity as tolerated, to maximize his caloric expenditure, and to improve his glucose control and body composition. Although Drew's BP is in the "prediabetes" category, his fasting glucose strongly suggests that he has a Type 2 diabetes. With his high body fat, he is at high risk for cardiovascular disease (CVD). By working to improve his body composition and glucose control through exercise and diet, Drew will also work to improve his BP.

## CASE STUDY CES.II(1)

### Multiple-Choice Answers for Case Study CES.II(1)

**1—B.** 6 MET

If exercise test data is available, exercise should be prescribed at a workload below the ischemic threshold (~1 MET).

*Resource:* Pescatello LS, senior editor. *ACSM's Guidelines for Exercise Testing and Prescription.* 9th ed. Baltimore (MD): Lippincott Williams and Wilkins; 2014.

**2—B.** <124 bpm

If exercise test data is available, exercise should be prescribed at an HR below the ischemic threshold (<10 bpm).

*Resource:* Pescatello LS, senior editor. *ACSM's Guidelines for Exercise Testing and Prescription.* 9th ed. Baltimore (MD): Lippincott Williams and Wilkins; 2014.

**3—D.** All of Greg's medication classes may have acute adverse side effects during exercise.

Statin drugs may commonly produce muscle soreness and/or patients can develop rhabdomyolysis (a muscle wasting condition), which would affect exercise performance.

*Resource:* Pescatello LS, senior editor. *ACSM's Guidelines for Exercise Testing and Prescription.* 9th ed. Baltimore (MD): Lippincott Williams and Wilkins; 2014.

**4—C.** Antiangina medications

Note that nitrates may cause an increase in HR, especially during rest.

*Resource:* Pescatello LS, senior editor. *ACSM's Guidelines for Exercise Testing and Prescription.* 9th ed. Baltimore (MD): Lippincott Williams and Wilkins; 2014.

**5—B.** 3.0 mph and 6.5% grade

Calculations:

The ACSM's metabolic equation for walking is most accurate for speeds of 1.9–3.7 mph. All speed units for equations should be in units of meter per minute, which is converted when you multiply miles per hour by the constant 26.8. All grades should be in decimal form, for example, 15% = 0.15.

The vertical component is only valid for estimating the metabolic cost of walking and running on a grade on a treadmill. The vertical component equation is NOT valid for the metabolic cost of ground walking or running on grades.

Workload Equivalent = 6 MET

Resting Component = $3.5$ mL $\cdot$ kg$^{-1}$ $\cdot$ min$^{-1}$

Walking Horizontal
Component = $0.1 \times$ speed
$= 0.1 \times (3.0$ mph $\times 26.8)$
$= 0.1 \times 80.4$ m $\cdot$ min$^{-1}$
$= 8.4$ mL $\cdot$ kg$^{-1}$ $\cdot$ min$^{-1}$

Walking Vertical
Component = $1.8 \times$ speed $\times$ grade
$= 1.8 \times 80.4$ m $\cdot$ min$^{-1}$ $\times$ .065
$= 9.4$ mL $\cdot$ kg$^{-1}$ $\cdot$ min$^{-1}$

$\dot{V}O_2$ mL $\cdot$ kg$^{-1}$ $\cdot$ min$^{-1}$ = Resting + Walking Horizontal + Vertical Components

$\dot{V}O_2$ mL $\cdot$ kg$^{-1}$ $\cdot$ min$^{-1}$ = 3.5 + 8.4 + 9.4
$= 21.3$ mL $\cdot$ kg$^{-1}$ $\cdot$ min$^{-1}$

MET $= \dot{V}O_2$ mL $\cdot$ kg$^{-1}$ $\cdot$ min$^{-1}$/3.5 mL $\cdot$ kg$^{-1}$ $\cdot$ min$^{-1}$
MET $= 21.3$ mL $\cdot$ kg$^{-1}$ $\cdot$ min$^{-1}$/3.5 mL $\cdot$ kg$^{-1}$ $\cdot$ min$^{-1}$
$= 6.08$ MET

**6—C.**    535 kgm $\cdot$ min$^{-1}$

Calculations:

If the initial GXT was completed on a treadmill, then the conversion to similar physiological aerobic stress will be approximately 10%–15% less on a cycle ergometer. Therefore, either the functional capacity (FC) or the workload in MET needs to be reduced by 10%–15%. The metabolic equation is most accurate for work rates of 300–1,200 kgm $\cdot$ min$^{-1}$.

Workload Equivalent
(Treadmill) = 6 MET
$= 6$ MET $\times 3.5$
$= 21.0$ mL $\cdot$ kg$^{-1}$ $\cdot$ min$^{-1}$

Workload Equivalent (Cycle
Ergometer) = 21.0 mL $\cdot$ kg$^{-1}$ $\cdot$ min$^{-1}$ $\times$ 0.90 (10% reduction)
$= 18.9$ mL $\cdot$ kg$^{-1}$ $\cdot$ min$^{-1}$

Greg's Body Weight = 178 lb $\times$ 0.454
$= 80.8$ kg

Resting Component = $3.5$ mL $\cdot$ kg$^{-1}$ $\cdot$ min$^{-1}$

Cycle Ergometer Horizontal Component = $3.5$ mL $\cdot$ kg$^{-1}$ $\cdot$ min$^{-1}$

Cycle Ergometer Resistance Component = (1.8 $\times$ Work Rate kgm $\cdot$ min$^{-1}$)/Body Mass kg

Cycle Ergometer Total Equation mL $\cdot$ kg $\cdot$ min$^{-1}$ = Resistance + Horizontal + Resting

18.9 mL $\cdot$ kg$^{-1}$ $\cdot$ min$^{-1}$ = (1.8 $\times$ Work Rate kgm $\cdot$ min$^{-1}$) / 80.8 kg + 3.5 + 3.5

11.9 mL $\cdot$ kg$^{-1}$ $\cdot$ min$^{-1}$ = (1.8 $\times$ Work Rate kgm $\cdot$ min$^{-1}$) / 80.8 kg

961 mL $\cdot$ kg$^{-1}$ $\cdot$ min$^{-1}$ = 1.8 $\times$ Work Rate kgm $\cdot$ min$^{-1}$

534.17 = Work Rate kgm $\cdot$ min$^{-1}$

**7—D.**    12–15 RM

*Resource:* Pescatello LS, senior editor. *ACSM's Guidelines for Exercise Testing and Prescription.* 9th ed. Baltimore (MD): Lippincott Williams and Wilkins; 2014.

**8—B.**    30%–40%

Initial load should allow 12–15 repetitions that can be lifted comfortably (~30%–40% of 1-RM for the upper body; ~50%–60% of 1-RM for the lower body).

*Resource:* Pescatello LS, senior editor. *ACSM's Guidelines for Exercise Testing and Prescription.* 9th ed. Baltimore (MD): Lippincott Williams and Wilkins; 2014.

**9—B.**    2–4 MET

Initial MET level of exercise for a patient with heart disease with no exercise or pharmacologic test available should be 2–4 MET.

*Resource:* Pescatello LS, senior editor. *ACSM's Guidelines for Exercise Testing and Prescription.* 9th ed. Baltimore (MD): Lippincott Williams and Wilkins; 2014.

**10—B.**    55%

Calculations:

Maximum FC = 10.1 MET

$\dot{V}O_2R$ = 10.1 MET − 1 MET
$= 9.1$ MET

Maximum Workload Question 1 = 6.0 MET

$\dot{V}O_2R\%$ = [(6.0 MET − 1.0 MET) / 9.1 MET]
$= 0.549$
$= 0.549 \times 100$
$= 54.9$ %

## Discussion Question Answers for Case Study CES.II(1)

1.  Outline of Discussion
    Effect of exercise alone on blood chemistries:
    *   Total cholesterol
    *   Cholesterol subfractions
        1.  VLDL
        2.  LDL
        3.  HDL
    *   Triglycerides
    *   Plasma glucose
    Effect of fat loss alone on blood chemistries:
    *   Total cholesterol
    *   Cholesterol subfractions
        1.  VLDL
        2.  LDL
        3.  HDL
    *   Triglycerides
    *   Plasma glucose

Drug effect on blood chemistries:
*   Total cholesterol
*   Cholesterol subfractions
    1.  VLDL
    2.  LDL
    3.  HDL
*   Triglycerides
*   Plasma glucose

Concerns of drug side effects on blood chemistries:
*   β-blockers' possible effect on plasma glucose
*   Statin drugs possible effect on liver enzymes

2.  Outline of Discussion
    *   Contributive indices to rate-pressure product (RPP) calculation
    *   Physiology of relationship of RPP to ischemic and/or anginal threshold
    *   Effect of exercise training on RPP indices
    *   Use of RPP for exercise mode changes
    *   Use of RPP for exercise progression

## CASE STUDY CES.II(2)

### Multiple-Choice Answers to Case Study CES.II(2)

**1—B.**  50%–85% of one's maximal oxygen uptake reserve

*Resource:* Pescatello LS, senior editor. *ACSM's Guidelines for Exercise Testing and Prescription.* 9th ed. Baltimore (MD): Lippincott Williams and Wilkins; 2014.

**2—B.**  3–5 d · wk$^{-1}$

*Resource:* Pescatello LS, senior editor. *ACSM's Guidelines for Exercise Testing and Prescription.* 9th ed. Baltimore (MD): Lippincott Williams and Wilkins; 2014.

**3—B.**  Moderate risk

Moderate risk with more than one risk factor but undiagnosed heart disease.

*Resource:* American College of Sports Medicine. *ACSM's Resource Manual for Guidelines for Exercise Testing and Prescription.* 7th ed. Baltimore (MD): Lippincott Williams and Wilkins; 2014.

**4—A.**  Metabolic syndrome

*Resource:* American College of Sports Medicine. *ACSM's Resource Manual for Guidelines for Exercise Testing and Prescription.* 7th ed. Baltimore (MD): Lippincott Williams and Wilkins; 2014.

**5—D.**  103–122 bpm (50%–85% of HRR)

**6—C.**  3.0 mph and 2% grade

**7—C.**  105,000 cal; 16,632 min

**8—C.**  2; moderate

*Resource:* Pescatello LS, senior editor. *ACSM's Guidelines for Exercise Testing and Prescription.* 9th ed. Baltimore (MD): Lippincott Williams and Wilkins; 2014.

### Discussion Question Answers for Case Study CES.II(2)

1.  Do you have SOB any other time other than walking up the hills?
    Are you interested in quitting smoking?
2.  Weight loss; gradually increasing duration and frequency with the goal of increasing energy expenditure for weight loss.

## CASE STUDY CES.II(3)

### Multiple-Choice Answers to Case Study CES.II(3)

**1—A.**   Weight reduction

*Resource:* Pescatello LS, senior editor. *ACSM's Guidelines for Exercise Testing and Prescription.* 9th ed. Lippincott Williams and Wilkins; 2014.

**2—D.**   The one your patient most enjoys

Assuming the equipment is available.

*Resource:* Pescatello LS, senior editor. *ACSM's Guidelines for Exercise Testing and Prescription.* 9th ed. Baltimore (MD): Lippincott Williams and Wilkins; 2014.

**3—A.**   Lowest risk; MET level of >7 MET

*Resource:* American College of Sports Medicine. *ACSM's Resource Manual for Guidelines for Exercise Testing and Prescription.* 7th ed. Baltimore (MD): Lippincott Williams and Wilkins; 2014.

**4—D.**   Very high risk

*Resource:* Pescatello LS, senior editor. *ACSM's Guidelines for Exercise Testing and Prescription.* 9th ed. Baltimore (MD): Lippincott Williams and Wilkins; 2014.

**5—C.**   83–104 bpm (40%–80% of HRR)

**6—C.**   25 W

**7—C.**   4.0 mph and 0% grade

4.0 mph and 0% grade comes closest to 4 MET: it's nearly impossible to determine grade on most roads, so it's important to give an approximate speed and have them use HR ranges or RPE as an adjunct method for monitoring at an appropriate exercise intensity.

### Discussion Question Answers for Case Study CES.II(3)

1.   No. The ACSM's equation is used by many metabolic systems but is designed to be used with steady-state exercise. The Bruce protocol equation is the most appropriate estimate of peak oxygen consumption while using this protocol. Remember to use a handrail equation if the client holds on to the handrail during the test for a more accurate estimation.

2.   He is not used to exercising especially on a lower leg ergometer. It is likely that the workload will need to be lower than on the treadmill especially at the onset of the program.

## CASE STUDY CES.II(4)

### Multiple-Choice Answers for Case Study CES.II(4)

**1—D.**   None of the above

No exercise intensity has been defined; however, 60%–80% of peak work rates are suggested or titration of oxygen saturation to HR monitoring or HR to dyspnea scale.

*Resource:* Pescatello LS, senior editor. *ACSM's Guidelines for Exercise Testing and Prescription.* 9th ed. Baltimore (MD): Lippincott Williams and Wilkins; 2014.

**2—A.**   Walking track

If a track is available and slow walking can be accomplished without desaturation; treadmill as a backup. Weight-bearing exercises (such as walking) helps to maintain the ability to perform ADL.

*Resource:* Pescatello LS, senior editor. *ACSM's Guidelines for Exercise Testing and Prescription.* 9th ed. Baltimore (MD): Lippincott Williams and Wilkins; 2014.

**3—C.**   Severe

*Resource:* Pescatello LS, senior editor. *ACSM's Guidelines for Exercise Testing and Prescription.* 9th ed. Baltimore (MD): Lippincott Williams and Wilkins; 2014.

**4—D.**   B and C

*Resource:* Pescatello LS, senior editor. *ACSM's Guidelines for Exercise Testing and Prescription.* 9th ed. Baltimore (MD): Lippincott Williams and Wilkins; 2014.

**5—C.**   25 W, 150 kg $\cdot$ m $\cdot$ min$^{-1}$

A.   Attempt to improve respiratory muscle dynamics

B.   For moderate-to-severe COPD

*Resource:* Pescatello LS, senior editor. *ACSM's Guidelines for Exercise Testing and Prescription.* 9th ed. Baltimore (MD): Lippincott Williams and Wilkins; 2014.

**6—B.**   Quadriceps, hamstrings, and gluteal muscles

**7—A.**   2–4 d $\cdot$ wk$^{-1}$

## Discussion Question Answers for Case Study CES.II(4)

1. It is likely that she will be able to work at a slightly higher intensity while walking because she has been walking but not using a lower leg ergometer. However, walking is a weight-bearing exercise and will require more work, so the bottom line is that the exercise intensity will need to be titrated to a workload that will allow her to exercise for a longer period of time without severe dyspnea or desaturation.

2. Rather than using HRR or oxygen consumption ($\dot{V}O_2R$) levels to prescribe intensity, workloads should be adjusted to make sure the patient can exercise for the duration of exercise without desaturating ≤88%. Use a pulse oximeter to monitor oxygen saturation during exercise. In this case, SOB seems to be the limiting factor, so allowing the patient to adjust to very low workload levels may be helpful at the beginning of the exercise program.

## CASE STUDY CES.II(5)

## Multiple-Choice Answers for Case Study CES.II(5)

**1—C.** Exercise testing was clinically nonessential because coronary anatomy has been documented.

There are several scenarios when exercise testing is not given prior to beginning outpatient cardiac rehabilitation. In these cases, the science of exercise prescription turns into the "art" of exercise programming at the clinical level.

According to McConnell and colleagues, patients without preentry exercise tests progressed as well as those with preentry exercise tests. More importantly, no events requiring emergency medical management occurred for those without preentry exercise testing.

Success of such practices depends on the knowledge and skill of the clinical exercise physiologists.

*Resource:* McConnell RR, Klinger TA, Gardner JK, Laubach CA, Herman CE, Hauck CA. Cardiac rehabilitation without exercise tests for post-myocardial infarction and post-bypass surgery patients. *J Cardiopulm Rehabil.* 1998;18:458–63.

**2—C.** 2–4 MET

How were these guidelines formed? The initial intensities were chosen based on an interview assessing activity in in-patient, activity after discharge, according to McConnell and colleagues. Their beginning intensity ranged from 2–3 MET and was titrated to exhibit an RPE of 11–14. HR, ECG, BP, RPE, and signs/symptoms were monitored throughout the exercise session to assure normal responses. The intensity was lowered if abnormal responses were detected. The progressions were 0.5–1 MET; also based on the signs/symptoms, ECG, and hemodynamic responses. The RPE stayed at 11–14 for the progressions.

*Resource:* McConnell RR, Klinger TA, Gardner JK, Laubach CA, Herman CE, Hauck CA. Cardiac rehabilitation without exercise tests for post-myocardial infarction and post-bypass surgery patients. *J Cardiopulm Rehabil.* 1998;18:458–63.

**3—B.** 6–8 MET

If you can document the patient's physical work capacity, the intensity Rx can be adjusted accordingly. The DASI estimates physical work capacity based on daily physical function.

The DASI: $\dot{V}O_{2peak}$ (mL · min · kg$^{-1}$) = 0.43 × (sum of weights for "yes") + 9.6

Thus, estimated $\dot{V}O_{2peak}$ (mL · min · kg$^{-1}$) = 44.5 mL · min · kg$^{-1}$ or 12.7 MET

In this case, estimated $\dot{V}O_{2peak}$ is high. Giving this individual an intensity of 2–4 MET would be only 15%–31% of his physical work capacity; too low for optimizing the limited exercise time he has with you in the outpatient setting. An intensity of 70%–85% was chosen based on Table 9.1 p. 214, as the patient was stable and asymptomatic.

It should be noted that the use of the DASI is not mentioned in the current edition of the *ACSM's GETP.* The DASI may represent another tool useful in programming for patients with heart disease.

*Resource:* Hlatky MA, Boineau RE, Higginbotham MB et al. A brief self-administered questionnaire to determine functional capacity (the Duke Activity Status Index). *Am J Cardiol.* 1989;64:651–4.

**4—C.** After a proper warm-up, monitor his RPE, ECG, HR/BP response, and signs/symptoms during exercise at the selected MET.

Use all the variables you have available in the outpatient setting to monitor the safety of the intensity you estimated for him. Your focus on these variables would be similar to how you monitor and interpret during the exercise testing. The RPE gives you an idea of his effort. The ECG is monitored for dysrhythmia and ischemia. The HR and BP will not exhibit the classic responses to graded exercise (increasing intensities). You can compare resting, warm-up, and target intensity responses, but you will not have increasing intensities up to 85% or max.

**5—C.** Give him a THR no higher than the HR he has been exercising at in outpatient rehabilitation.

The purpose of the exercise test is to determine a safe exercise intensity minimizing dysrhythmia, ischemia, and abnormal hemodynamic responses. In this scenario, estimated target intensity was given, based on his medical history and an estimated FC. Then, ECG, RPE, HR and BP, and signs and symptoms were observed when the patient exercised at that estimated intensity. In other words, the same variables observed in an exercise test were observed without the formal exercise test. Normal responses mean that the exercise is safe up to the intensity of the workouts in outpatient rehabilitation. You can give him this intensity for activities outside of the outpatient setting or you can give him an intensity 10% lower. *You should never give him a THR higher than what you've documented to be safe.* (Not in guidelines)

It is not unusual for a single THR range be given for every physical activity a patient with CVD does in and out of the cardiac rehabilitation program. Giving a single THR range for a diversity of physical activity is not a good for controlling exercise intensity and probably should not be done in a nonclinical population. However, it is often done with the patient with CVD. In this case, the THR is given because it reflects the work of the heart and is given as an upper limit for heart work in any situation.

Knowledge and understanding of the HR–$\dot{V}O_2$ curve is an essential consideration when giving a general THR for all activities. HR are given to guide intensity because the HR is linear with $\dot{V}O_2$. That is, 50% intensity is 50% of HRR. However, this relationship only holds true for dynamic whole body cardiovascular exercise. The less aerobic the exercise and the smaller the muscle mass, the relationship changes, as illustrated in the following figures. As illustrated in the figure to the right, 50% as calculated with HR (black dashed line) is

related to lower exercise intensities (gray and light red dashed lines) than expected (dark red dashed line).

**HEART RATE - VO₂ RELATIONSHIP: RESERVE**

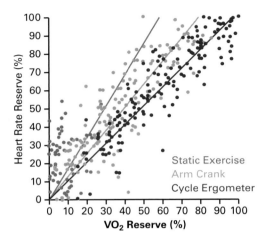

**HEART RATE - VO₂ RELATIONSHIP: RESERVE**

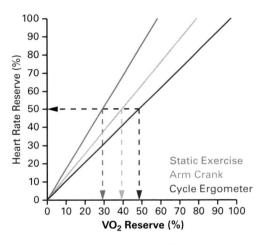

Reprinted with permission from http://www.iub.edu/~k561/revo2.html.

**6—D.** 2–4 MET

Dipyridamole does not produce a linear increase in HR in which a THR to guide the intensity can be determined. Therefore, 2–4 MET intensity is appropriate for exercise intensity when the chemical exercise test doesn't provide enough information for an exercise prescription.

Had she been given a dobutamine stress echocardiogram, there would have been a linear HR increase, which a THR could be given. In this case, the THR should be set at an HR lower than the ST segment depression or +1 angina exhibited.

**7—D.**  2–4 MET (Table 9.1)

How can that be? 2–4 MET is the intensity whether she shows abnormalities on a myocardial perfusion imaging or doesn't have any preentry exercise test.

Intensities of 2–4 MET are conservative and a good starting place. Each exercise prescription is then titrated based on the HR, ECG, BP, and signs/symptoms response.

**8—B.**  2–3 MET

Because the line is drawn in the 3 MET category, 3 MET is the intensity of her daily functioning. Giving her an exercise prescription at 3.5 MET would be maximal work for her and 4 MET would be higher than her predicted exercise capacity. (See next question.)

**9—B.**  3.5 MET

Draw a line from her age to the MET from the questionnaire and extend the line to the predicted exercise capacity to find her physical work capacity. Her predicted exercise capacity or physical work capacity is 3.5 MET.

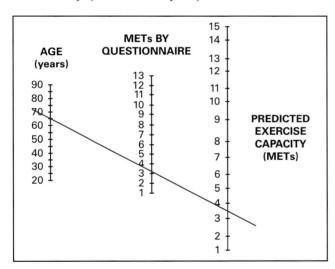

Adapted with permission from Meyer J, Do D, Herbert W, Ribisl P, Froelicher VF. A nomogram to predict exercise capacity from a Specific Activity Questionnaire and Clinical Data. *Am J Cardiol*. 1994;73:591–6.

**10—A.**  Keep her RPE at 11–14 but increase her absolute intensity 1–2 MET.

An increase of 1–2 MET is recommended in the *ACSM's GETP* (Table 9.1, p. 214) for a progression in the outpatient setting. Because her exercise capacity is so low, the MET increase should be closer to the 1 MET than the 2 MET.

A good question regarding progression in cardiac rehabilitation — Should a progression represent an increase in absolute intensity or relative intensity? Absolute intensity is the MET expenditure of the activity, whereas relative intensity is the percent intensity for the individual patient.

For example, a patient with a physical work capacity of 5 MET was given an exercise intensity of 60% or 3 MET. After 6 wk, her physical work capacity increases it to 7 MET. The 3 MET work rate is now 42% (3 MET / 7 MET) of her physical work capacity. If the relative exercise intensity is maintained at 60%, the absolute work rate needs to increase to 4.2 MET (7 MET × 60%) to be 60% relative intensity. So, do we increase absolute exercise intensity, keeping the relative intensity constant? Or do we increase both relative and absolute exercise intensities?

The progressions depend on the performance. Observe her HR, RPE, BP, ECG, and signs/symptoms before making any decisions on increasing intensity. The more normal the responses, the more aggressive the progression can be.

On the other hand, increasing the MET intensity is not always reflected by an increase in THR. For example, the HR range of this patient was 90 (rest) to 150 (max) when her physical work capacity was at 5 MET. Now that she is 7 MET, her HR range is 70 (rest) to 150 (max). If we keep her exercise intensity at 60%, her THR may decrease, not increase. See the calculations in the following table.

| Variable | Initial | Training |
|---|---|---|
| HR$_{rest}$ (/min) | 90 | 70 |
| HR$_{max}$ (/min) | 150 | 150 |
| HR range (max − rest) | 60 | 80 |
| HR range × 60% | 36 | 48 |
| (HR range × 60%) + resting HR | 126 | 118 |
| THR at 60% (/10 s) | 21 | 19 |

Although HR$_{max}$ does not change in most populations, the symptom-limited HR$_{max}$ can increase in cardiac rehabilitated patients.

CES

## CASE STUDY CES.III

### Multiple-Choice Answers for Case Study CES.III

**1—B.** Call Earl's pulmonologist and discuss his 6MWT results with the medical staff.

*Resource:* Pescatello LS, senior editor. *ACSM's Guidelines for Exercise Testing and Prescription.* 9th ed. Baltimore (MD): Lippincott Williams and Wilkins; 2014.

**2—A.** Be deferred until Earl's pulmonologist provides follow-up recommendations based upon his initial assessment.

*Resource:* Pescatello LS, senior editor. *ACSM's Guidelines for Exercise Testing and Prescription.* 9th ed. Baltimore (MD): Lippincott Williams and Wilkins; 2014.

**3—C.** Help shrink the swelling and inflammation of the airways.

*Resource:* Pescatello LS, senior editor. *ACSM's Guidelines for Exercise Testing and Prescription.* 9th ed. Baltimore (MD): Lippincott Williams and Wilkins; 2014.

**4—B.** 150

*Resource:* Pescatello LS, senior editor. *ACSM's Guidelines for Exercise Testing and Prescription.* 9th ed. Baltimore (MD): Lippincott Williams and Wilkins; 2014.

**5—C.** Collect as much information as possible in your initial assessment about these issues and contact his physician with this information.

*Resource:* Pescatello LS, senior editor. *ACSM's Guidelines for Exercise Testing and Prescription.* 9th ed. Baltimore (MD): Lippincott Williams and Wilkins; 2014.

**6—A.** The University of California at San Diego Shortness of Breath Questionnaire

*Resource:* Pescatello LS, senior editor. *ACSM's Guidelines for Exercise Testing and Prescription.* 9th ed. Baltimore (MD): Lippincott Williams and Wilkins; 2014.

**7—A.** Underweight

*Resource:* Pescatello LS, senior editor. *ACSM's Guidelines for Exercise Testing and Prescription.* 9th ed. Baltimore (MD): Lippincott Williams and Wilkins; 2014.

**8—B.** Vitamin B and D supplementation to help improve his $FEV_{1.0}$ and FVC values

*Resource:* Pescatello LS, senior editor. *ACSM's Guidelines for Exercise Testing and Prescription.* 9th ed. Baltimore (MD): Lippincott Williams and Wilkins; 2014.

**9—A.** 6MWT, 30-s sit-to-stand test, grip dynamometer test, dyspnea survey

*Resource:* Pescatello LS, senior editor. *ACSM's Guidelines for Exercise Testing and Prescription.* 9th ed. Baltimore (MD): Lippincott Williams and Wilkins; 2014.

**10—D.** Bronchiectasis is structural damage to airway cartilage and muscle tissue involving one or more lobes of the lung.

*Resource:* Pescatello LS, senior editor. *ACSM's Guidelines for Exercise Testing and Prescription.* 9th ed. Baltimore (MD): Lippincott Williams and Wilkins; 2014.

### Discussion Question Answers to Case Study CES.III

1. The following are some of the short- and long-term goals that Earl should be trying to achieve throughout his pulmonary program:

Short-term goals of pulmonary rehabilitation program

- Maintain smoking cessation
- Incorporate nutrition education
- Decrease depression/stress
- Decrease level of dyspnea
- Have physician look at his depression issues
- Have physician evaluate his SaO2 desaturation issues

Long-term goals of pulmonary rehabilitation program

- Increase upper body strength
- Increase lower body strength
- Increase overall body weight/BMI
- Increase lean body mass
- Increase FC and 6MWT distance
- Increase QOL
- Decrease level of dyspnea
- Decrease joint pain with exercise prescription and stretching program for osteoarthritis
- Decrease leg pain with exercise prescription for peripheral artery disease (PAD)

2. Earl might have problems with program participation, compliance, and completion related to the following:
   a. Travel distance
   b. Low compliance if he continues smoking
   c. Low body weight (increase upper respiratory infections)

d. His depression
e. His level of dyspnea
f. Leg pain from PAD
g. Joint pain from osteoarthritis
h. Daily fatigue

3. To develop Earl's exercise prescription from the results of his 6MWT,

- Determine the speed that he is walking in mph (901 / 6 min = X / 60 min) = 2.5 mph
- Find the MET equivalent for 2.5 mph, 0% grade

OR

To calculate METS:

Step 1: $901 \times 0.3048 = 274.62$ m
Step 2: $274.62$ m / 6 min = $45.77$ m $\cdot$ min$^{-1}$
Step 3: $[0.1 (45.77) + 3.5] = 8.1$ mL $\cdot$ kg$^{-1}$ $\cdot$ min$^{-1}$
Step 4: $8.1 / 3.5 = 2.3$ MET

Then, prescribe exercise anywhere from 30%–80% of this MET level (depending upon one's philosophy — no solid evidence to support an actual entry starting MET level). Determine his workload levels on the treadmill, NuStep, arm ergometer, etc. from the ACSM's metabolic equations.

Use target RPE: 12–14 (Borg category scale)

Use target dyspnea: 3–4 (Borg 10-point dyspnea scale)

Determine THR: Take 60%–80% of peak HR achieved during 6MWT for THR range — this is one technique (not validated at this time)

To calculate his average walking speed:

Step 1: 1 mph = $26.8$ m $\cdot$ min$^{-1}$
Step 2: Walking speed = m $\cdot$ min$^{-1}$ / 26.8
Step 3: $67$ m $\cdot$ min$^{-1}$ / 26.8 = 2.5 mph

OR

Step 1: Convert feet to miles and minutes to hours
Step 2: He walked 901 ft in 6 min
Step 3: (X feet $\times$ 10) / 5280 ft (1 mi) = mph

---

## CASE STUDY CES.IV

### Multiple-Choice Answers for Case Study CES.IV

**1—F.** All of the above

**2—E.** A and C

**3—B.** Social cognitive theory

**4—D.** Challenging self with difficult goals

**5—C.** Goals should be challenging.

### Discussion Question Answers for Case Study CES.IV

1. The following are the three barriers and its impact on exercise compliance:

a. Time

A full-time job and primary child care responsibilities place a time crunch on the client. Discontinuous bouts of activity with a focus on walking may alleviate the burden of time as a significant barrier. In addition, this mode of activity can be completed in various convenient settings, thereby matching the work and commuter schedule.

b. Fatigue/pain

Patients with FMS often complain of multiple tender points, undue fatigue, and morning stiffness. In addition, the client's sleep disturbances coupled with chronic soft tissue discomfort may make some exercise intensities and types of exercise difficulty. Consideration of using low-intensity exercise with shorter bouts may reduce the fatigue and pain response. Remind the client that discomfort during exercise may occur, but that pain may require exercise termination or selection of various modalities of exercise.

c. Depression/motivation

Due to the primary symptoms associated with FMS and life demands currently placed on Kimberly, it is not uncommon to see a significant reduction in motivation toward physical activity. In addition, the incidence of depression is higher in patients with FMS as compared to their apparently healthy counterparts.

2. Selecting types of exercise that Kimberly enjoys and has easy access to may alleviate some of the barriers that she presents. Little skill and equipment (good walking shoes, pedometer, polar heart monitor) are necessary to implement an effective exercise program.

In addition, shorter, discontinuous bouts of exercise may be warranted considering the numerous demands on Kimberly's time. Suggestions to include her children in the exercise plan (biking alongside) would increase her social support, which has been demonstrated to increase adherence.

CES

3. The client should be part of the goal-setting process with the health care team to develop realistic goals, time line for implementation, periodic measures, and revisions to goals as warranted. Developing a goal-setting contract with signature for client and CES provides a public proclamation, which often may enhance the effectiveness of the goal setting plan. In addition, both short- and long-terms goals should be included with regular assessment to allow for new strategies if necessary.

## CASE STUDY CES.V(1)

### True or False and Multiple-Choice Answers for Case Study CES.V(1)

**1—False.**

A patient's health information should only be shared with those involved in the case and have a clear need to know. You should question the woman about her need to read this patient's record.

If you need to give a patient's health information to individuals who are not directly involved in the patient's care, you must obtain written permission from the patient to do so. If the patient cannot give you permission because of a mental or physical condition, you must get authorization from the patient's legal representative.

A patient's family members and close friends, other than those who have legal authority to make decisions for a patient, cannot view the patient's information without written permission. Even minors who live in states, such as Virginia and Washington, have rights to privacy and confidentiality from their parents when they receive treatment for sexually transmitted diseases or desire to start birth control. Make sure that you know what your state laws require for the release of health information to others.

**2—D.** Tell the visitor that you are very sorry, but you cannot release any patient-related information without written consent from the patient to do so.

You cannot share personal health information with anyone without written permission from the patient. In some instances, such as mandatory reporting, federal laws do not require patients' permission for release of their health information.

- For example, if patients or employees are exposed to communicable diseases, such as HIV or TB, your organization does not need to obtain permission from an individual before giving health information to the state health department.
- Other examples of mandatory reporting include cases of abuse.

**3—False.**

Federal law requires an organization to contact the state health department when patients are diagnosed with, or have been exposed to, TB.

Civil and criminal penalties can be imposed on individuals who do not follow the HIPAA laws. HIPAA laws set the minimum requirements for privacy and confidentiality across the United States. However, if your state privacy laws, professional practice standards, or your organization's policies and procedures are stricter than the HIPAA laws, you must follow the stricter rules.

| Penalties for Noncompliance | | |
|---|---|---|
| **Type of Noncompliance** | **Type of Penalty** | **Penalty** |
| Organizations that violate HIPAA laws | Civil | • $100 per violation<br>• Up to $25,000 per calendar year<br>• If the violation occurs and an organization is using reasonable means to protect a patient's health information and if actions to correct the problem are started within 30 d of the violation, no civil penalties are filed. |
| A health care worker who purposely shares or releases a patient's health information in violation of the HIPAA laws | Criminal | • $50,000<br>• Up to 1 yr in prison |
| Individuals who sell, transfer, or use a patient's health information to harm a patient or for personal gain | Criminal | • Fines up to $250,000<br>• 10 yr in prison |

Adapted from Summary of HIPAA Privacy Rule at http://www.hhs.gov/ocr/privacy/hipaa/understanding/summary/index.html

**4—D.**  Criminal penalties of up to $250,000 and 10 yr in prison

Individuals who willfully violate the privacy and confidentiality laws will be prosecuted by the U.S. Department of Justice, receiving penalties of up to $250,000 and 10 yr in prison.

HIPAA laws require that health care organizations, such as hospitals and clinics, set policies and procedures to prevent use or release of health information. Your organization is also required to provide education to you about its privacy and confidentiality policies and procedures. Make sure that you read and understand your organization's policies to prevent accidentally breaking these important rules.

Ensuring privacy and confidentiality is important when building a trusting relationship with patients whom you serve. Therefore,

- Never discuss a patient's health information with anyone who does not have permission to know it.
- Don't discuss patient information in public areas, such as the hallway and cafeteria.
- If you are unsure about what information you can give, contact your supervisor or manager before giving information to others.

Employees, like patients, have the right to privacy and confidentiality of their employment information. If you receive a call about the employment status of another employee, transfer the call to one of your human resources personnel.

**5—B.**  Do not answer any questions and transfer the call to the human resources department or resources manager.

The human resources department can best handle this type of call to avoid breaking confidentiality rules.

**6—C.**  Tell your friend that it would be a violation of the law to discuss the patient's case with her.

You should tell your friends of why this is a violation of all patients' right to confidentiality and privacy, and refuse these requests.

**7—C.**  Only the employees of the hospital who are directly involved with the care of that employee may view the medical records on a need-to-know basis.

*Resources:*
1. Health Insurance Portability and Accountability Act of 1996 http://www.hhs.gov/ocr/privacy/
2. Centers for Medicaid and Medicare Services. https://www.cms.gov/HIPAAGenInfo/

## CASE STUDY CES.V(2)

### True or False and Multiple-Choice Answers for Case Study CES.V(2)

**1—False.**

The purpose of the Exposure Control Plan is to eliminate or minimize health care workers' exposure to bloodborne pathogens in the workplace, not radiation.

**2—False.**

Health care organizations are required by OSHA to develop an exposure control plan that eliminates or reduces the risk of exposure to bloodborne pathogens.

### Personal Protective Equipment

Your health care organization is required to provide free PPE to you if you are at risk for exposure to bloodborne pathogens. This requirement is enforced by OSHA for all health care workers who may have contact with blood, body fluids, or any other hazardous materials.

Under normal conditions of use and for the time that it is used, PPE should prevent blood and other possibly infectious materials from passing through to your
- Work clothes, street clothes, and undergarments; and
- Skin, eyes, mouth, and other mucous membranes.

The sequence for donning PPE is very important to be adequately protected. Equally as important is the appropriate removal and disposal sequence for PPE. For specific details of these methods, please see this CDC instruction: http://www.cdc.gov/ncidod/dhqp/pdf/ppe/ppeposter1322.pdf

Examples of PPE include the following:
- Gowns
- Face shields, or masks
- Laboratory coats
- Eye protection
- Gloves
- Mouthpieces
- Resuscitation bags
- Pocket masks and other ventilation devices

## CASE STUDY CES.V(3)

### Multiple-Choice Answers for Case Study CES.V(3)

**1—A.** Standard precautions include using gloves when handling blood or body fluids to prevent exposure to bloodborne pathogens and washing hands between patient contacts.

**2—A.** Bloodborne pathogens are germs carried in the blood that can cause disease.

**3—C.** Hepatitis B virus, hepatitis C virus, and HIV are bloodborne pathogens.

**4—D.** An accidental needlestick while changing a patient's bed linens is called an exposure incident.

**5—D.** Placing used or contaminated needles and sharps in a puncture-resistant container is an example of an effective work practice control.

**6—C.** OSHA requires health care organizations to include nonmanagerial employees responsible

for direct patient care in the decision-making process regarding safety devices.

**7—A.** A health care organization's exposure control plan must describe your risk for exposure to bloodborne pathogens.

**8—B.** Standard precautions should be used for every patient whom you come in contact with.

**9—D.** The purpose of an exposure control plan is to eliminate or decrease the exposure of health care workers to bloodborne pathogens.

**10—A.** Bloodborne pathogens are spread from an infected person to a noninfected person when blood and body fluids come in contact with broken skin or mucous membranes.

*Resource:* Occupational Safety and Health Administration.*Bloodborne Pathogen Standard, 29 CFR 1910.1030.* 1992.

## ECG CASE STUDIES ANSWERS AND EXPLANATIONS

### CES.ECG(1)

#### Short Answers for CES.ECG(1)
1. Rate is approximately 70 bpm
2. Irregular rhythm
3. Atrial fibrillation

#### Multiple-Choice Answers for CES.ECG(1)

**1—B.** Warfarin

**2—D.** None of the above

**3—A.** RPE

**Teaching points:** Warfarin is often prescribed in patients with atrial fibrillation to prevent the formation of and to treat existing thrombi that result

due to the unorganized and weak contractions of the atria. It is important to confirm that the patient is on some type of anticoagulation therapy. Patients presenting with new onset atrial fibrillation should see a physician before resuming cardiac rehabilitation. Regarding exercise training, while $VO_{2peak}$ is compromised with this condition because of the reduced "atrial kick," patients can still improve fitness. Although HR does increase with exercise, the HR method is not reliable because of the irregular nature of this arrhythmia. Because of the irregular rhythm, when measuring the HR with atrial fibrillation, the number of cardiac cycles should be counted from a 6- or 10-s strip.

### CES.ECG(2)

#### Short Answers for CES.ECG(2)
1. Sinus
2. Ventricular bigeminy

#### Multiple-Choice Answers for CES.ECG(2)

**1—A.** Continue to monitor.

**2—D.** All of the above.

**Teaching points:** Ventricular bigeminy is a stable and non–life-threatening dysrhythmia. Patients

with this may or may not report feeling "skipped beats". Regardless, as with any new onset arrhythmias, the referring physician should be notified, but this does not warrant withholding exercise. Although emotional distress and stimulants, such as caffeine, can lead to increased rates and ectopic beats, some patients may regularly have frequent ventricular activity without precipitating factors. Regardless, the clinician should first "rule out" medication noncompliance before considering secondary causes in a new onset.

## CES.ECG(3)

### Short Answers for CES.ECG(3)

1. 98 bpm
2. Regular
3. Sinus rhythm with left ventricular hypertrophy (LVH) and an LBBB

### True or False and Multiple-Choice Answers for CES.ECG(3)

**1—D.** Contact referring physician to verify the test ordered.

**2—True.**

**Teaching points:** Both LVH as well as LBBB can mask changes due to myocardial ischemia that are typically seen on a standard 12-lead ECG. Therefore, a symptom-limited exercise stress test with ECG only is typically not administered due to the inability to diagnose ischemia. However, new onset LBBB in the presence of angina may indicate an acute coronary event. Regardless of the presence (or lack) of angina, a new occurrence of LBBB should be reported to a physician to determine the underlying cause.

## CES.ECG(4)

### Short Answers for CES.ECG(4)

1. 176 bpm
2. Regular
3. Sinus tachycardia

### Multiple-Choice Answers for CES.ECG(4)

**1—B.** Supraventricular tachycardia (SVT)

**2—D.** β-blocker

**3—B.** No

**Teaching points:** The HR response in the earlier ECG is normal for someone during stage IV of the Bruce protocol. Although his HR is close to his age-predicted maximum, percentage of age-predicted maximum HR is not a criterion for stopping at test. If this ECG were obtained at rest, it would be abnormal and likely an SVT, not emanating from the sinoatrial (SA) node. Finally, because of the normal HR response during exercise, if this individual was on antihypertensive medications, it would likely not be a type of β-blocker because they attenuate the chronotropic response to exercise.

## CES.ECG(5)

### Short Answers for CES.ECG(5)

1. 115 bpm
2. Irregular
3. Sinus tachycardia with a PVC and a ventricular triplet

### Multiple-Choice Answers for CES.ECG(5)

**1—B.** Continue with the test.

**2—A.** They are multifocal.

**Teaching points:** An isolated ventricular triplet, although associated with a greater likelihood of ventricular tachycardia, is not by itself dangerous. Therefore, although an isolated triplet should be noted, it is not an indication for stopping a test, according to *ACSM's GETP*. The fact that these are multifocal PVC, thus originating at different ventricular areas does not change these guidelines. More than one observed ventricular triplet, however, is listed as a relative contraindication for stopping a stress test.

## CES.ECG(6)

### Short Answers for CES.ECG(6)

1. 78 bpm
2. Regular
3. Sinus rhythm with a right bundle-branch block (RBBB)

### Multiple-Choice Answers for CES.ECG(6)

**1—D.** The athlete will likely undergo additional evaluation before returning to play.

**Teaching points:** RBBB is not an uncommon finding in athletes. As long as there is no underlying structural heart disease, most athletes are cleared to return to play.

CES

## CES.ECG(7)

### Short Answers for CES.ECG(7)

1. 50 bpm
2. Regular
3. Sinus bradycardia with a first-degree AV block and PVC

### True or False and Multiple-Choice Answers for CES.ECG(7)

**1—False.**

**2—D.**   There is a slight risk for atrial reentry tachycardia.

**Teaching points:** First-degree AV block is a benign finding in healthy individuals. There is no known risk for individuals who have a first-degree AV block to develop more severe AV nodal disruptions that necessitate a pacemaker. The bradycardia is caused by enhanced vagal tone (*i.e.*, parasympathetic influence), which is common in endurance athletes. Isolated PVC are also benign.

## CES.ECG(8)

### Short Answers for CES.ECG(8)

1. 83 bpm
2. Regular
3. Sinus with ventricular-paced rhythm (notice pacemaker spike before QRS complex)

### Multiple-Choice Answers for CES.ECG(8)

**1—C.**   Third-degree AV block

**2—C.**   If present, ischemia would not be undetectable by ECG alone because of the pacemaker depolarization.

**Teaching points:** Pacemakers are indicated when the heart's natural pacemaker (*i.e.*, SA node) does not depolarize properly, as in sick sinus syndrome, or complete AV nodal block (*i.e.*, third-degree block). Due to the fact that this ECG is only ventricular paced, the cause was likely not sick sinus syndrome, otherwise there would also be a pacer spike before the P wave. Similar to LVH and LBBB, ventricular pacemakers can hide ECG changes due to myocardial ischemia.

## CES.ECG(9)

### Short Answer Answers for CES.ECG(9)

1. 120 bpm
2. Regular
3. Sinus tachycardia with 2 mm of ST segment depression in the inferior and lateral leads.

### Multiple-Choice Answers for CES.ECG(9)

**1—A.**   Nitroglycerine

**2—D.**   Both A and C

**Teaching points:** This is an example of classic ST segment depression due to myocardial ischemia. The ECG reveals 2 mm of ST segment depression in both the inferior leads (II, III, and aVF) and the lateral leads ($V_4$, $V_5$, and $V_6$). Although left-sided chest pressure along with concomitant left arm pain is considered classic angina by many, pain in the jaw, between the shoulder blades, indigestion-type sensation, or just excessive SOB can be anginal equivalents. If discontinuing exercise and rest do not relieve the angina, then the drug of choice would be nitroglycerin. Typically, given sublingually for rapid absorption, the main mechanism of nitroglycerin in reducing the ischemic burden is the reduction of preload on the heart from dilation of the veins.

## CES.ECG(10)

### Short Answers for CES.ECG(10)

1. 125 bpm
2. Regular
3. Ventricular tachycardia

### Multiple-Choice Answers for CES.ECG(10)

**1—D.** All of the above.

**2—D.** Low CO

**Teaching points:** Ventricular tachycardia can be a lethal arrhythmia and is an indication for stopping a stress test. When a patient loses consciousness and a pulse cannot be obtained, immediate defibrillation is indicated. Although transient changes leading to wide QRS complexes are also seen with rate-dependent bundle-branch blocks and aberrancies, the clinician should always rule out ventricular tachycardia first because of its serious implications.

CES

*Note: CES certification candidates should also review the knowledge, skills, and abilities (KSAs) found in Part 1, ACSM Certified Personal Trainer (CPT) and Part 2, ACSM Certified Health Fitness Specialist (HFS).*

## DOMAIN I: PATIENT/CLIENT ASSESSMENT

| A. Determine and obtain the necessary physician referral and medical records to assess the potential participant. | | |
|---|---|---|
| **Knowledge or Skill Statement** | **Explanation/Examples** | **Resources** |
| **Knowledge** of the procedure to obtain informed consent from participant to meet legal requirements | • Participant and/or guardian should have verbal explanation and questions answered.<br>• If the participant is a minor, a legal guardian must sign the consent.<br>• Various components of informed consent (*e.g.*, purpose, risks, participant responsibilities, freedom to withdraw, etc.)<br>• Purpose, legal concerns, content, administration | *ACSM's Guidelines for Exercise Testing and Prescription* (GETP), 9th edition (6)<br>• Chapter 3 |
| **Knowledge** of information and documentation required for program participation<br>**Knowledge** of the procedure to obtain physician referral and medical records required for program participation<br>**Knowledge** of the procedure to obtain participant's medical history through available documentation | • American Heart Association (AHA)/ American College of Sports Medicine (ACSM) Health/Fitness Facility Preparticipation Screening Questionnaire, Physical Activity Readiness Questionnaire (PAR-Q), medical history, informed consent<br>• Must be treated as confidential and privileged information<br>• Understand policy and procedures for obtaining medical records and Health Insurance Portability and Accountability Act (HIPAA) regulations. | *ACSM's Guidelines for Exercise Testing and Prescription* (GETP), 9th edition (6)<br>• Chapter 2<br>*ACSM's Guidelines for Exercise Testing and Prescription* (GETP), 9th edition (6)<br>• Chapter 3 |
| **Skill** in assessing participant physician referral and medical records to determine program participation status | • Assess appropriateness of referral and classify risk based on medical records/ physician referral. | *ACSM's Guidelines for Exercise Testing and Prescription* (GETP), 9th edition (6)<br>• Chapter 2 |

**B.  Perform a preparticipation health screening including review the participant's medical history and knowledge, their needs and goals, the program's potential benefits, and additional required testing and data.**

| Knowledge or Skill Statement | Explanation/Examples | Resources |
|---|---|---|
| **Knowledge** of normal cardiovascular, pulmonary, and metabolic anatomy and physiology<br>**Knowledge** of cardiovascular, pulmonary, and metabolic pathologies; clinical progression; diagnostic testing; and medical regimens/procedures<br>**Knowledge** of instructional techniques to assess participant's expectations and goals<br>**Knowledge** of commonly used medication for cardiovascular, pulmonary, and metabolic diseases<br>**Knowledge** of the effects of physical inactivity, including bed rest, and methods to counteract these changes<br>**Knowledge** of normal physiologic responses to exercise<br>**Knowledge** of abnormal responses/signs and symptoms to exercise associated with different pathologies (*e.g.*, cardiovascular, pulmonary, metabolic)<br>**Knowledge** of anthropometric measurements and their interpretation<br>**Knowledge** of normal 12-lead and telemetry electrocardiogram (ECG) interpretation<br>**Knowledge** of interpretation of ECGs for abnormalities (*e.g.*, arrhythmias, blocks, ischemia, infarction)<br>**Knowledge** of normal and abnormal heart and lung sounds<br>**Knowledge** of pertinent areas of a participant's medical history (*e.g.*, any symptoms since their procedure, description of discomfort/pain, orthopedic issues)<br>**Knowledge** of validated tools for measurement of psychosocial health status<br>**Knowledge** of various behavioral assessment tools (*e.g.*, SF-36, health-related quality of life, Chronic Respiratory Disease Questionnaire) and strategies for their use<br>**Knowledge** of psychological issues associated with acute and chronic illness (*e.g.*, anxiety, depression, social isolation, suicidal ideation)<br>**Knowledge** of participant-centered goal setting | • Understand resting and exercise cardiovascular, pulmonary, and metabolic anatomy and physiology<br>• Understanding of how diagnostic testing and medical regimens/procedures can assess clinical progression of disease and/or exercise effects<br>• Coaching techniques to set achievable goals and overcome potential obstacles<br>• Understanding medication effects on resting and exercise related to cardiovascular, pulmonary, and metabolic diseases<br>• Understanding of deconditioning effects of bed rest and inactivity on the various body systems (*e.g.*, cardiovascular, pulmonary, muscular)<br>• Metabolic energy equivalent (MET) requirements for various physical activities; arm vs. leg exercise differences in hemodynamics; volume of oxygen consumed per unit of time ($\dot{V}O_2$); myocardial oxygen consumption; neuromuscular, vascular, and metabolic adaptations; muscle hypertrophy<br>• Knowledge of absolute and relative contraindications to exercise and abnormal responses/signs and symptoms for cardiovascular, pulmonary, and metabolic disease states<br>• Height, weight, circumferences, and body composition testing (*e.g.*, skinfolds, body mass index [BMI]); understand the difference between BMI and body fat percentage.<br>• Know the anatomical landmarks for ECG lead placement, identify/minimize artifact, identify normal resting ECG and exercise ECG changes, and know/identify dangerous arrhythmias.<br>• Understanding clinical descriptions and auscultation sounds for normal and abnormal heart and lung sounds<br>• Issues that may alter exercise testing selection and/or the exercise prescription (*e.g.*, knee osteoarthritis may limit weight-bearing activity, previous injury, or surgery)<br>• Five factor model of personality, transtheoretical model, *Diagnostic and Statistical Manual of Mental Disorders* (*DSM*), classes of mood disorders, subtypes of anxiety disorders | *ACSM's Resource Manual for Guidelines for Exercise Testing and Prescription*, 7th edition (7)<br>• Chapter 3<br>*ACSM's Resource Manual for Guidelines for Exercise Testing and Prescription*, 7th edition (7)<br>• Chapters 6–8 and 24–26<br>*ACSM's Resource Manual for Guidelines for Exercise Testing and Prescription*, 7th edition (7)<br>• Chapter 45<br>*ACSM's Guidelines for Exercise Testing and Prescription* (GETP), 9th edition (6)<br>• Appendix A<br>*ACSM's Resource Manual for Guidelines for Exercise Testing and Prescription*, 7th edition (7)<br>• Chapter 5<br>*ACSM's Resource Manual for Guidelines for Exercise Testing and Prescription*, 7th edition (7)<br>• Chapter 3<br>*ACSM's Exercise Management for Persons with Chronic Diseases and Disabilities*, 3rd edition (2)<br>• Chapters 6–26<br>*ACSM's Resource Manual for Guidelines for Exercise Testing and Prescription*, 7th edition (7)<br>• Chapter 18<br>*ACSM's Resource Manual for Guidelines for Exercise Testing and Prescription*, 7th edition (7)<br>• Chapter 29<br>*ACSM's Resource Manual for Guidelines for Exercise Testing and Prescription*, 7th edition (7)<br>• Chapter 24<br>*ACSM's Resource Manual for Guidelines for Exercise Testing and Prescription*, 7th edition (7)<br>• Chapter 11<br>*ACSM's Resource Manual for Guidelines for Exercise Testing and Prescription*, 7th edition (7)<br>• Chapters 16 and 17 |

**B. Perform a preparticipation health screening including review the participant's medical history and knowledge, their needs and goals, the program's potential benefits, and additional required testing and data. (cont.)**

| Knowledge or Skill Statement | Explanation/Examples | Resources |
|---|---|---|
| **Knowledge** of functional and diagnostic exercise testing methods, including symptom-limited maximal and submaximal aerobic testing<br>**Knowledge** of indications and contraindications to exercise testing<br>**Knowledge** of normal and abnormal (*i.e.*, signs/symptoms) endpoints for termination of exercise testing<br>**Knowledge** of testing and interpretation of muscle strength/endurance and flexibility<br>**Knowledge** of current published guidelines for treatment of cardiovascular, pulmonary, and metabolic pathologies (*e.g.*, American College of Cardiology [ACC]/American Heart Association [AHA] Joint Guidelines, Global Initiative for Chronic Obstructive Lung Disease [GOLD], American Diabetes Association [ADA] guidelines) | • Knowledge of health-related quality-of-life tools, their target populations, strategies for their use, and how results may effect program participation<br>• Know how these conditions may affect exercise adherence and motivation; social support groups; referral to other health care professionals.<br>• Set goals that are specific, measurable, and challenging but realistic (*e.g.*, specific, measurable, attainable, realistic, and time-bound [SMART] goals).<br>• Knowledge of exercise test modalities, test protocols, disease diagnosis, severity and prognosis, functional testing, and return-to-work testing<br>• Clinical understanding of absolute and relative indications for terminating exercise testing<br>• Clinical understanding of what exercise testing termination does to normal (*i.e.*, target heart rate achieved) or abnormal (*i.e.*, signs/symptoms) physiological markers<br>• One repetition maximum bench press and leg press, push-up test, curl up (crunch test), Young Men's Christian Association (YMCA) bench press test, sit and reach (trunk flexion), range of motion in select single joints<br>• Clinical understanding, application, and basis synthesis of multiple national scientific/medical guidelines and position stands | *ACSM's Resource Manual for Guidelines for Exercise Testing and Prescription*, 7th edition (7)<br>• Chapters 16 and 17<br>*ACSM's Resource Manual for Guidelines for Exercise Testing and Prescription*, 7th edition (7)<br>• Chapters 16 and 17<br>*ACSM's Resource Manual for Guidelines for Exercise Testing and Prescription*, 7th edition (7)<br>• Chapter 46<br>*ACSM's Guidelines for Exercise Testing and Prescription* (GETP), 9th edition (7)<br>• Chapter 5<br>*ACSM's Guidelines for Exercise Testing and Prescription* (GETP), 9th edition (6)<br>• Chapters 3 and 5<br>"Exercise Standards for Testing and Training: A Statement for Health Care Professionals from the American Heart Association" (11)<br>*ACSM's Guidelines for Exercise Testing and Prescription* (GETP), 9th edition (6)<br>• Chapter 4<br>*ACSM's Guidelines for Exercise Testing and Prescription* (GETP), 9th edition (6)<br>• Chapter 4 |
| **Skill** in auscultation methods for common cardiopulmonary abnormalities<br>**Skill** in data collection during baseline intake assessment<br>**Skill** in assessment and interpretation of information collected during the baseline intake assessment<br>**Skill** in formulating an exercise program based upon the information collected during the baseline intake assessment<br>**Skill** in selection, application, and monitoring of exercise testing for healthy and patient populations | • Evaluate arteries for adequate pulses and bruits, lungs for emphysema, the heart for heart failure, murmurs, etc.<br>• Techniques to appropriately acquire individual patient information that may influence patient participation status<br>• Interpretation of graded exercise tests, blood pressure and heart rate response, ECG interpretation, oxygen saturation, and gas exchange and ventilatory responses<br>• Practice the frequency, intensity, time, and type, volume and progression (FITT-VP) principle for aerobic, muscle strength and endurance, and flexibility exercise based upon the goals, limitations, and ability of the patient.<br>• Determine testing protocols that are safe and effective for the individual; know the procedure and be able to effectively explain it to the individual; know testing termination criteria. | *ACSM's Resource Manual for Guidelines for Exercise Testing and Prescription*, 7th edition (7)<br>• Chapters 24 and 25<br>*ACSM's Guidelines for Exercise Testing and Prescription* (GETP), 9th edition (6)<br>• Chapter 6<br>*ACSM's Guidelines for Exercise Testing and Prescription* (GETP), 9th edition (6)<br>• Chapter 6<br>*ACSM's Guidelines for Exercise Testing and Prescription* (GETP), 9th edition (6)<br>• Chapters 4 and 5<br>*ACSM's Resource Manual for Guidelines for Exercise Testing and Prescription*, 7th edition (7)<br>• Chapters 21–23 |

CES

## B.  Perform a preparticipation health screening including review the participant's medical history and knowledge, their needs and goals, the program's potential benefits, and additional required testing and data. (cont.)

| Knowledge or Skill Statement | Explanation/Examples | Resources |
|---|---|---|
| **Skill** in muscle strength, endurance, and flexibility assessments for healthy and patient populations<br>**Skill** in patient preparation and ECG electrode application for resting and exercise ECG | • Practice one repetition maximum bench press and leg press, push-up test, curl up (crunch test), YMCA bench press test, sit and reach (trunk flexion), range of motion in select single joints<br>• Practice finding the anatomical landmarks for ECG lead placement; dry the skin, alcohol prep the landmarks, and shave body hair (if necessary). | *ACSM's Guidelines for Exercise Testing and Prescription* (GETP), 9th edition (6)<br>• Chapter 4<br>*ACSM's Resource Manual for Guidelines for Exercise Testing and Prescription*, 7th edition (7)<br>• Chapter 29 |

## C.  Evaluate the participant's risk to ensure safe participation and determine level of monitoring/supervision in a preventive or rehabilitative exercise program.

| Knowledge or Skill Statement | Explanation /Examples | Resources |
|---|---|---|
| **Knowledge** of applied exercise physiology principles<br>**Knowledge** of cardiovascular, pulmonary, and metabolic pathologies; their clinical progression; diagnostic testing; and medical regimens/procedures to treat<br>**Knowledge** of American College of Sports Medicine (ACSM) preparticipation screening algorithm<br>**Knowledge** of the participant's risk factor profile (*i.e.*, cardiovascular, pulmonary, and metabolic) to determine level of exercise supervision using ACSM, American Heart Association (AHA), and American Association of Cardiovascular and Pulmonary Rehabilitation (AACVPR) risk stratification criteria<br>**Knowledge** of indications and contraindications to exercise testing<br>**Knowledge** of functional and diagnostic exercise testing methods, including symptom-limited maximal and submaximal aerobic testing<br>**Knowledge** of interpretation of electrocardiograms (ECGs) for abnormalities (*e.g.*, arrhythmias, blocks, ischemia, infarction)<br>**Knowledge** of normal and abnormal (*i.e.*, signs/symptoms) endpoints for termination of exercise testing<br>**Knowledge** of testing and interpretation of muscle strength/endurance and flexibility<br>**Knowledge** of commonly used medication for cardiovascular, pulmonary, and metabolic diseases | • Understand the acute and chronic responses and adaptations exercise has on the body. These include the cardiorespiratory responses, metabolic responses, neuromuscular responses, and muscular fatigue.<br>• Understanding of clinical information necessary to assess disease status, indications of clinical progression, and possible methods of treatment<br>• Understanding of self-guided screening for physical activity, risk stratification, and exercise testing recommendations based on risk category<br>• Understanding of self-guided screening for physical activity, risk stratification, exercise testing recommendations, and level of supervision based on risk category<br>• Understanding of cardiovascular, pulmonary, and metabolic disorder variables that affect the decisions regarding administration of and exercise test<br>• Knowledge of parameters of exercise test modalities, test protocols, disease diagnosis, severity and prognosis, functional testing, and return-to-work testing<br>• Be able to identify resting and exercise abnormalities including, but not limited to, bundle-branch blocks, sinus bradycardia and tachycardia, sinus arrest, atrial fibrillation and flutter, ventricular tachycardia and fibrillation, ST depression and elevation, and premature ventricular and atrial contractions. | *ACSM's Resource Manual for Guidelines for Exercise Testing and Prescription*, 7th edition (7)<br>• Chapter 3<br>*ACSM's Resource Manual for Guidelines for Exercise Testing and Prescription*, 7th edition (7)<br>• Chapters 6–8 and 24–26<br>*ACSM's Guidelines for Exercise Testing and Prescription* (GETP), 9th edition (6)<br>• Chapter 2<br>*ACSM's Guidelines for Exercise Testing and Prescription* (GETP), 9th edition (6)<br>• Chapter 2<br>*ACSM's Guidelines for Exercise Testing and Prescription* (GETP), 9th edition (6)<br>• Chapters 2, 3, and 5<br>*ACSM's Guidelines for Exercise Testing and Prescription* (GETP), 9th edition (6)<br>• Chapter 5<br>*ACSM's Resource Manual for Guidelines for Exercise Testing and Prescription*, 7th edition (7)<br>• Chapter 29<br>*ACSM's Guidelines for Exercise Testing and Prescription* (GETP), 9th edition (6)<br>• Chapter 5 |

## C. Evaluate the participant's risk to ensure safe participation and determine level of monitoring/supervision in a preventive or rehabilitative exercise program. (cont.)

| Knowledge or Skill Statement | Explanation/Examples | Resources |
|---|---|---|
| **Knowledge** of current published guidelines for treatment of cardiovascular, pulmonary, and metabolic pathologies (*e.g.*, American College of Cardiology [ACC]/AHA Joint Guidelines, Global Initiative for Chronic Obstructive Lung Disease [GOLD], American Diabetes Association [ADA] guidelines) | • Clinical understanding of absolute and relative indications for terminating exercise testing<br>• Knowledge of one repetition maximum bench press and leg press, push-up test, curl up (crunch test), Young Men's Christian Association (YMCA) bench press test, sit and reach (trunk flexion), and range of motion in select single joints to evaluate muscle strength/endurance and flexibility<br>• Understanding medications' normal and abnormal effects on resting and exercise cardiovascular, pulmonary, and metabolic diseases<br>• Clinical understanding, application, and basis of multiple national scientific/medical guidelines and position stands | *ACSM's Guidelines for Exercise Testing and Prescription* (GETP), 9th edition (6)<br>• Chapter 4<br>*ACSM's Guidelines for Exercise Testing and Prescription* (GETP), 9th edition (6)<br>• Appendix A |
| **Skill** in risk stratification using established guidelines (ACSM, AHA vs. informal)<br>**Skill** in selection, application, and monitoring of exercise tests for apparently healthy participants and those with chronic disease<br>**Skill** in ECG interpretation and interpreting exercise test results | • Determine level of risk to evaluate who requires physician supervision during exercise testing.<br>• Understanding of and management of testing protocols that are safe and effective for the individual; know the procedure and be able to effectively explain it to the individual; know testing termination criteria and data collection during test stages.<br>• Understand clinical significance in identifying normal resting ECGs, normal changes with ECGs during exercise, abnormal ECG changes during exercise, know dangerous arrhythmias, and exercise termination criteria. | *ACSM's Guidelines for Exercise Testing and Prescription* (GETP), 9th edition (6)<br>• Chapter 2<br>*ACSM's Resource Manual for Guidelines for Exercise Testing and Prescription*, 7th edition (7)<br>• Chapter 10<br>*ACSM's Guidelines for Exercise Testing and Prescription* (GETP), 9th edition (6)<br>• Chapters 4 and 5<br>*ACSM's Resource Manual for Guidelines for Exercise Testing and Prescription*, 7th edition (7)<br>• Chapters 21–23<br>*ACSM's Resource Manual for Guidelines for Exercise Testing and Prescription*, 7th edition (7)<br>• Chapter 29 |

CES

# DOMAIN II: EXERCISE PRESCRIPTION

## A. Develop a clinically appropriate exercise prescription using all available information (*e.g.*, clinical and physiological status, goals, and behavioral assessment).

| Knowledge or Skill Statement | Explanation/Examples | Resources |
|---|---|---|
| **Knowledge** of applied exercise physiology principles<br>**Knowledge** of the frequency, intensity, time, and type (FITT) principle for cardiovascular, muscular fitness/resistance training, and flexibility exercise prescription<br>**Knowledge** of cardiovascular, pulmonary, and metabolic pathologies; their clinical progression; diagnostic testing; and medical regimens/procedures to treat<br>**Knowledge** of the effects of physical inactivity, including bed rest, and methods to counteract these changes<br>**Knowledge** of normal physiologic responses to exercise<br>**Knowledge** of abnormal responses/signs and symptoms to exercise associated with different pathologies (*e.g.*, cardiovascular, pulmonary, metabolic)<br>**Knowledge** of validated tools of measurement of psychosocial health status<br>**Knowledge** of functional and diagnostic exercise testing methods, including symptom-limited maximal and submaximal aerobic testing<br>**Knowledge** of normal and abnormal (*i.e.*, signs/symptoms) endpoints for termination of exercise testing<br>**Knowledge** of tests to assess and interpret muscle strength/endurance and flexibility<br>**Knowledge** of commonly used medication for cardiovascular, pulmonary, and metabolic diseases and their effect on exercise prescription<br>**Knowledge** of exercise principles (prescription, progression/maintenance, and supervision) for apparently healthy participants and participants with cardiovascular, pulmonary, and/or metabolic diseases<br>**Knowledge** of appropriate mode, volume, and intensity of exercise to produce desired outcomes for apparently healthy participants and those with cardiovascular, pulmonary, and metabolic diseases<br>**Knowledge** of the application of metabolic calculations<br>**Knowledge** of goal development strategies | • Understand the acute and chronic responses and adaptations exercise has on the body. These include the cardiorespiratory responses, metabolic, and neuromuscular responses and muscular fatigue.<br>• Understanding of FITT-VP principles and how to manipulate each principle to achieve desired exercise volume and response<br>• Understanding of how diagnostic testing and medical regimens/procedures can assess clinical progression of disease and/or exercise effects<br>• Understanding of deconditioning effects of bed rest and inactivity on the various body systems (*e.g.*, cardiovascular, pulmonary, muscular)<br>• Metabolic energy equivalent (MET) requirements for various physical activities; arm vs. leg exercise differences in hemodynamics; volume of oxygen consumed per unit of time ($\dot{V}O_2$); myocardial oxygen consumption; neuromuscular, vascular, and metabolic adaptations; muscle hypertrophy<br>• Knowledge of absolute and relative contraindications to exercise and abnormal responses/signs and symptoms for cardiovascular, pulmonary, and metabolic disease stated<br>• Five factor model of personality, transtheoretical model, *Diagnostic and Statistical Manual of Mental Disorders* (*DSM*), classes of mood disorders, subtypes of anxiety disorders<br>• Knowledge of parameters of exercise test modalities, test protocols, disease diagnosis, severity and prognosis, functional testing, and return-to-work testing<br>• Clinical understanding of absolute and relative indications for terminating exercise testing<br>• One repetition maximum bench press and leg press, push-up test, curl up (crunch test), Young Men's Christian Association (YMCA) bench press test, sit and reach (trunk flexion), range of motion in select single joints<br>• Understanding medications' normal and abnormal effects on resting and exercise cardiovascular, pulmonary, and metabolic diseases | *ACSM's Resource Manual for Guidelines for Exercise Testing and Prescription*, 7th edition (7)<br>• Chapter 3<br>*ACSM's Guidelines for Exercise Testing and Prescription* (GETP), 9th edition (6)<br>• Chapter 7<br>*ACSM's Resource Manual for Guidelines for Exercise Testing and Prescription*, 7th edition (7)<br>• Chapters 6–8 and 24–26<br>*ACSM's Resource Manual for Guidelines for Exercise Testing and Prescription*, 7th edition (7)<br>• Chapter 5<br>*ACSM's Resource Manual for Guidelines for Exercise Testing and Prescription*, 7th edition (7)<br>• Chapter 3<br>*ACSM's Guidelines for Exercise Testing and Prescription* (GETP), 9th edition (6)<br>• Chapter 2<br>*ACSM's Resource Manual for Guidelines for Exercise Testing and Prescription*, 7th edition (7)<br>• Chapters 16 and 17<br>*ACSM's Guidelines for Exercise Testing and Prescription* (GETP), 9th edition (6)<br>• Chapter 5<br>*ACSM's Guidelines for Exercise Testing and Prescription* (GETP), 9th edition (6)<br>• Chapter 5<br>*ACSM's Guidelines for Exercise Testing and Prescription* (GETP), 9th edition (6)<br>• Chapter 4<br>*ACSM's Guidelines for Exercise Testing and Prescription* (GETP), 9th edition (6)<br>• Appendix A<br>*ACSM's Guidelines for Exercise Testing and Prescription* (GETP), 9th edition (6)<br>• Chapters 7–10 |

## A. Develop a clinically appropriate exercise prescription using all available information (*e.g.*, clinical and physiological status, goals, and behavioral assessment). (cont.)

| Knowledge or Skill Statement | Explanation/Examples | Resources |
|---|---|---|
| **Knowledge** of behavioral assessment tools (*e.g.*, SF-36, health-related quality of life, Chronic Respiratory Disease Questionnaire) and strategies for use **Knowledge** of psychological issues associated with acute and chronic illness (*e.g.*, anxiety, depression, social isolation, suicidal ideation) | • Knowledge of the FITT-VP principle and the components of a single exercise session: warm-up, stretching, conditioning phase (or sports-related exercise) and cool-down <br> • Exercise program design specific to the individual (novice vs. advanced exerciser) and their goals; exercise program design to help manage chronic disease (hypertension, diabetes, dyslipidemia, obesity, asthma, chronic obstructive pulmonary disease [COPD], etc.) <br> • Understanding how to calculate and apply $\dot{V}O_2$ equations for walking, running, leg cycling, arm cranking, and stepping <br> • Set goals that are specific, measurable and challenging but realistic (*e.g.*, specific, measurable, attainable, realistic, and time-bound [SMART] goals). <br> • Application of health-related quality-of-life, their target populations, strategies for their use, and how results may affect exercise prescription <br> • Know how these conditions may affect exercise program adherence and motivation; social support groups; referral to other health care professionals. | *ACSM's Guidelines for Exercise Testing and Prescription* (GETP), 9th edition (6) <br> • Chapters 7–10 <br> *ACSM's Metabolic Calculations Handbook* (3) <br> *ACSM's Resource Manual for Guidelines for Exercise Testing and Prescription*, 7th edition (7) <br> • Chapter 46 <br> *ACSM's Resource Manual for Guidelines for Exercise Testing and Prescription*, 7th edition (7) <br> • Chapters 16 and 17 <br> *ACSM's Resource Manual for Guidelines for Exercise Testing and Prescription*, 7th edition (7) <br> • Chapters 16 and 17 |
| **Skill** in interpretation of functional and diagnostic exercise testing with applications to exercise prescription <br> **Skill** in interpretation of muscular strength/endurance testing with applications to exercise prescription <br> **Skill** in developing an exercise prescription based on a participant's clinical status | • Design and implement an exercise program that is safe and effective for the individual based on their functional ability, risk classification, and known risk factors/disease(s). <br> • Design and implement a resistance training program that is safe and effective for the individual based on their functional ability, risk classification, and known risk factors/disease(s). <br> • Develop an exercise program that is safe for the individual based on their clinical status yet effective to manage/treat their risk factors/disease(s). | *ACSM's Resource Manual for Guidelines for Exercise Testing and Prescription*, 7th edition (7) <br> • Chapters 23–26 and 37–41 <br> *ACSM's Guidelines for Exercise Testing and Prescription* (GETP), 9th edition (6) <br> • Chapters 4 and 7–10 <br> *ACSM's Guidelines for Exercise Testing and Prescription* (GETP), 9th edition (6) <br> • Chapters 9 and 10 |

**B.** Review the exercise prescription and exercise program with the participant, including home exercise, compliance, and participant's expectations and goals.

| Knowledge or Skill Statement | Explanation/Examples | Resources |
|---|---|---|
| **Knowledge** of applied exercise physiology principles<br>**Knowledge** of normal physiologic responses to exercise<br>**Knowledge** of abnormal responses/signs and symptoms to exercise associated with different pathologies (*e.g.*, cardiovascular, pulmonary, metabolic)<br>**Knowledge** of anthropometric measurements and their interpretation<br>**Knowledge** of participant-centered goal setting<br>**Knowledge** of exercise principles (prescription, progression/maintenance, and supervision) for apparently healthy participants and participants with cardiovascular, pulmonary, and/or metabolic diseases<br>**Knowledge** of the frequency, intensity, time, and type (FITT) principle for cardiovascular, muscular fitness/resistance training, and flexibility exercise prescription<br>**Knowledge** of appropriate mode, volume, and intensity of exercise to produce desired outcomes for apparently healthy participants and those with cardiovascular, pulmonary, and metabolic diseases<br>**Knowledge** of the application of metabolic calculations<br>**Knowledge** of goal development strategies<br>**Knowledge** of terminology appropriate to provide the client with education regarding their exercise prescription<br>**Knowledge** of instructional techniques for safe and effective prescription implementation and understanding by participant<br>**Knowledge** of the timing of daily activities with exercise (*e.g.*, medications, meals, insulin/glucose monitoring)<br>**Knowledge** of disease-specific strategies and tools to improve tolerance of exercise (*e.g.*, breathing techniques, insulin pump use and adjustments, prophylactic nitroglycerin)<br>**Knowledge** of instructional strategies for improving exercise adoption and maintenance | • Understand the acute and chronic responses and adaptations exercise has on the body. These include the cardiorespiratory responses, neuromuscular responses, and muscular fatigue.<br>• Metabolic energy equivalent (MET) requirements for various physical activities; arm vs. leg exercise differences in hemodynamics; volume of oxygen consumed per unit of time ($\dot{V}O_2$); myocardial oxygen consumption; neuromuscular adaptations; muscle hypertrophy<br>• Knowledge of absolute and relative contraindications to exercise and abnormal responses/signs and symptoms for cardiovascular, pulmonary, and metabolic disease stated<br>• Body mass index (BMI), circumferences, skinfold measurements, hydrodensitometry, dual-energy x-ray absorptiometry, bioimpedance and their clinical significance<br>• Set goals that are specific, measurable, and challenging but realistic (*e.g.*, specific, measurable, attainable, realistic, and time-bound [SMART] goals)<br>• Knowledge of the FITT-VP principle and the components of a single exercise session: warm-up, stretching, conditioning phase (or sports-related exercise), and cool-down<br>• Understanding of FITT-VP principles and how manipulation of each affects the exercise prescription for cardiovascular strength/endurance, muscular fitness/resistance training, and flexibility<br>• Exercise program design specific to the individual (novice vs. advanced exerciser) and their goals; exercise program design to help manage chronic disease (hypertension, diabetes, dyslipidemia, obesity, asthma, chronic obstructive pulmonary disorder [COPD], etc.)<br>• Knowledge of calculating $\dot{V}O_2$/MET equations for walking, running, leg cycling, arm cranking, and stepping to design the exercise program based on the patient's ability (*e.g.*, MET level)<br>• Set goals that are specific, measurable, and challenging but realistic (*e.g.*, SMART goals). | *ACSM's Resource Manual for Guidelines for Exercise Testing and Prescription*, 7th edition (7)<br>• Chapter 3<br>*ACSM's Resource Manual for Guidelines for Exercise Testing and Prescription*, 7th edition (7)<br>• Chapter 3<br>*ACSM's Guidelines for Exercise Testing and Prescription* (GETP), 9th edition (6)<br>• Chapter 2<br>*ACSM's Guidelines for Exercise Testing and Prescription* (GETP), 9th edition (6)<br>• Chapter 4<br>*ACSM's Resource Manual for Guidelines for Exercise Testing and Prescription*, 7th edition (7)<br>• Chapter 46<br>*ACSM's Guidelines for Exercise Testing and Prescription* (GETP), 9th edition (6)<br>• Chapters 7–10<br>*ACSM's Guidelines for Exercise Testing and Prescription* (GETP), 9th edition (6)<br>• Chapter 7<br>"Pulmonary Rehabilitation: Joint ACCP/AACVPR Evidence-Based Guidelines" (9)<br>*ACSM's Guidelines for Exercise Testing and Prescription* (GETP), 9th edition (6)<br>• Chapters 7–10<br>*ACSM's Metabolic Calculations Handbook* (3)<br>*ACSM's Resource Manual for Guidelines for Exercise Testing and Prescription*, 7th edition (7)<br>• Chapter 46<br>*ACSM's Guidelines for Exercise Testing and Prescription* (GETP), 9th edition (6)<br>• Appendix A<br>*ACSM's Resource Manual for Guidelines for Exercise Testing and Prescription*, 7th edition (7)<br>• Chapters 19 and 40 |

## B. Review the exercise prescription and exercise program with the participant, including home exercise, compliance, and participant's expectations and goals. (cont.)

| Knowledge or Skill Statement | Explanation/Examples | Resources |
| --- | --- | --- |
| **Knowledge** of common barriers to exercise compliance and strategies to address these (*e.g.*, physical, psychological, environmental, demographic)<br>**Knowledge** of instructional techniques to assess participant's expectations and goals<br>**Knowledge** of risk factor reduction programs and alternative community resources (*e.g.*, dietary counseling, weight management/Weight Watchers, smoking cessation, stress management, physical therapy/back care) | • Ability to educate individuals on a practical level. Avoid "technical" terms and choose basic terms (*e.g.*, chest instead of pectoralis major).<br>• Communicating to participant via various methods (*e.g.*, verbal, visual, written), proper technique, theory, and rational for implementation of an effective exercise prescription<br>• Optimal times to exercise with relation to eating and blood sugar (energy levels), medication peak times and their effects on exercise performance, insulin use/injection site recommendations, evening exercise, and hypoglycemia risk<br>• Be able to respond/recommend the appropriate strategy to maximize exercise safety and the conditioning effect and minimize any adverse reactions.<br>• Patient education on the benefits of exercise specific to the patient; developing exercise programs that meet the needs of the patient; patient-centered approaches that consider the patient's priorities, risk factors, and psychosocial status<br>• Develop patient-centered strategies to overcome exercise barriers.<br>• Set goals that are specific, measurable, and challenging but realistic (*e.g.*, SMART goals).<br>• Be familiar with various programs and services that assist with improving cardiac, pulmonary, and metabolic health. | *ACSM's Resource Manual for Guidelines for Exercise Testing and Prescription*, 7th edition (7)<br>• Chapter 46<br>*ACSM's Resource Manual for Guidelines for Exercise Testing and Prescription*, 7th edition (7)<br>• Chapter 35 |
| **Skill** in communicating with participants from a wide variety of educational backgrounds<br>**Skill** in effectively communicating exercise prescription and exercise techniques<br>**Skill** in applying various models to optimize patient compliance and adherence in order to achieve patient goals | • Practice communicating in a way that the patient will understand and will not be intimidated.<br>• Describe/explain the exercise program so the patient will understand what they are doing and why.<br>• Consider personal factors, behavioral factors, enjoyment, incentives, social support, environmental factors, conveniences, etc. | *ACSM's Resource Manual for Guidelines for Exercise Testing and Prescription*, 7th edition (7)<br>• Chapter 47<br>*ACSM's Resource Manual for Guidelines for Exercise Testing and Prescription*, 7th edition (7)<br>• Chapter 47<br>*ACSM's Resource Manual for Guidelines for Exercise Testing and Prescription*, 7th edition (7)<br>• Chapter 45 |

## C. Instruct the participant in the safe and effective use of exercise modalities, exercise plan, reporting symptoms, and class organization.

| Knowledge or Skill Statement | Explanation/Examples | Resources |
|---|---|---|
| **Knowledge** of applied exercise physiology principles<br>**Knowledge** of normal physiologic responses to exercise<br>**Knowledge** of abnormal responses/ signs and symptoms to exercise associated with different pathologies (*e.g.*, cardiovascular, pulmonary, metabolic)<br>**Knowledge** of the timing of daily activities with exercise (*e.g.*, medications, meals, insulin/glucose monitoring)<br>**Knowledge** of commonly used medication for cardiovascular, pulmonary, and metabolic diseases<br>**Knowledge** of lay terminology for explanation of exercise prescription<br>**Knowledge** of the operation of various exercise equipment/modalities<br>**Knowledge** of proper biomechanical technique for exercise (*e.g.*, gait assessment, proper weightlifting form)<br>**Knowledge** of muscle strength/ endurance and flexibility modalities and their safe application and instruction<br>**Knowledge** of tools to measure exercise tolerance (heart rate/pulse, blood pressure, glucometry, oximetry, rating of perceived exertion, dyspnea scale, pain scale)<br>**Knowledge** of principles and application of exercise session organization | • Understand the acute and chronic responses and adaptations exercise has on the body. These include the cardiorespiratory responses, neuromuscular responses, and muscular fatigue.<br>• Metabolic energy equivalent (MET) requirements for various physical activities; arm vs. leg exercise differences in hemodynamics; volume of oxygen consumed per unit of time ($\dot{V}O_2$); myocardial oxygen consumption; neuromuscular adaptations; muscle hypertrophy<br>• Knowledge of absolute and relative contraindications to exercise and abnormal responses/signs and symptoms for cardiovascular, pulmonary, and metabolic disease stated<br>• Optimal times to exercise with relation to eating and blood sugar (energy levels), medication peak times and their effects on exercise performance, insulin use/ injection site recommendations, evening exercise, and hypoglycemia risk<br>• Understanding medications' normal and abnormal effects on resting and exercise cardiovascular, pulmonary, and metabolic diseases<br>• Ability to educate individuals on a practical level. Avoid "technical" terms and choose basic terms (*e.g.*, chest instead of pectoralis major).<br>• Be familiar with equipment settings and adjustments; demonstrate proper technique; know common errors when using various exercise modalities.<br>• Knowledge of proper anatomical positioning to aerobic and resistance training modalities<br>• Be familiar with numerous resistance training exercises and stretches, their proper applications, and common mistakes.<br>• Understand how to use and interpret these tools; know how the measurements relate to exercise tolerance (*e.g.*, blood glucose readings that are too low or too high for exercise).<br>• Warm-up, stretching, conditioning exercise, cool-down | *ACSM's Resource Manual for Guidelines for Exercise Testing and Prescription*, 7th edition (7)<br>• Chapter 3<br>*ACSM's Resource Manual for Guidelines for Exercise Testing and Prescription*, 7th edition (7)<br>• Chapter 3<br>*ACSM's Guidelines for Exercise Testing and Prescription* (GETP), 9th edition (6)<br>• Chapter 2<br>*ACSM's Guidelines for Exercise Testing and Prescription* (GETP), 9th edition (6)<br>• Chapter 10<br>• Appendix A<br>*ACSM's Guidelines for Exercise Testing and Prescription* (GETP), 9th edition (6)<br>• Appendix A<br>*ACSM's Resource Manual for Guidelines for Exercise Testing and Prescription*, 7th edition (7)<br>• Chapters 38–40<br>*ACSM's Resource Manual for Guidelines for Exercise Testing and Prescription*, 7th edition (7)<br>• Chapter 2<br>*Essentials of Strength Training and Conditioning*, 3rd edition (13)<br>• Chapters 13 and 14<br>*ACSM's Guidelines for Exercise Testing and Prescription* (GETP), 9th edition (6)<br>• Chapters 4, 5, and 10<br>*ACSM's Guidelines for Exercise Testing and Prescription* (GETP), 9th edition (6)<br>• Chapter 7 |

## C. Instruct the participant in the safe and effective use of exercise modalities, exercise plan, reporting symptoms, and class organization. (cont.)

| Knowledge or Skill Statement | Explanation/Examples | Resources |
|---|---|---|
| **Skill** in the observational assessment of participants<br>**Skill** in communicating with participants from a wide variety of educational backgrounds<br>**Skill** in communicating with participants regarding the proper organization of exercise sessions | • Ability to assess a patient's exercise technique, posture, movements, balance, etc<br>• Communicate in a way that the patient will understand and will not be intimidated.<br>• Describe/explain the exercise program so the patient will understand what they are doing and why. | *ACSM's Resource Manual for Guidelines for Exercise Testing and Prescription*, 7th edition (7)<br>• Chapter 47<br>*ACSM's Resource Manual for Guidelines for Exercise Testing and Prescription*, 7th edition (7)<br>• Chapter 47 |

# DOMAIN III: PROGRAM IMPLEMENTATION AND ONGOING SUPPORT

## A. Implement the program (*e.g.*, exercise prescription, education, counseling, and goals).

| Knowledge or Skill Statement | Explanation/Examples | Resources |
|---|---|---|
| **Knowledge** of abnormal responses/signs and symptoms to exercise associated with different pathologies (*i.e.*, cardiovascular, pulmonary, metabolic)<br>**Knowledge** of normal and abnormal 12-lead and telemetry electrocardiogram (ECG) interpretation<br>**Knowledge** of the frequency, intensity, time, and type (FITT) principle for cardiovascular, muscular fitness/resistance training, and flexibility exercise prescription<br>**Knowledge** of exercise progression/maintenance and supervision for apparently healthy participants and participants with cardiovascular, pulmonary, and/or metabolic diseases<br>**Knowledge** of disease-specific strategies and tools to improve tolerance of exercise (*e.g.*, breathing techniques, insulin pump use and adjustments, prophylactic nitroglycerin)<br>**Knowledge** of instructional strategies for improving exercise adoption and maintenance<br>**Knowledge** of strategies to maximize exercise compliance (*e.g.*, overcoming barriers, values clarification, goals setting)<br>**Knowledge** of the operation of various exercise equipment/modalities<br>**Knowledge** of proper biomechanical technique for exercise (*e.g.*, gait, weightlifting form) | • Knowledge of absolute and relative contraindications to exercise and abnormal responses/signs and symptoms for cardiovascular, pulmonary, and metabolic disease stated<br>• Determine and identify normal resting ECG, normal changes with ECG during exercise, abnormal ECG changes during exercise, and identify various arrhythmias.<br>• Clinical understanding of the FITT-VP principle and how to manipulate it based on changes in participants' disease status, progression/regression, maintenance, and supervision<br>• Knowledge and clinical understanding of the effect of participants disease status (cardiovascular, pulmonary, and/or metabolic) on exercise progression/maintenance and supervision<br>• Be able to respond/recommend the appropriate strategy to maximize exercise safety and the conditioning effect and minimize any adverse reactions.<br>• Patient education on the benefits of exercise specific to the patient; developing exercise programs that meet the needs of the patient; patient-centered approaches that consider the patient's priorities, risk factors, and psychosocial status<br>• Develop patient-centered strategies to overcome exercise barriers; develop specific, measurable, attainable, realistic, and time-bound (SMART) goals with the patient; consider what is most important to the patient. | *ACSM's Guidelines for Exercise Testing and Prescription* (GETP), 9th edition (6)<br>• Chapter 2<br>"Position Stand: Exercise and Hypertension" (4)<br>*ACSM's Resource Manual for Guidelines for Exercise Testing and Prescription*, 7th edition (7)<br>• Chapter 29<br>*ACSM's Guidelines for Exercise Testing and Prescription* (GETP), 9th edition (6)<br>• Chapter 7<br>*ACSM's Guidelines for Exercise Testing and Prescription* (GETP), 9th edition (6)<br>• Chapters 7 and 10<br>*ACSM's Resource Manual for Guidelines for Exercise Testing and Prescription*, 7th edition (7)<br>• Chapters 19 and 40<br>*ACSM's Resource Manual for Guidelines for Exercise Testing and Prescription*, 7th edition (7)<br>• Chapter 46<br>*ACSM's Resource Manual for Guidelines for Exercise Testing and Prescription*, 7th edition (7)<br>• Chapters 38–40<br>*ACSM's Resource Manual for Guidelines for Exercise Testing and Prescription*, 7th edition (7)<br>• Chapter 2 |

## A. Implement the program (*e.g.*, exercise prescription, education, counseling, and goals). (cont.)

| Knowledge or Skill Statement | Explanation/Examples | Resources |
|---|---|---|
| **Knowledge** of tools to measure clinical exercise tolerance (*e.g.*, heart rate, glucometry, oximetry, subjective assessments) **Knowledge** of the principles and application of exercise session organization **Knowledge** of commonly used medications for cardiovascular, pulmonary, and metabolic diseases **Knowledge** of exercise program monitoring (*e.g.*, telemetry, oximetry, glucometry) **Knowledge** of principles and application of muscular strength/ endurance and flexibility training **Knowledge** of methods to assess participant's educational goals **Knowledge** of counseling techniques to optimize participant's disease management, risk reduction, and goal attainment | • Be familiar with equipment settings and adjustments; demonstrate proper technique; know common errors when using various exercise modalities. <br>• Knowledge of proper anatomical positioning to aerobic and resistance training modalities <br>• Understand how to use and interpret these tools; know how the measurements relate to exercise tolerance (*e.g.*, blood glucose readings that are too low or too high for exercise). <br>• Warm-up, stretching, conditioning exercise, cool-down <br>• Understanding medications' normal and abnormal effects on resting and exercise cardiovascular, pulmonary, and metabolic diseases <br>• Knowledge and clinical understanding of various exercise monitoring tools/techniques with specific attention to individual patient safety parameters <br>• Understanding of various resistance exercises and stretches: understand proper technique, body alignment and posture, muscles/joints involved, and common mistakes. <br>• Knowledge and understanding of various methods (*e.g.*, questionnaires, surveys, tests) to assess participants educational goals/needs <br>• Establish rapport, show interest and empathy, listen actively, then provide information and advice. | *ACSM's Guidelines for Exercise Testing and Prescription* (GETP), 9th edition (6) <br>• Chapters 4, 5, and 10 <br>*ACSM's Guidelines for Exercise Testing and Prescription* (GETP), 9th edition (6) <br>• Chapter 7 <br>*ACSM's Guidelines for Exercise Testing and Prescription* (GETP), 9th edition (6) <br>• Appendix A <br>*ACSM's Resource Manual for Guidelines for Exercise Testing and Prescription*, 7th edition (7) <br>• Chapter 29 <br>*ACSM's Guidelines for Exercise Testing and Prescription* (GETP), 9th edition (6) <br>• Chapters 9 and 10 <br>*ACSM's Guidelines for Exercise Testing and Prescription* (GETP), 9th edition (6) <br>• Chapter 7 <br>*Essentials of Strength Training and Conditioning*, 3rd edition (13) <br>• Chapters 13 and 14 <br>*ACSM's Resource Manual for Guidelines for Exercise Testing and Prescription*, 7th edition (7) <br>• Chapter 46 |
| **Skill** in educating participants on the use and effects of medications **Skill** in the application of metabolic calculations **Skill** in communicating the exercise prescription and related exercise programming techniques **Skill** in observation of clients for problems associated with comprehension and performance of their exercise program **Skill** in muscular strength/endurance and flexibility training | • Provide patients with an understanding of how their medications work, what the benefits are, and the importance of medication compliance; speak to the patient in lay terms. <br>• Knowledge of calculating ($\dot{V}O_2$)/metabolic energy equivalent (MET) equations for walking, running, leg cycling, arm cranking, and stepping to design the exercise program based on the patient's ability (*e.g.*, MET level) <br>• Describe/explain the exercise program so the patient will understand what they are doing and why. <br>• Ask for patient feedback to ensure they understand what they are doing and how to do it; follow up with observation; re-educate when necessary. <br>• Understanding of various resistance exercises and stretches: practice proper technique, body alignment, and posture; be familiar with muscles/joints involved and common mistakes. | *ACSM's Guidelines for Exercise Testing and Prescription* (GETP), 9th edition (6) <br>• Appendix A <br>*ACSM's Metabolic Calculations Handbook* (3) <br>*ACSM's Resource Manual for Guidelines for Exercise Testing and Prescription*, 7th edition (7) <br>• Chapter 47 <br>*ACSM's Guidelines for Exercise Testing and Prescription* (GETP), 9th edition (6) <br>• Chapter 7 <br>*Essentials of Strength Training and Conditioning*, 3rd edition (13) <br>• Chapters 13 and 14 |

**B.  Continually assess participant feedback, clinical signs and symptoms, and exercise tolerance, and provide feedback to the participant about their exercise, general program participation, and clinical progress.**

| Knowledge or Skill Statement | Explanation/Examples | Resources |
|---|---|---|
| **Knowledge** of cardiovascular, pulmonary, and metabolic pathologies; their clinical progression; diagnostic testing; and medical regimens/procedures to treat<br>**Knowledge** of normal and abnormal exercise responses and signs and symptoms associated with different pathologies (*i.e.*, cardiovascular, pulmonary, metabolic)<br>**Knowledge** of normal and abnormal 12-lead and telemetry ECG interpretation<br>**Knowledge** of normal and abnormal heart and lung sounds<br>**Knowledge** of the components of a participant's medical history necessary to screen during program participation<br>**Knowledge** of appropriate mode, volume, and intensity of exercise to produce desired outcomes for apparently healthy participants and those with cardiovascular, pulmonary, and metabolic diseases<br>**Knowledge** of psychological issues associated with acute and chronic illness (*e.g.*, depression, social isolation, suicidal ideation)<br>**Knowledge** of the timing of daily activities with exercise (*e.g.*, medications, meals, insulin/glucose monitoring)<br>**Knowledge** of how medications or missed dose(s) of medications impact exercise and its progression<br>**Knowledge** of methods to provide participant feedback relative to their exercise, general program participation, and clinical progress | • Understanding of how diagnostic testing and medical regimens/procedures can assess clinical progression of disease and/or effects of exercise<br>• Knowledge of absolute and relative contraindications to exercise and abnormal responses/signs and symptoms for cardiovascular, pulmonary, and metabolic disease stated<br>• Know the anatomical landmarks for electrocardiogram (ECG) lead placement and skill to identify/minimize artifact, identify normal resting ECG and exercise ECG changes and know/identify dangerous arrhythmias.<br>• Understand the clinical descriptions and auscultation sounds for normal and abnormal heart and lung sounds.<br>• Knowledge of and interpretation of established exercise screening tools (*e.g.*, Physical Activity Readiness Questionnaire [PAR-Q], American Heart Association (AHA)/American College of Sports Medicine (ACSM) Health/Fitness Facility Participation Screening Questionnaire) and individual medical history for program participation<br>• Exercise program design specific to the individual (novice vs. advanced exerciser) and their goals; exercise program design to help manage chronic disease (hypertension, diabetes, dyslipidemia, obesity, asthma, chronic obstructive pulmonary disease [COPD], etc.)<br>• Know how these conditions may affect exercise adherence and motivation; social support groups; referral to other health care professionals.<br>• Optimal times to exercise in relation to eating and blood sugar (energy levels), medication peak times and their effects on exercise performance, insulin use/injection site recommendations, evening exercise, and hypoglycemia risk<br>• Understand the dangers of missed doses of medication and the possible effects on exercise participation<br>• Make necessary adjustments to the patients exercise program based on feedback (*e.g.*, increase exercise variety) for optimal outcomes | *Guidelines for Cardiac Rehabilitation and Secondary Prevention Programs*, 4th edition (8)<br>• Chapter 9<br>*ACSM's Guidelines for Exercise Testing and Prescription* (GETP), 9th edition (6)<br>• Chapter 2<br>*ACSM's Resource Manual for Guidelines for Exercise Testing and Prescription*, 7th edition (7)<br>• Chapter 29<br>*ACSM's Resource Manual for Guidelines for Exercise Testing and Prescription*, 7th edition (7)<br>• Chapter 24<br>*ACSM's Guidelines for Exercise Testing and Prescription* (GETP), 9th edition (6)<br>• Chapter 2<br>*ACSM's Guidelines for Exercise Testing and Prescription* (GETP), 9th edition (6)<br>• Chapters 7–10<br>*ACSM's Resource Manual for Guidelines for Exercise Testing and Prescription*, 7th edition (7)<br>• Chapters 16 and 17<br>*ACSM's Guidelines for Exercise Testing and Prescription* (GETP), 9th edition (6)<br>• Chapter 10<br>• Appendix A<br>*ACSM's Guidelines for Exercise Testing and Prescription* (GETP), 9th edition (6)<br>• Appendix A<br>*ACSM's Resource Manual for Guidelines for Exercise Testing and Prescription*, 7th edition (7)<br>• Chapter 46 |

**B. Continually assess participant feedback, clinical signs and symptoms, and exercise tolerance, and provide feedback to the participant about their exercise, general program participation, and clinical progress. (cont.)**

| Knowledge or Skill Statement | Explanation/Examples | Resources |
|---|---|---|
| **Skill** in auscultation methods for common cardiovascular and pulmonary abnormalities<br>**Skill** in the assessment of normal and abnormal response to exercise<br>**Skill** in adjusting the exercise program based on participant's signs and symptoms, feedback, and exercise response<br>**Skill** in communicating exercise techniques, program goals, and clinical monitoring and progress<br>**Skill** in applying and interpreting tools for clinical assessment (*e.g.*, telemetry, oximetry and glucometry, perceived rating scales) | • Evaluate arteries for adequate pulses and bruits, lungs for emphysema, the heart for heart failure, murmurs, etc.<br>• Identify any of the nine major symptoms of cardiovascular, pulmonary, or metabolic disease; identify normal responses to exercise (*e.g.*, heart rate, blood pressure, respirations, peripheral fatigue, etc.)<br>• Make necessary adjustments to the patients' exercise program based on feedback for optimal outcomes and safety (*e.g.*, reduce or increase exercise intensity or duration).<br>• Educate the patients in lay terminology on proper exercise technique, setting realistic goals, and how you assess their progress.<br>• Understand the practice and use of these tools for measurements related to exercise tolerance (*e.g.*, blood glucose readings that are too low or too high for exercise, exercise intensity based on rating of perceived exertion [RPE] scales). | *ACSM's Resource Manual for Guidelines for Exercise Testing and Prescription*, 7th edition (7)<br>• Chapters 24 and 25<br>*ACSM's Resource Manual for Guidelines for Exercise Testing and Prescription*, 7th edition (7)<br>• Chapter 3<br>*ACSM's Guidelines for Exercise Testing and Prescription* (GETP), 9th edition (6)<br>• Chapter 2<br>*ACSM's Resource Manual for Guidelines for Exercise Testing and Prescription*, 7th edition (7)<br>• Chapter 46<br>*ACSM's Resource Manual for Guidelines for Exercise Testing and Prescription*, 7th edition (7)<br>• Chapters 46 and 47<br>*ACSM's Resource Manual for Guidelines for Exercise Testing and Prescription*, 7th edition (7)<br>• Chapter 29<br>*ACSM's Guidelines for Exercise Testing and Prescription* (GETP), 9th edition (6)<br>• Chapters 9 and 10 |

**C. Reassess and update the program (*e.g.*, exercise, education, and client goals) based on the participant's progress and feedback.**

| Knowledge or Skill Statement | Explanation/Examples | Resources |
|---|---|---|
| **Knowledge** of techniques to determine participant's medical history through available documentation<br>**Knowledge** of normal physiologic responses to exercise<br>**Knowledge** of abnormal responses/signs and symptoms to exercise associated with different pathologies (*e.g.*, cardiovascular, pulmonary, metabolic)<br>**Knowledge** of participant's educational and behavioral goals and methods to obtain them<br>**Knowledge** of counseling techniques focusing on participant goal attainment<br>**Knowledge** of exercise progression/maintenance and supervision for apparently healthy participants and participants with cardiovascular, pulmonary, and/or metabolic diseases | • Self-guided, professionally guided screenings for physical activity; risk stratify<br>• Know the normal responses to exercise (*e.g.*, heart rate, blood pressure, respirations, peripheral fatigue, etc.).<br>• Knowledge of absolute and relative contraindications to exercise and abnormal responses/signs and symptoms for cardiovascular, pulmonary, and metabolic disease states<br>• Active listening, ask open-ended questions, clarify and summarize their statements<br>• Establish rapport, show interest and empathy, listen actively, provide information and advice; help set specific, measurable, attainable, realistic, and time-bound (SMART) goals. | *ACSM's Guidelines for Exercise Testing and Prescription* (GETP), 9th edition (6)<br>• Chapter 2<br>*ACSM's Resource Manual for Guidelines for Exercise Testing and Prescription*, 7th edition (7)<br>• Chapter 3<br>*ACSM's Guidelines for Exercise Testing and Prescription* (GETP), 9th edition (6)<br>• Chapter 2<br>*ACSM's Resource Manual for Guidelines for Exercise Testing and Prescription*, 7th edition (7)<br>• Chapter 46 |

CES

## C. Reassess and update the program (*e.g.*, exercise, education, and client goals) based on the participant's progress and feedback. (cont.)

| Knowledge or Skill Statement | Explanation/Examples | Resources |
|---|---|---|
| **Knowledge** of appropriate mode, volume, and intensity of exercise to produce desired outcomes for apparently healthy participants and those with cardiovascular, pulmonary, and metabolic diseases<br>**Knowledge** of strategies to maximize exercise compliance (*e.g.*, overcoming barriers, values clarification, goals setting)<br>**Knowledge** of risk factor reduction programs and alternative community resources (*e.g.*, dietary counseling/Weight Watchers, smoking cessation, physical therapy/back care)<br>**Knowledge** of proper biomechanical technique for exercise (*e.g.*, gait, weightlifting form)<br>**Knowledge** of clinical monitoring of the exercise program (*e.g.*, telemetry, oximetry and glucometry, adjusting exercise intensity)<br>**Knowledge** of commonly used medication for cardiovascular, pulmonary, and metabolic diseases<br>**Knowledge** of the application and instruction of muscle strength/endurance and flexibility modalities<br>**Knowledge** of modification of the exercise prescription for clinical changes and attainment of participant's goals<br>**Knowledge** of community resources available to the participant following discharge from the program | • Appropriate rate of progression based on health status, exercise tolerance, and exercise goals; monitor for adverse effects once when exercises are progressed; know recommendations to enhance exercise adherence<br>• Exercise program design specific to the individual (novice vs. advanced exerciser) and their goals and desired physiological outcome; exercise program design to help manage chronic disease (hypertension, diabetes, dyslipidemia, obesity, asthma, chronic obstructive pulmonary disease [COPD], etc.)<br>• Develop patient-centered strategies to overcome exercise barriers; develop SMART goals with the patient; consider what is most important to the patient.<br>• Be familiar with various methods of improving cardiac, pulmonary, and metabolic health.<br>• Knowledge of proper anatomical positioning to aerobic and resistance training modalities<br>• Knowledge and clinical understanding of various exercise monitoring tools/techniques to establish exercise programming with attention to individual patient safety parameters<br>• Understanding medications' normal and abnormal effects on resting and exercise cardiovascular, pulmonary, and metabolic diseases<br>• For various resistance exercises and stretches: understand proper technique, body alignment and posture, muscles/joints involved, and common mistakes.<br>• Make necessary adjustments to the patients' exercise program based on feedback and exercise responses for optimal outcomes and safety (*e.g.*, reduce or increase exercise intensity or duration).<br>• Help facilitate a smooth transition from rehabilitation to continuing health behavior changes (*e.g.*, joining a fitness club, social support groups). | *ACSM's Resource Manual for Guidelines for Exercise Testing and Prescription*, 7th edition (7)<br>• Chapter 46<br>*ACSM's Guidelines for Exercise Testing and Prescription* (GETP), 9th edition (6)<br>• Chapters 7 and 10<br>*ACSM's Guidelines for Exercise Testing and Prescription* (GETP), 9th edition (6)<br>• Chapters 7 and 10<br>*ACSM's Resource Manual for Guidelines for Exercise Testing and Prescription*, 7th edition (7)<br>• Chapter 46<br>*ACSM's Resource Manual for Guidelines for Exercise Testing and Prescription*, 7th edition (7)<br>• Chapters 35 and 48<br>*ACSM's Resource Manual for Guidelines for Exercise Testing and Prescription*, 7th edition (7)<br>• Chapter 2<br>*ACSM's Resource Manual for Guidelines for Exercise Testing and Prescription*, 7th edition (7)<br>• Chapter 29<br>*ACSM's Guidelines for Exercise Testing and Prescription* (GETP), 9th edition (6)<br>• Chapters 9 and 10<br>"Resistance Exercise Update in Individuals With and Without Cardiovascular Disease: 2007 Update: A Scientific Statement from the American Heart Association" (15)<br>*ACSM's Guidelines for Exercise Testing and Prescription* (GETP), 9th edition (6)<br>• Appendix A<br>*ACSM's Guidelines for Exercise Testing and Prescription* (GETP), 9th edition (6)<br>• Chapter 7<br>*Essentials of Strength Training and Conditioning*, 3rd edition (13)<br>• Chapters 13 and 14<br>*ACSM's Resource Manual for Guidelines for Exercise Testing and Prescription*, 7th edition (7)<br>• Chapters 38–41 |

CES

## C. Reassess and update the program (*e.g.,* exercise, education, and client goals) based on the participant's progress and feedback. (cont.)

| Knowledge or Skill Statement | Explanation/Examples | Resources |
|---|---|---|
| **Skill** in modifying the exercise program based on participant's signs and symptoms, feedback, and exercise responses<br>**Skill** in using metabolic calculations and clinical data to adjust the exercise prescription<br>**Skill** in observation of participant for problems associated with comprehension and performance of their exercise program<br>**Skill** in communicating exercise techniques, program goals, and clinical monitoring and progress<br>**Skill** in applying and interpreting tools for clinical assessment (*e.g.,* telemetry, oximetry and glucometry, perceived rating scales) | • Exercise program modifications based on the patient's exercise tolerance, their likes/dislikes with the program, and their adaptations/responses to the program<br>• Practice adjusting exercise prescriptions to meet the physical abilities and desired energy expenditure (*e.g.,* current metabolic energy equivalent [MET] level) of the patient (*e.g.,* appropriate exercise mode, intensity level).<br>• Practice talking with the patient/obtaining patient feedback to ensure they understand the program, know proper exercise technique and understand progression; educate the patient in a manner that they understand, the principles of exercise (*e.g.,* FITT-VP), proper exercise technique, and the goals of the exercise program; and practice monitoring applicable clinical data (*e.g.,* electrocardiogram [ECG], blood pressure).<br>• Educate the patients in lay terminology on proper exercise technique, setting realistic goals, and how you assess their progress.<br>• Understand the practice and use of these tools for measurements related to exercise tolerance (*e.g.,* blood glucose readings that are too low or too high for exercise, exercise intensity based on rating of perceived exertion [RPE] scales). | *ACSM's Guidelines for Exercise Testing and Prescription* (GETP), 9th edition (6)<br>• Chapters 7 and 10<br>"Compendium of Physical Activities: An Update of Activity Codes and MET intensities" (1)<br>*ACSM's Resource Manual for Guidelines for Exercise Testing and Prescription*, 7th edition (7)<br>• Chapter 48<br>*ACSM's Resource Manual for Guidelines for Exercise Testing and Prescription*, 7th edition (7)<br>• Chapter 29<br>*ACSM's Guidelines for Exercise Testing and Prescription* (GETP), 9th edition (6)<br>• Chapters 9 and 10 |

## D.  Maintain participant records to document progress and clinical status.

| Knowledge or Skill Statement | Explanation/Examples | Resources |
| --- | --- | --- |
| **Knowledge** of participant's medical history through available documentation<br>**Knowledge** of cardiovascular, pulmonary, and metabolic pathologies; diagnostic testing; and medical management regimens and procedures<br>**Knowledge** of commonly used medication for cardiovascular, pulmonary, and metabolic diseases<br>**Knowledge** of Health Insurance Portability and Accountability Act (HIPAA) regulations relative to documentation<br>**Knowledge** of medical documentation (*e.g.*, progress notes, SOAP notes) | • Self-guided, professionally guided screenings for physical activity; risk stratification<br>• Understanding of how diagnostic testing and medical regimens/procedures can assess clinical status progression of disease<br>• Understanding medication effects on resting and exercise vitals; cardiovascular, pulmonary, and metabolic diseases as well as side effects<br>• Promotion of access for consumers to health insurance, privacy protection of health care data, standardize billing, and insurance claims processing in the health care industry<br>• Know how to document all data collected during assessments, testing and training, and goal setting; SOAP notes — subjective, objective, assessment, and plan. | *ACSM's Guidelines for Exercise Testing and Prescription* (GETP), 9th edition (6)<br>• Chapter 2<br>*ACSM's Resource Manual for Guidelines for Exercise Testing and Prescription*, 7th edition (7)<br>• Chapters 6–8 and 24–26<br>*ACSM's Guidelines for Exercise Testing and Prescription* (GETP), 9th edition (6)<br>• Appendix A<br>*Drugs for the Heart*, 6th edition (14)<br>*ACSM's Resource Manual for Guidelines for Exercise Testing and Prescription*, 7th edition (7)<br>• Chapter 10 |
| **Skill** in applying knowledge of medical documentation and regulations<br>**Skill** in summarizing participants' exercise sessions, outcomes, and clinical issues into an appropriate medical record | • Contract law, informed consent, Tort law, negligence, malpractice, standards of practice (*e.g.*, practice peer-developed guidelines, report incidents, communicate critical information in a timely manner)<br>• Practice documenting the details (mode, intensity, duration) of the exercises performed, any issues, abnormal responses, or significant findings during the session. | *ACSM's Resource Manual for Guidelines for Exercise Testing and Prescription*, 7th edition (7)<br>• Chapter 10 |

# DOMAIN IV: LEADERSHIP AND COUNSELING

## A.  Educate the participant about performance and progression of aerobic, strength, and flexibility exercise programs.

| Knowledge or Skill Statement | Explanation/Examples | Resources |
| --- | --- | --- |
| **Knowledge** of physiological responses and signs and symptoms to exercise associated with different pathologies (*i.e.*, cardiovascular, pulmonary, metabolic)<br>**Knowledge** of exercise (as written previously) principles (prescription, progression/maintenance, and supervision) for apparently healthy participants and participants with cardiovascular, pulmonary, and/or metabolic diseases<br>**Knowledge** of exercise progression, maintenance, and supervision for apparently healthy participants and participants with cardiovascular, pulmonary, and/or metabolic diseases | • Help the patient understand abnormal responses/signs and symptoms for cardiovascular, pulmonary, and metabolic disease.<br>• Explain the FITT-VP principle and the components of a single exercise session: warm-up, stretching, conditioning phase (or sports-related exercise), and cool-down; special exercise considerations for various clinical populations.<br>• Knowledge and use of the FITT-VP principle and components for exercise progression of various patient population | *ACSM's Guidelines for Exercise Testing and Prescription* (GETP), 9th edition (6)<br>• Chapter 2<br>*ACSM's Guidelines for Exercise Testing and Prescription* (GETP), 9th edition (6)<br>• Chapters 7–10<br>*ACSM's Guidelines for Exercise Testing and Prescription* (GETP), 9th edition (6)<br>• Chapters 4, 5, and 10 |

## A. Educate the participant about performance and progression of aerobic, strength, and flexibility exercise programs. (cont.)

| Knowledge or Skill Statement | Explanation/Examples | Resources |
|---|---|---|
| **Knowledge** of tools for measuring clinical exercise tolerance (*e.g.*, heart rate, glucometry, subjective rating scales) <br> **Knowledge** of the application and instruction of muscle strength/endurance and flexibility modalities <br> **Knowledge** of exercise modalities and the operation of associated equipment <br> **Knowledge** of proper biomechanical techniques (*e.g.*, gait assessment, resistance training form) <br> **Knowledge** of methods to educate participant in proper exercise programming and progression <br> **Knowledge** of the timing of daily activities with exercise (*e.g.*, medications, meals, insulin/glucose monitoring) <br> **Knowledge** of disease-specific strategies and tools to improve exercise tolerance (*e.g.*, breathing techniques, insulin pump use, prophylactic nitroglycerin) <br> **Knowledge** of behavioral strategies for improving exercise adoption and maintenance <br> **Knowledge** of barriers to exercise compliance and associated strategies (*e.g.*, physical, psychological, environmental) | • Understand how to use and interpret these tools; know how the measurements relate to exercise tolerance (*e.g.*, blood glucose readings that are too low or too high for exercise). <br> • Demonstrate numerous resistance training exercises and stretches, their proper applications, and common mistakes. <br> • Demonstrate various exercise machines/modalities, proper setup, adjustments, proper technique, and common errors. <br> • Explain proper anatomical positioning for aerobic and resistance training modalities. <br> • Knowledge of techniques to educate patients on the benefits of exercise specific to the patient; discuss how the exercise program meet the needs of the patient; patient-centered approaches that consider the patient's priorities, risk factors and psychosocial status; use terminology that they will understand. <br> • Optimal times to exercise with relation to eating and blood sugar (energy levels), medication peak times and their effects on exercise performance, insulin use/injection site recommendations, evening exercise, and hypoglycemia risk <br> • Explain how disease-specific adjunct therapies and techniques can improve exercise tolerance (*e.g.*, breathing retraining, insulin pump use and adjustment, prophylactic nitroglycerin). <br> • Knowledge and implementation of behavioral strategies (*e.g.*, counseling, education, scheduling) to improve adoption of exercise and maintenance <br> • Knowledge of and skill in developing patient-centered strategies to overcome exercise barriers | *ACSM's Resource Manual for Guidelines for Exercise Testing and Prescription*, 7th edition (7) <br> • Chapter 29 <br> *ACSM's Guidelines for Exercise Testing and Prescription* (GETP), 9th edition (6) <br> • Chapters 9 and 10 <br> *Essentials of Strength Training and Conditioning*, 3rd edition (13) <br> • Chapters 13 and 14 <br> *Essentials of Strength Training and Conditioning*, 3rd edition (13) <br> • Chapter 14 <br> *ACSM's Resource Manual for Guidelines for Exercise Testing and Prescription*, 7th edition (7) <br> • Chapter 2 <br> *ACSM's Guidelines for Exercise Testing and Prescription* (GETP), 9th edition (6) <br> • Chapter 10 <br> • Appendix A <br> *ACSM's Resource Manual for Guidelines for Exercise Testing and Prescription*, 7th edition (7) <br> • Chapters 19 and 40 <br> *ACSM's Resource Manual for Guidelines for Exercise Testing and Prescription*, 7th edition (7) <br> • Chapter 37 <br> *ACSM's Resource Manual for Guidelines for Exercise Testing and Prescription*, 7th edition (7) <br> • Chapter 46 <br> *Pollock's Textbook of Cardiovascular Disease and Rehabilitation* (10) |
| **Skill** in communication of exercise techniques, prescription, and progression <br> **Skill** in the assessment of participant symptoms, biomechanics, and exercise effort | • Describe/explain the exercise program so the patient will understand what they are doing and why (*e.g.*, proper technique, FITT-VP principle, how and when to progress); use a terminology that they will understand. <br> • Practice in recognizing adverse symptoms from exercise, proper movement and gait patterns, and subjective/objective exercise monitoring (*e.g.*, rating of perceived exertion [RPE], heart rate). | *ACSM's Resource Manual for Guidelines for Exercise Testing and Prescription*, 7th edition (7) <br> • Chapter 47 <br> *ACSM's Resource Manual for Guidelines for Exercise Testing and Prescription*, 7th edition (7) <br> • Chapter 2 <br> *ACSM's Guidelines for Exercise Testing and Prescription* (GETP), 9th edition (6) <br> • Chapter 4 |

## B. Provide disease management and risk factor reduction education based on the participant's medical history, needs, and goals.

| Knowledge or Skill Statement | Explanation/Examples | Resources |
|---|---|---|
| **Knowledge** of education program development based on participant's medical history, needs, and goals<br>**Knowledge** of methods to educate participant in risk factor reduction<br>**Knowledge** of published national standards on risk factors for cardiovascular, pulmonary, and metabolic disease<br>**Knowledge** of risk factor reduction programs and alternative community resources (*e.g.*, dietary counseling/Weight Watchers, smoking cessation, physical therapy/back care)<br>**Knowledge** of strategies to improve participant compliance to risk factor reduction<br>**Knowledge** of goal development strategies<br>**Knowledge** of counseling techniques<br>**Knowledge** of validated tools for measurement of psychosocial health status (*e.g.*, SF-36, strait-trait anxiety, Beck depression)<br>**Knowledge** of psychological issues associated with acute and chronic illness (*e.g.*, anxiety, depression, social isolation, suicidal ideation)<br>**Knowledge** of outcome evaluation methods (*e.g.*, American Association of Cardiovascular and Pulmonary Rehabilitation [AACVPR] outcomes model) | • Patient-centered approach to counseling and educating patients; establish rapport, listen actively, show interest, recognize their stage of readiness to change, provide education that is applicable and timely for the patient<br>• Knowledge and implementation of various methods of patient education (*e.g.*, videos, handouts, consultations) methods to assess and educate participant on risk factor reduction<br>• Knowledge and attainment of national standards of risk factor reduction for cardiovascular, pulmonary, and metabolic diseases; their target populations; strategies for their use; and how results may effect program participation<br>• Be familiar with various methods of improving cardiac, pulmonary, and metabolic health.<br>• Skill and knowledge to recognize possible "high-risk" situations that may cause a relapse in healthy behavior change (*e.g.*, vacations, bad weather); suggest alternatives, refer to other health care professional when appropriate<br>• Set goals that are specific, measurable, and challenging but realistic (*e.g.*, specific, measurable, attainable, realistic, and time-bound [SMART] goals).<br>• Understand the key components of counseling for health behavior: listen actively, show empathy, ask open-ended questions, establish rapport, know stages of change, etc.<br>• Knowledge of health-related quality-of-life, their target populations, strategies for their use, and how results may affect program participation<br>• Understanding of how these conditions may affect exercise adherence and motivation; social support groups; and referral to other health care professionals<br>• Understand the core components of rehabilitation and assessment/outcomes for each component. | *ACSM's Resource Manual for Guidelines for Exercise Testing and Prescription*, 7th edition (7)<br>• Chapter 46<br>*ACSM's Guidelines for Exercise Testing and Prescription* (GETP), 9th edition (6)<br>• Chapters 3 and 10<br>*ACSM's Resource Manual for Guidelines for Exercise Testing and Prescription*, 7th edition (7)<br>• Chapter 38<br>*ACSM's Resource Manual for Guidelines for Exercise Testing and Prescription*, 7th edition (7)<br>• Chapter 46<br>*ACSM's Resource Manual for Guidelines for Exercise Testing and Prescription*, 7th edition (7)<br>• Chapter 46<br>*ACSM's Resource Manual for Guidelines for Exercise Testing and Prescription*, 7th edition (7)<br>• Chapter 46<br>*ACSM's Resource Manual for Guidelines for Exercise Testing and Prescription*, 7th edition (7)<br>• Chapters 16 and 17<br>*ACSM's Resource Manual for Guidelines for Exercise Testing and Prescription*, 7th edition (7)<br>• Chapters 16 and 17<br>*ACSM's Resource Manual for Guidelines for Exercise Testing and Prescription*, 7th edition (7)<br>• Chapter 48 |
| **Skill** in communicating with participants from a wide variety of backgrounds<br>**Skill** in selection of participant outcome parameters | • Understanding how to communicate in a way that the patient will understand and will not be intimidated<br>• Knowledge and understanding the selection of appropriate participant outcome parameters. Select outcomes that are relevant to the patient and measurable (*e.g.*, achieve a resting blood pressure of <120/80 mm Hg). | *ACSM's Resource Manual for Guidelines for Exercise Testing and Prescription*, 7th edition (7)<br>• Chapter 47<br>*ACSM's Resource Manual for Guidelines for Exercise Testing and Prescription*, 7th edition (7)<br>• Chapter 46 |

CES

## C. Create a positive environment for participant adherence and outcomes by incorporating effective motivational skills, communication techniques, and behavioral strategies.

| Knowledge or Skill Statement | Explanation/Examples | Resources |
|---|---|---|
| **Knowledge** of current behavior facilitation theories (*e.g.*, health-belief model, transtheoretical model)<br>**Knowledge** of behavioral strategies and coaching methods for improving exercise adoption and maintenance<br>**Knowledge** of communication strategies that foster a positive environment<br>**Knowledge** of methods to educate participant in motivational skills and behavioral strategies<br>**Knowledge** of barriers to exercise compliance (*e.g.*, physical, psychological, environmental)<br>**Knowledge** of community resources available for participant use following discharge from the program | • Understand stages of change, processes of change, motivational readiness for change<br>• Knowledge and skill in choosing appropriate behavioral strategies (*e.g.*, patient education on the benefits of exercise specific to the patient; developing exercise programs that meet the needs of the patient; patient-centered approaches that consider the patient's priorities, risk factors, and psychosocial status)<br>• Knowledge and use of communication strategies that provide the patient with social support, rewards/incentives; find activities or an environment that will be enjoyable for the patient (*e.g.*, exercise in groups)<br>• Knowledge of educational methods for participant motivation and implementation of behavioral strategies (*e.g.*, counseling, education, scheduling)<br>• Identify potential barriers to consistent exercise and apply strategies to overcome them; develop patient-centered strategies to overcome exercise barriers<br>• Help facilitate a smooth transition from rehabilitation to continuing health behavior changes (*e.g.*, joining a fitness club, social support groups) | *ACSM's Resource Manual for Guidelines for Exercise Testing and Prescription*, 7th edition (7)<br>• Chapter 44<br>*ACSM's Resource Manual for Guidelines for Exercise Testing and Prescription*, 7th edition (7)<br>• Chapters 17 and 46<br>*Behavior Modification: What It Is and How To Do It*, 9th edition (12)<br>• xvii, p. 462<br>*ACSM's Resource Manual for Guidelines for Exercise Testing and Prescription*, 7th edition (7)<br>• Chapter 45<br>*ACSM's Resource Manual for Guidelines for Exercise Testing and Prescription*, 7th edition (7)<br>• Chapter 45<br>*ACSM's Resource Manual for Guidelines for Exercise Testing and Prescription*, 7th edition (7)<br>• Chapters 44–46<br>*ACSM's Resource Manual for Guidelines for Exercise Testing and Prescription*, 7th edition (7)<br>• Chapter 46 |

## D.  Collaborate and consult with health care professionals to address clinical issues and provide referrals to optimize participant outcomes.

| Knowledge or Skill Statement | Explanation/Examples | Resources |
|---|---|---|
| **Knowledge** of cardiovascular, pulmonary, and metabolic pathologies; clinical progression; diagnostic testing; medical regimens; and treatment procedures<br>**Knowledge** of techniques to determine participant's medical history through available documentation<br>**Knowledge** of commonly used medication for cardiovascular, pulmonary, and metabolic diseases<br>**Knowledge** of tools for measuring clinical exercise tolerance (*e.g.*, heart rate, glucometry, subjective rating scales)<br>**Knowledge** of risk factor reduction programs and alternative community resources (*e.g.*, dietary counseling/Weight Watchers, smoking cessation, physical therapy/back care)<br>**Knowledge** of psychological issues associated with acute and chronic illness (*e.g.*, anxiety, depression, suicidal ideation)<br>**Knowledge** of assessment tools to measure psychosocial health status<br>**Knowledge** of accepted methods of referral<br>**Knowledge** of community resources available for participant use following program discharge | • Understand how exercise effects cardiovascular, pulmonary, and metabolic pathologies. Understand how diagnostic testing and medical regimens/procedures can assess clinical progression of disease and/or exercise effects.<br>• Self-guided, professionally guided screenings for physical activity; risk stratification<br>• Understanding medication effects on resting and exercise vitals; cardiovascular, pulmonary, and metabolic diseases as well as side effects<br>• Understand how to use and interpret these tools; know how the measurements relate to exercise tolerance (*e.g.*, blood glucose readings that are too low or too high for exercise).<br>• Be familiar with various methods of improving cardiac, pulmonary, and metabolic health.<br>• How these conditions may affect exercise adherence and motivation; social support groups; referral to other health care professionals<br>• Five factor model of personality, transtheoretical model, *Diagnostic and Statistical Manual of Mental Disorders* (*DSM*), classes of mood disorders, subtypes of anxiety disorders<br>• Recognize signs and symptoms of various issues (*e.g.*, eating disorders, mental health states) that may require referral to another health care professional; know who to refer to and suggest appropriate professional; understand the appropriate protocol for referral including documentation and staff involved.<br>• Help facilitate a smooth transition from rehabilitation to continuing health behavior changes (*e.g.*, joining a fitness club, social support groups). | *ACSM's Resource Manual for Guidelines for Exercise Testing and Prescription*, 7th edition (7)<br>• Chapters 6–8 and 24–26<br>*ACSM's Guidelines for Exercise Testing and Prescription* (GETP), 9th edition (6)<br>• Chapter 2<br>*ACSM's Guidelines for Exercise Testing and Prescription* (GETP), 9th edition (6)<br>• Appendix A<br>*ACSM's Guidelines for Exercise Testing and Prescription* (GETP), 9th edition (6)<br>• Chapter 35<br>*ACSM's Resource Manual for Guidelines for Exercise Testing and Prescription*, 7th edition (7)<br>• Chapters 16 and 17<br>*ACSM's Resource Manual for Guidelines for Exercise Testing and Prescription*, 7th edition (7)<br>• Chapters 16 and 17<br>*ACSM's Resource Manual for Guidelines for Exercise Testing and Prescription*, 7th edition (7)<br>• Chapters 9 and 27<br>*ACSM's Resource Manual for Guidelines for Exercise Testing and Prescription*, 7th edition (7)<br>• Chapter 46 |
| **Skill** in collaborative decision making<br>**Skill** in interpretation of psychosocial assessment tools | • Practice making decisions with the patient; decision-making theory, decisional balance.<br>• Practice determining and understanding a patient's psychosocial status based on the results of assessments tools (*e.g.*, *DSM-IV*; make appropriate referral when necessary. | *ACSM's Resource Manual for Guidelines for Exercise Testing and Prescription*, 7th edition (7)<br>• Chapters 44 and 46<br>*ACSM's Resource Manual for Guidelines for Exercise Testing and Prescription*, 7th edition (7)<br>• Chapters 16 and 17 |

# DOMAIN V: LEGAL AND PROFESSIONAL CONSIDERATIONS

## A. Evaluate the exercise environment to minimize risk and optimize safety by following routine inspection procedures based on established facility and industry standards and guidelines.

| Knowledge or Skill Statement | Explanation/Examples | Resources |
|---|---|---|
| **Knowledge** of government and industry standards and guidelines (*e.g.,* American Association of Cardiovascular and pulmonary Rehabilitation [AACVPR], Health Insurance Portability and Accountability Act [HIPAA], Occupational Health and Safety Administration (OHSA)<br>**Knowledge** of the operation, calibration, and maintenance of exercise equipment | • Make sure you and your facility are following proper protocols, minimizing risk, and maximizing safety.<br>• Understand how to maintain the equipment, be able to recognize problems with the equipment (*e.g.,* a treadmill that needs to be calibrated), and know to fix the problem or contact the appropriate personnel. | *ACSM's Resource Manual for Guidelines for Exercise Testing and Prescription*, 7th edition (7)<br>• Chapter 10<br>*ACSM's Resource Manual for Guidelines for Exercise Testing and Prescription*, 7th edition (7)<br>• Chapters 20 and 29 |

## B. Perform regular inspections of emergency equipment and practice emergency procedures (*e.g.,* crash cart, advanced cardiac life support procedures, activation of emergency medical system).

| Knowledge or Skill Statement | Explanation/Examples | Resources |
|---|---|---|
| **Knowledge** of standards of practice during emergency situations (*e.g.,* American Heart Association [AHA])<br>**Knowledge** of local and institutional procedures for activation of the emergency medical system<br>**Knowledge** of standards for inspection of emergency medical equipment | • Cardiopulmonary resuscitation (CPR), automated external defibrillator (AED), advanced cardiac life support (ACLS), activating emergency medical service (EMS), assisting the code team, basic first aid, proper documentation<br>• Knowledge of institutional policy and procedures for activation of emergency response (*i.e.,* Code Team, EMS, etc.)<br>• Knowledge of and skill to be able to perform periodic reviews of the emergency equipment to ensure it is operational | *ACSM's Resource Manual for Guidelines for Exercise Testing and Prescription*, 7th edition (7)<br>• Chapter 19<br>*ACSM's Resource Manual for Guidelines for Exercise Testing and Prescription*, 7th edition (7)<br>• Chapter 19<br>*ACSM's Resource Manual for Guidelines for Exercise Testing and Prescription*, 7th edition (7)<br>• Chapter 19 |
| **Skill** in the application of basic life support procedures and external defibrillator use | • Obtain and maintain CPR/AED certification; participate in announced and unannounced emergency drills. | *ACSM's Resource Manual for Guidelines for Exercise Testing and Prescription*, 7th edition (7)<br>• Chapter 19 |

## C. Promote awareness and accountability and minimize risk by informing participants of safety procedures, self-monitoring of exercise, and related symptoms.

| Knowledge or Skill Statement | Explanation/Examples | Resources |
|---|---|---|
| **Knowledge** of signs and symptoms of exercise intolerance<br>**Knowledge** of the timing of daily activities with exercise (*e.g.*, medications, meals, insulin/glucose monitoring)<br>**Knowledge** of commonly used medications for cardiovascular, pulmonary, and metabolic diseases<br>**Knowledge** of communication techniques to ensure safety in participant's self-monitoring and symptom management<br>**Knowledge** of contraindicated and higher risk exercises and proper exercise form to minimize risk | • Knowledge of absolute and relative contraindications to exercise and abnormal responses/signs and symptoms for cardiovascular, pulmonary, and metabolic disease states<br>• Optimal times to exercise with relation to eating and blood sugar (energy levels), medication peak times and their effects on exercise performance, insulin use/injection site recommendations, evening exercise, and hypoglycemia risk.<br>• Understanding medication effects on resting and exercise vitals; cardiovascular, pulmonary, and metabolic diseases as well as side effects<br>• Educate patients in a way that they understand you (*e.g.*, lay terminology); ask for feedback to confirm that they understand how to self-monitor themselves.<br>• Know common exercise errors, and how to correct them; identify high risk exercises and offer alternative, safer ones. | *ACSM's Guidelines for Exercise Testing and Prescription* (GETP), 9th edition (6)<br>• Chapter 5<br>*ACSM's Guidelines for Exercise Testing and Prescription* (GETP), 9th edition (6)<br>• Chapter 10<br>• Appendix A<br>*ACSM's Guidelines for Exercise Testing and Prescription* (GETP), 9th edition (6)<br>• Chapter 10<br>• Appendix A<br>*Essentials of Strength Training and Conditioning*, 3rd edition (13)<br>• Chapter 14 |
| **Skill** in the instruction and modification of exercises to minimize risk of injury | • Educate participant in proper exercise technique, body alignment, and overall form for safe and effective exercise training; demonstrate alternative exercises when needed for safe participation. | *Essentials of Strength Training and Conditioning*, 3rd edition (13)<br>• Chapters 13 and 14 |

## D. Comply with Health Insurance Portability and Accountability Act (HIPAA) laws and industry-accepted professional, ethical, and business standards in order to maintain confidentiality, optimize safety, and reduce liability.

| Knowledge or Skill Statement | Explanation/Examples | Resources |
|---|---|---|
| **Knowledge** of HIPAA regulations relative to documentation and protecting patient privacy (*e.g.*, written and electronic medical records)<br>**Knowledge** of the use and limitations of informed consent<br>**Knowledge** of advanced directives and implications for rehabilitation programs<br>**Knowledge** of professional responsibilities and their implications related to liability and negligence | • Educate and knowledge of institutional and federal regulations regarding HIPAA and protecting patient privacy.<br>• Conveys an understanding of the tests/exercises, risks, option to choose to participate<br>• Living will, personal directive<br>• Follow peer-reviewed guidelines, maintain professional credentials, understand your scope of practice, instruct patients, document your services, report incidents, and maintain equipment. | *ACSM's Resource Manual for Guidelines for Exercise Testing and Prescription*, 7th edition (7)<br>• Chapter 10<br>*ACSM's Resource Manual for Guidelines for Exercise Testing and Prescription*, 7th edition (7)<br>• Chapter 10<br>*ACSM's Resource Manual for Guidelines for Exercise Testing and Prescription*, 7th edition (7)<br>• Chapter 10 |

## E.  Promote a positive image of the program by engaging in healthy lifestyle practices.

| Knowledge or Skill Statement | Explanation/Examples | Resources |
|---|---|---|
| **Knowledge** of common sources of health information, education, and promotion techniques | • Be familiar with various, credible sources of information and professional organizations that will educate patients on health and well-being (*e.g.*, American Heart Association [AHA]). | *ACSM's Resource Manual for Guidelines for Exercise Testing and Prescription*, 7th edition (7)<br>• Chapter 47 |
| **Skill** in the practice and demonstration of a healthy lifestyle | • Practice what you "preach"; exercise and be active regularly; eat a healthy diet; set a good example. | |

## F.  Select and participate in continuing education programs that enhance knowledge and skills on a continuing basis, maximize effectiveness, and increase professionalism in the field.

| Knowledge or Skill Statement | Explanation/Examples | Resources |
|---|---|---|
| **Knowledge** of continuing education opportunities as required for maintenance of professional credentials<br>**Knowledge** of total quality management (TQM) and continuous quality improvement (CQI) concepts and application to personal professional growth | • Know what is required (*e.g.*, how many Continuing Education Credits [CECs]) to maintain professional certification(s); focus on areas for professional growth/areas of current practice.<br>• Continuously improve the quality of your knowledge and skills through continuing education. | ACSM's Web site (5)<br>• Especially see Certification section |

# REFERENCES

## ACSM REFERENCES:

1. Ainsworth BE, Haskell WL, Whitt MC, et al. Compendium of physical activities: an update of activity codes and MET intensities. *Med Sci Sports Exerc.* 2000;32:S498–S504.
2. American College of Sports Medicine. *ACSM's Exercise Management for Persons with Chronic Diseases and Disabilities.* 3rd ed. Champaign (IL): Human Kinetics; 2009. 440 p.
3. American College of Sports Medicine. *ACSM's Metabolic Calculations Handbook.* Baltimore (MD): Lippincott Williams & Wilkins 2006. 111 p.
4. American College of Sports Medicine. Position stand: exercise and hypertension. *Med Sci Sports Exerc.* 2004;36:533–553.
5. American College of Sports and Medicine Web site [Internet]. Indianapolis (IN): American College of Sports Medicine; [cited 2012 Jul 13]. Available from: http://www.acsm.org
6. Pescatello LS, senior editor. *ACSM's Guidelines for Exercise Testing and Prescription.* 9th ed. Baltimore (MD): Lippincott Williams & Wilkins; 2014.
7. Swain DP, senior editor. *ACSM's Resource Manual for Guidelines for Exercise Testing and Prescription.* 7th ed. Baltimore (MD): Lippincott Williams & Wilkins 2014.

## NON-ACSM REFERENCES:

8. American Association of Cardiovascular and Pulmonary Rehabilitation. *Guidelines for Cardiac Rehabilitation and Secondary Prevention Programs.* 4th ed. Champaign (IL): Human Kinetics; 2004. 280 p.
9. American College of Chest Physicians/American Association of Cardiovascular and Pulmonary Rehabilitation Guidelines Panel. Pulmonary rehabilitation: joint ACCP/AACVPR evidence-based guidelines. *Chest.* 1997;112:1363–96.
10. Durstine JL, Moore GE, LaMonte MJ, Franklin BA, eds. *Pollock's Textbook of Cardiovascular Disease and Rehabilitation.* Champaign (IL): Human Kinetics; 2008. 411 p.
11. Fletcher GF, Balady GJ, Amsterdam EA, et al. Exercise standards for testing and training: a statement for healthcare professionals from the American Heart Association. *Circulation.* 2001;104(14):1694–1740.
12. Martin G, Pear J. *Behavior Modification: What It Is and How To Do It.* 9th ed. Boston (MA): Pearson Education/Allyn & Bacon; 2011. xvii, 462 p.
13. National Strength and Conditioning Association. *Essentials of Strength Training and Conditioning.* 3rd ed. Champaign (IL): Human Kinetics; 2008.
14. Opie LH. *Drugs for the Heart.* 6th ed. Philadelphia (PA): Saunders; 2004. 437 p.
15. Williams MA, Haskell WL, Ades PA, et al. Resistance exercise update in individuals with and without cardiovascular disease: 2007 update: A scientific statement from the American Heart Association. *Circulation.* 2007;116: 572–584.

CES

*Note: CES certification candidates should also review the practice examinations found in Part 1, ACSM Certified Personal Trainer (CPT) and Part 2, ACSM Certified Health Fitness Specialist (HFS).*

DIRECTIONS: Each of the numbered items or incomplete statements in this section is followed by answers or by completions of the statement. Select the ONE lettered answer or completion that is BEST in each case.

1. During a medical emergency, which of the following medications is an endogenous catecholamine that can be used to increase blood flow to the heart and brain?
   A) Lidocaine
   B) Oxygen
   C) Atropine
   D) Epinephrine

2. If a healthy young man who weighs 80 kg exercises at an intensity of 45 mL $\cdot$ kg$^{-1}$ $\cdot$ min$^{-1}$ for 30 min, five times per week, how long (assuming an isocaloric diet) would it take him to lose 10 lb?
   A) 9 wk
   B) 11 wk
   C) 13 wk
   D) 15 wk

3. Which of the following techniques can be used to diagnose coronary artery disease and assess heart wall motion abnormalities, ejection fraction, and cardiac output?
   A) Electrocardiography
   B) Radionuclide imaging
   C) Echocardiography
   D) Cardiac spirometry

4. Which of the following would be an adequate initial exercise prescription for a patient who has had a heart transplant?
   A) High intensity, short duration, small muscle groups, and high frequency
   B) High intensity, long duration, small muscle groups, and high frequency
   C) Moderate intensity, 6 d $\cdot$ wk$^{-1}$, large muscle groups, and moderate duration
   D) Low intensity, 3 d $\cdot$ wk$^{-1}$, large muscle groups, and moderate duration

5. Individuals with diabetes should follow exercise guidelines to avoid unnecessary risks. The following list of recommendations should include all of the following EXCEPT
   A) Avoiding injection of insulin into an exercising muscle.
   B) Exercising with a partner.
   C) Exercising only when temperature and humidity are moderate.
   D) Avoiding exercise during peak insulin activity.

6. Which of the following is a reversible pulmonary condition caused by some type of irritant (*e.g.*, dust, pollen) and characterized by bronchial airway narrowing, dyspnea, coughing, and, possibly, hypoxia and hypercapnia?
   A) Emphysema
   B) Bronchitis
   C) Asthma
   D) Pulmonary vascular disease

7. A supraventricular ectopic rhythm that results from a focus of automaticity located in the bundle of His is an example of
   A) Ventricular arrhythmia.
   B) Junctional arrhythmia.
   C) Atrioventricular (AV) block.
   D) Premature ventricular contraction.

8. Which of the following statements regarding contraindications to graded exercise testing is accurate?
   A) Some individuals have risk factors that outweigh the potential benefits from exercise testing and the information that may be obtained.
   B) Absolute contraindications refer to individuals for whom exercise testing should not be performed until the situation or condition has stabilized.
   C) Relative contraindications include patients who might be tested if the potential benefit from exercise testing outweighs the relative risk.
   D) All of the above statements are true.

9. Cardiac impulses originating in the sinoatrial node and then spreading to both atria, causing atrial depolarization, is represented on the electrocardiogram (ECG) as a
A) P wave.
B) QRS complex.
C) ST segment.
D) T wave.

10. For previously sedentary individuals, a 20%–30% reduction in all-cause mortality can be obtained from physical activity with a daily energy expenditure of
A) 50–80 kcal · d$^{-1}$.
B) 80–100 kcal · d$^{-1}$.
C) 150–200 kcal · d$^{-1}$.
D) >400 kcal · d$^{-1}$.

11. Exercise has been shown to reduce mortality in people with coronary artery disease. Which of the following mechanisms is NOT responsible?
A) The effect of exercise on other risk factors
B) Reduced myocardial oxygen demand at rest and at submaximal workloads
C) Reduced platelet aggregation
D) Decreased endothelial-mediated vasomotor tone

12. Which of the following may be an INAPPROPRIATE strategy for permanent weight loss?
A) Dietary changes
B) Increased exercise
C) Rapid weight loss
D) Dietary changes and exercise

13. Which of the following treatment strategies are most commonly used in patients with multiple vessel disease who are not responding to other treatments?
A) Percutaneous transluminal coronary angioplasty (PTCA)
B) Coronary artery stent
C) Coronary artery bypass graft (CABG) surgery
D) Pharmacologic therapy

14. Which of the following statements BEST describes the exercise precautions for patients with an automatic implantable cardioverter defibrillator (AICD)?
A) Persons with AICD must be monitored closely during exercise, keeping the heart rate (HR) 10 beats or more below the activation rate for a shock.
B) Persons with AICD are not at risk for an inappropriate shock because most AICDs are set to an HR of 300 bpm.
C) Persons with AICD can inactivate the AICD before high-intensity exercise to avoid the risk of shock.
D) Persons with an AICD can exercise at or above the cutoff HR but only if monitored by instantaneous ECG telemetry.

15. Healthy, untrained individuals have an anaerobic threshold at approximately what percentage of their maximal oxygen consumption ($\dot{V}O_{2max}$)?
A) 25%
B) 55%
C) 75%
D) 95%

16. Which of the following medications reduces myocardial ischemia by lowering myocardial oxygen demand, is used to treat typical and variant angina, but has NOT been shown to reduce postmyocardial infarction mortality?
A) β-Adrenergic blockers
B) Niacin
C) Aspirin
D) Nitrates

17. A 35-yr-old female client asks the exercise specialist to estimate her energy expenditure. She weighs 110 lb and pedals the cycle ergometer at 50 rpm with a resistance of 2.5 kp for 60 min. The specialist should report which of the following caloric values?
A) 250 cal
B) 510 cal
C) 770 cal
D) 1,700 cal

18. The cardiac rehabilitation's medical director orders a prerehabilitation ECG on a 50-yr-old man. The exercise specialist performing the ECG notes the machine error message reads artifact in the precordial lead $V_4$. To correct the artifact, an exercise specialist would check which of the following lead positions for adhesive contact?
A) Fourth intercostal space, left sternal border
B) Fourth intercostal space, right sternal border
C) Midaxillary line, fifth intercostal space
D) Midclavicular line, fifth intercostal space

19. Which of the following cardiac indices increases curvilinearly with the work rate until it reaches near maximum at a level equivalent to approximately 50% of aerobic capacity, increasing only slightly thereafter?
A) Stroke volume
B) HR
C) Cardiac output
D) Systolic blood pressure

20. A 55-yr-old cardiac rehabilitation patient returned from vacation with the following complaints: elevation in blood pressure, slight chest pain, shortness of breath with chest wheezing, and dryness and burning of the mouth and throat. Based on this information, the exercise specialist would suspect that the patient was exposed to which of the following environments?
    A) Extreme cold
    B) Extreme heat
    C) High altitude
    D) High humidity

21. All of the following are major signs and symptoms suggestive of cardiac or metabolic disease EXCEPT
    A) Ankle edema.
    B) Claudication.
    C) Orthopnea.
    D) Bronchitis.

22. Which of the following best describes an irreversible necrosis of the heart muscle resulting from prolonged coronary artery blockage?
    A) Thrombosis
    B) Ischemia
    C) Infarction
    D) Thrombolysis

23. An exercise specialist monitoring the ECG of a cardiac rehabilitation patient observes QT-interval shortening and ST-segment scooping during exercise. Based on this observation, the specialist can suspect that the patient is treated with which of the following medications?
    A) β-Blockers
    B) Calcium channel blockers
    C) Potassium
    D) Digitalis

24. The exercise specialist is orienting a 60-yr-old patient entering cardiac rehabilitation after having CABG 3 wk ago. All of the following statements are correct EXCEPT
    A) The patient should avoid upper body resistance training because of sternal and leg wounds for 4–6 mo.
    B) The clinician should observe for infection or discomfort along the incision.
    C) The patient should be monitored for chest pain, dizziness, and dysrhythmias.
    D) The patient should avoid high-intensity exercise early in the rehabilitation period.

25. All of the following are nonmodifiable risk factors for the development of coronary artery disease EXCEPT
    A) Increasing age.
    B) Male gender.
    C) Family history.
    D) Tobacco smoking.

26. An aerobic exercise prescription of 5 d · wk$^{-1}$ at 50%–85% of $\dot{V}O_{2max}$ for 45 min will most favorably affect which of the following blood lipid profiles?
    A) Lipoprotein (a)
    B) Triglycerides (TG)
    C) Total cholesterol
    D) Low-density lipoprotein (LDL) cholesterol

27. The exercise specialist is asked to risk stratify a 65-yr-old patient for exercise testing. The patient has shortness of breath with mild exertion, orthopnea, smokes two packs of cigarettes a day and has a body mass index (BMI) of 32 kg · m$^{-2}$. Based on this information, in which risk stratification category would this individual fall?
    A) No risk
    B) Low risk
    C) Moderate risk
    D) High risk

28. While monitoring the ECG of a cardiac rehabilitation patient, a progressive lengthening of the PR interval until a dropped QRS complex is observed. Based on this observation, what kind of AV block are you observing?
    A) First degree
    B) Mobitz type I
    C) Mobitz type II
    D) Third degree

29. You are asked to review an ECG strip for evidence of myocardial ischemia and/or injury. On what areas of the ECG should you focus?
    A) Q wave
    B) PR interval
    C) ST segment
    D) T wave

30. All of the following are classifications of obesity and result in an increased risk for coronary artery disease in males EXCEPT
    A) BMI ≥30 kg · m$^{-2}$.
    B) Waist-to-hip ratio >0.95.
    C) Body fat >25%.
    D) Waist circumference >35 in.

31. In an ECG recording, the presence of certain combinations of ST-segment abnormalities (*i.e.*, elevation and/or depression) and significant Q waves may be suggestive of what condition?
    A) Acute myocardial infarction
    B) Left ventricular hypertrophy
    C) Right bundle-branch block
    D) Ventricular aneurysm

32. What is the relative oxygen consumption rate for walking on a treadmill at 3.5 mph with a 10% grade?
    A) $18.17 \ \text{mL} \cdot \text{kg}^{-1} \cdot \text{min}^{-1}$
    B) $27.96 \ \text{mL} \cdot \text{kg}^{-1} \cdot \text{min}^{-1}$
    C) $29.76 \ \text{mL} \cdot \text{kg}^{-1} \cdot \text{min}^{-1}$
    D) $31.28 \ \text{mL} \cdot \text{kg}^{-1} \cdot \text{min}^{-1}$

33. Which of the following individuals DO NOT need a physician's evaluation before initiating a vigorous exercise program?
    A) Men >50 yr of age with fewer than two risk factors
    B) Women <50 yr of age with fewer than two risk factors
    C) Men <40 yr of age with two risk factors
    D) Women <50 yr of age with known disease

34. For persons free of absolute contraindications to exercise, the health and medical benefits of exercise clearly outweigh any associated risks. To ensure a safe environment during exercise testing and training, the clinical exercise specialist must be prepared to do all the following EXCEPT
    A) Explain the risks associated with exercise and exercise testing.
    B) Implement preventive measures.
    C) Perform emergency medical procedures.
    D) Take care of an injury or medical emergency.

35. Although certification of clinical exercise rehabilitation programs is a relatively new concept, it involves many already established components of the exercise program. Which of the following is NOT an important component of a clinical exercise rehabilitation program certification?
    A) A policies and procedures manual
    B) Program health outcomes and quality measures
    C) Staff certification and/or licensure
    D) Adherence to insurance codes for billing

36. A burning, constricting, heavy, or squeezing sensation of the chest, neck, shoulders, or arms, provoked by physical work or stress, is characteristic of which of the following?
    A) Angina
    B) Aortic aneurysms
    C) Exercise-induced asthma
    D) Atherosclerosis

37. Health screening before participation in a graded exercise test is indicated for all of the following reasons EXCEPT
    A) To determine the presence of disease.
    B) To evaluate contraindications for exercise testing or training.
    C) To determine the need for referral to a medically supervised exercise program.
    D) To evaluate aerobic capacity.

38. Which of the following is the proper emergency response for a patient who has experienced a cardiac arrest but now is breathing and has a palpable pulse?
    A) Continue the exercise test to determine why the patient had this response.
    B) Place the patient in the recovery position with the head to the side to prevent airway obstruction.
    C) Place the patient in a comfortable seated position.
    D) Start phase I cardiac rehabilitation.

39. A patient weighing 200 lb sets the treadmill at 4.0 mph with a 5% grade. At peak exercise, his blood pressure is 150/90 mm Hg, HR is 150 bpm, and respiratory quotient is 1.0. What is his estimated absolute energy expenditure?
    A) $1.07 \ \text{L} \cdot \text{min}^{-1}$
    B) $2.17 \ \text{L} \cdot \text{min}^{-1}$
    C) $4.28 \ \text{L} \cdot \text{min}^{-1}$
    D) $8.56 \ \text{L} \cdot \text{min}^{-1}$

40. Which of the following procedures provides the LEAST sensitivity and specificity in the diagnosis of coronary artery disease?
    A) Coronary angiography
    B) Echocardiography
    C) Electrocardiography
    D) Radionuclide imaging

41. What does flow-resistive training (a type of breathing retraining) teach patients with pulmonary disease?
    A) To effectively breathe through a progressively smaller airway
    B) Coordinate breathing with activities of daily living
    C) Increase respiratory muscle endurance and strength
    D) Increase ventilatory threshold

42. Which of the following is a NONMODIFIABLE risk factor for the development of coronary artery disease?
    A) Tobacco use
    B) Dyslipidemia
    C) Family history
    D) Hypertension

43. Which of the following is NOT an example of a capital expense?
    A) Renovations
    B) Staff salaries
    C) Exercise equipment purchases
    D) Furniture and fixtures

44. Which of the following is the thickest, middle layer of the artery wall that is composed predominantly of smooth muscle cells and is responsible for vasoconstriction and vasodilation?
    A) Endothelium
    B) Intima
    C) Media
    D) Adventitia

45. Which ECG electrode is positioned at the fourth intercostal space just to the left of the sternal border?
    A) $V_1$
    B) $V_2$
    C) $V_3$
    D) $V_4$

46. What is the total energy expenditure for a 70-kg man doing an exercise session composed of 5 min of warm-up at 2.0 metabolic equivalent (MET), 20 min of treadmill running at 9 MET, 20 min of leg cycling at 8 MET, and 5 min of cool-down at 2.5 MET?
    A) 162 kcal
    B) 868 kcal
    C) 444 kcal
    D) 1,256 kcal

47. How should the exercise prescription be initially altered for a patient exercising in the heat or in a humid environment?
    A) Increasing the intensity and increasing the duration
    B) Decreasing the intensity and increasing the duration
    C) Decreasing the intensity and decreasing the duration
    D) Increasing the intensity and decreasing the duration

48. Which of the following statements regarding an emergency plan is TRUE?
    A) The emergency plan does not need to be written down as long as everyone understands it.
    B) As long as everyone knows his or her individual responsibilities during an emergency, a list of each staff member's responsibilities is not needed.
    C) All emergency situations must be documented with dates, times, actions, people involved, and outcomes.
    D) There is no need to practice emergencies as long as the staff members fully understand their responsibilities.

49. Which of the following is NOT considered to be an orthopedic condition that can lead to limitation of regular exercise (physical conditioning)?
    A) Osteoarthritis
    B) Rheumatoid arthritis
    C) Osteoporosis
    D) Multiple sclerosis

50. Which of the following is characterized by an inflammation and edema of the trachea and bronchial tubes, hypertrophy of the mucous glands that narrows the airway, arterial hypoxemia that leads to vasoconstriction of smooth muscle in the pulmonary arterioles and venules, and in the presence of continued vasoconstriction results in pulmonary hypertension?
    A) Emphysema
    B) Bronchitis
    C) Pulmonary hypertension
    D) Asthma

51. Which of the following would be prudent for any high-risk patient who wishes to exercise?
    A) Skip both the warm-up and the cool-down entirely.
    B) Increase the intensity of the warm-up and decrease the intensity of the cool-down.
    C) Decrease the intensity of the warm-up and increase the intensity of the cool-down.
    D) Prolong both the warm-up and the cool-down.

52. Which of the following is NOT a characteristic of ventricular tachycardia?
    A) Wide QRS complex ($\geq 120$ ms)
    B) AV dissociation (P waves and QRS complexes have no relationship)
    C) Flutter waves at a rate of 250–350 atrial depolarizations per minute
    D) Three or more consecutive ventricular beats at 100 beats $\cdot$ min$^{-1}$

53. Which exercise intensity is used for training muscular endurance?
    A) 10%–40% of one repetition maximum
    B) 20%–40% of one repetition maximum
    C) 40%–60% of one repetition maximum
    D) 60%–80% of one repetition maximum

54. Which type of AV block occurs with a PR interval that progressively lengthens beyond 0.20 s until a P wave fails to conduct?
    A) First degree
    B) Second degree, Mobitz type I
    C) Second degree, Mobitz type II
    D) Third degree

CES

55. Which type of infarction is indicated if Q waves are detected by an ECG in leads $V_1$ and $V_2$ along with abnormal R waves?
    A) Anterolateral
    B) Localized anterior
    C) Posterior
    D) High lateral

56. What is an appropriate LDL goal for a patient with a very high risk for coronary artery disease?
    A) $<120$ mg $\cdot$ dL$^{-1}$
    B) $>100$ mg $\cdot$ dL$^{-1}$
    C) $<70$ mg $\cdot$ dL$^{-1}$
    D) $100-120$ mg $\cdot$ dL$^{-1}$

57. Which of the following graded exercise test protocols is NOT appropriate for previously sedentary individuals?
    A) Cooper 12-min test
    B) Step test
    C) Treadmill test
    D) Cycle ergometer test

58. For patients with congestive heart failure, which of the following statements is TRUE?
    A) Patients may not exceed a workload of 5 MET.
    B) Warm-up and cool-down periods should be limited to 5 min.
    C) Patients should expect no significant improvement in exercise capacity.
    D) Peripheral adaptations are largely responsible for an increase in exercise tolerance.

59. Which of the following populations would benefit MOST from regular muscular strength and endurance training?
    A) Postmenopausal women
    B) Athletes $<14$ yr of age
    C) Stroke survivors
    D) Hypertensive adults

60. Which of the following ECG interpretations involves a QRS complex duration that exceeds 0.11 s and a P wave precedes the QRS complex if it is present?
    A) AV conduction delay
    B) Normal cardiac function
    C) Supraventricular aberrant conduction
    D) Acute myocardial infarction

61. What is the incidence of cardiac arrest during clinical exercise testing?
    A) 1 in 10,000
    B) 1 in 2,500
    C) 1.4 in 10,000
    D) Minimal to nonexistent

62. In the "Readiness to Change Model," which stage is it recommended to use multiple resources to stress the importance of a desired change?
    A) Precontemplation
    B) Contemplation
    C) Preparation
    D) Instruction

63. Which should be lowered as an effective strategy in limiting the progression and promoting regression of atherosclerosis?
    A) LDL cholesterol
    B) High-density lipoprotein (HDL) cholesterol
    C) TGs
    D) Blood platelets

64. Which of the following medications does NOT affect exercise HR response?
    A) Angiotensin-converting enzyme (ACE) inhibitors and angiotensin II blockers
    B) Calcium channel blockers
    C) Thyroid medications
    D) β-Blockers

65. Which of the following treadmill protocols would be appropriate for an individual with intermittent claudication?
    A) Bruce
    B) Modified Åstrand
    C) Naughton
    D) Balke and Ware

66. Medications may directly alter the ECG response during exercise and result in false-positive tests. The drug MOST likely to have this effect is
    A) Lidocaine (Xylocaine).
    B) Propranolol (Inderal).
    C) Digitalis (Lanoxin).
    D) Reserpine (Serpasil).

67. Compared with data obtained during a previous graded exercise test when no medications were taken, a patient now taking Inderal (propranolol) would have the following response to the same submaximal exercise intensity during a second test
    A) A higher rate-pressure product (RPP)
    B) A larger QRS duration
    C) A lower HR
    D) Greater ST-segment depression

68. Two persons, one weighing 50 kg and the other weighing 80 kg, have maximal oxygen uptakes of 52 mL $\cdot$ kg $\cdot$ min$^{-1}$. They both exercise at 2.5 mph and 12% grade on a treadmill. Which variable will be approximately the same for each of the two subjects?
    A) MET
    B) Kilocalorie per minute
    C) Oxygen pulse ($\dot{V}O_2$/HR)
    D) $\dot{V}O_2$ (L $\cdot$ min$^{-1}$)

69. False-negative test results limit the diagnostic value of an exercise test. The incidence of false negatives is related to all but one of the following. Which is NOT related to false-negative results?
    A) Insufficient level of stress
    B) Single vessel coronary artery disease
    C) Monitoring an insufficient number of ECG leads
    D) Lack of metabolic determination (*i.e.*, $\dot{V}O_{2max}$)

70. Sounds heard during measurement of blood pressure are produced by
    A) The closing of the mitral valve.
    B) The closing of the aortic valve and pulmonary valves.
    C) The contraction of the ventricle.
    D) Turbulent blood flow.

71. Which of the following conditions would NOT necessarily indicate termination of an exercise stress test?
    A) ST-segment depression greater than 3.0 min
    B) A systolic blood pressure greater than 200 mm Hg
    C) Ventricular tachycardia
    D) Syncope

72. The 2001 National Committee Education Program (NCEP) guidelines state desirable lipid values for healthy adults as all of the following EXCEPT
    A) LDL cholesterol level <100 mg · dL$^{-1}$.
    B) Total cholesterol level <200 mg · dL$^{-1}$.
    C) HDL cholesterol level ≥40 mg · dL$^{-1}$.
    D) TG level ≤200 mg · dL$^{-1}$.

73. At a set workload (*e.g.*, 4 MET), myocardial oxygen consumption of a patient with coronary artery disease is reduced following endurance training as evidenced by a decrease in
    A) Systolic ejection period.
    B) Rating of perceived exertion (RPE).
    C) HR.
    D) Whole-body oxygen consumption.

74. When prescribing exercise for patients with atherosclerosis, which of the following is TRUE?
    A) Training HR among patients who are status post myocardial infarction are altered by α-blocking agents.
    B) Patients with peripheral arterial disease should exercise to leg pain level 3 (on 4-point scale), with intermittent rest periods.
    C) Most patients with stable angina who are cleared to participate in outpatient exercise programs (*i.e.*, Young Men's Christian Association [YMCA]) can exercise safely with moderate angina levels (2+).
    D) During the initial phase (1–3 d after the event) of inpatient programs, activities should be restricted to moderate intensity (3–5 MET).

75. Studies show the least physically active populations to include all of the following EXCEPT
    A) Obese.
    B) Elderly.
    C) Less educated.
    D) Upper middle class.

76. ST-segment elevation may occur in all of the following EXCEPT
    A) Coronary artery spasm.
    B) A ventricular aneurysm.
    C) An acute myocardial infarction.
    D) Subendocardial ischemia.

77. Which of the following statements are FALSE concerning stroke volume in healthy adults?
    A) A greater preload will increase stroke volume.
    B) Increased arterial blood pressure and greater ventricular outflow resistance will reduce stroke volume.
    C) During exercise, stroke volume increases to 50%–60% of maximal capacity, after which increases in cardiac output are largely caused by further increases in HR.
    D) Stroke volume is equal to the ratio of end-diastolic volume to end-systolic volume.

78. Long-term conditioning results in adaptations of the cardiovascular system. When measured at the same submaximal exercise intensity, these adaptations result in a decrease in
    A) Stroke volume.
    B) HR.
    C) Cardiac output.
    D) Arteriovenous oxygen difference.

79. An increase in maximal attainable RPP following successful CABG surgery for severe angina suggests
    A) Decreased myocardial oxygen demand.
    B) Increased cardiac output during submaximal exercise.
    C) Increase maximum coronary blood flow.
    D) Increased extraction of oxygen by the myocardium.

80. Greater oxygen delivery is provided to the myocardium in all of the following situations EXCEPT
    A) Severe coronary artery disease.
    B) Increase HR.
    C) Increase coronary blood flow.
    D) Increase cardiac output.

81. Which of the following would you not expect to occur with increased workload?
    A) Increased $\dot{V}O_2$
    B) Increased peripheral resistance
    C) Increased cardiac output
    D) Increased mean arterial pressure

CES

82. Which of the following is NOT associated with exercise-induced myocardial ischemia?
    A) Angina pectoris
    B) ST-segment depression
    C) Impaired left ventricular function
    D) Decreased RPP

83. While at rest, physically inactive men compared to physically active men of the same weight and age typically have a
    A) Higher blood pressure.
    B) Higher metabolic rate.
    C) Higher cardiac output.
    D) Lower stroke volume.

84. Myocardial oxygen consumption is highly correlated with RPP. Which variables are used to determine RPP?
    A) Systolic blood pressure and stroke volume
    B) Mean arterial pressure and HR
    C) Systolic pressure and HR
    D) Pulse pressure and HR

85. Which of the following would be the BEST marker of ischemic threshold?
    A) HR
    B) Blood pressure
    C) Oxygen uptake
    D) RPP

86. Long-term participation by healthy persons in activities such as running, cycling, and swimming result in the following adaptations during maximum exercise except one. The EXCEPTION is
    A) Increased oxidative capacity of a given mass of muscle.
    B) Increased venous return.
    C) Increased HR.
    D) Increased blood flow through active muscles.

87. The major determinant(s) of myocardial oxygen consumption is (are)
    A) Contractility.
    B) HR.
    C) Intramyocardial tension.
    D) All of the above.

88. Which of the following muscle groups is a prime mover for extension of the knee?
    A) Biceps femoris
    B) Biceps brachii
    C) Quadriceps femoris
    D) Gastrocnemius

89. During aerobic exercise, which of the following responses would NOT be considered normal?
    A) Increased systolic blood pressure
    B) Increased pulse pressure
    C) Increased mean arterial pressure
    D) Increased diastolic blood pressure

90. Which of the following statements regarding blood pressure and resistance exercise (weightlifting) is correct?
    A) People with even mild cardiovascular disease should never perform resistance exercise.
    B) Blood pressure elevations are highest during isometric muscular actions.
    C) Blood pressure elevations during resistance exercise are independent of the muscle mass involved.
    D) Typically, blood pressure elevations seen during maximal resistance exercise are less than those observed during maximal aerobic exercise.

91. Which of the following statements regarding osteoarthritis in older adults is FALSE?
    A) Exercise training improves function.
    B) Osteoarthritis is common in older adults.
    C) Exercise training slows down the progression of osteoarthritis.
    D) Exercise training does not exacerbate pain.

92. The primary effects of chronic exercise training on blood lipids include
    A) Decreased TG and increased HDL.
    B) Decreased total cholesterol and LDL.
    C) Decreased HDL and increased LDL.
    D) Decreased total cholesterol and increased HDL.

93. Which of the following statements concerning the surgical treatment of coronary artery disease is TRUE?
    A) A coronary artery stent carries a lower rate of revascularization than does PTCA.
    B) Atherectomy is a prerequisite requirement for PTCA.
    C) Venous grafts are significantly superior to arterial grafts in terms of patency.
    D) Long-term outcome of laser angioplasty is unknown and thus rarely used.

94. A cardiac patient is taking a β-blocker medication. During an exercise test, you would expect
    A) An ST-segment depression because β-blockers depress the ST segment on the resting ECG.
    B) An increase in the anginal threshold compared with a test without the medication.
    C) No change in HR or blood pressure compared with a test without the medication.
    D) A slight decrease or no effect on blood pressure compared with a test without the medication.

95. If an individual is in the action stage of the "Stages of Motivational Readiness," he or she
    A) Has been physically active on a regular basis for <6 mo.
    B) Participates in some exercise but does so irregularly.
    C) Intends to start exercising in the next 6 mo.
    D) Has been physically active on a regular basis for >6 mo.

96. Following termination of a graded exercise (stress) test, a 12-lead ECG is
    A) Monitored immediately, then every 1–2 min for 5 min of recovery or until exercise-induced changes are at baseline.
    B) Monitored immediately, then at 2 and 5 min after the test.
    C) Monitored immediately only.
    D) Monitored and recorded only if any signs or symptoms arise during recovery.

97. What is the best test to help determine ejection fraction at rest and during exercise?
    A) Angiogram
    B) Thallium stress test
    C) Single photo emission computed tomography test
    D) Multiple-gated acquisition (MUGA) (blood pool imagery) study

98. Which of the following is NOT part of an emergency plan?
    A) The plan should list the schedule of each staff member so that they can all be accounted for during an emergency.
    B) The plan must be written.
    C) The plan should outline each specific action.
    D) The staff should be prepared and trained in the plan.

99. Which of the following is NOT an appropriate treatment activity for inpatient rehabilitation of a patient on the second day after CABG surgery?
    A) Limit activities as tolerated to the development of self-care activities, range of motion (ROM) for extremities, and low-resistance activities.
    B) Limit upper body activities to bicep curls, horizontal arm adduction, and overhead press using 5-lb weights while sitting on the side of the bed.
    C) Progress all activities performed from supine to sitting to standing.
    D) Measure vital signs, symptoms, RPE, fatigue, and skin color and perform electrocardiography before, during, and after treatments to assess activity tolerance.

100. Which of the following statements about confidentiality is NOT correct?
    A) All records must be kept by the program director/manager under lock and key.
    B) Data must be available to all individuals who need to see it.
    C) Data should be kept on file for at least 1 yr before being discarded.
    D) Sensitive information (*e.g.*, participant's name) needs to be protected.

# CES EXAMINATION ANSWERS AND EXPLANATIONS

**1—D.** Epinephrine
Epinephrine is an endogenous catecholamine that optimizes blood flow to the heart and brain by increasing aortic diastolic pressure and preferentially shunting blood to the internal carotid artery. Lidocaine is an antiarrhythmic agent that can decrease automaticity in the ventricular myocardium as well as raise the fibrillation threshold. Supplemental oxygen ensures adequate arterial oxygen content and greatly enhances tissue oxygenation. Atropine is a parasympathetic blocking agent used to treat bradyarrhythmias.

**2—C.** 13 wk
The steps are as follows:

a. Convert relative $\dot{V}O_2$ to absolute $\dot{V}O_2$ by multiplying relative $\dot{V}O_2$ ($mL \cdot kg^{-1} \cdot min^{-1}$) by his body weight.

b. The young man weights 80 kg. Therefore,

$$\text{Absolute } \dot{V}O_2 = \text{relative } \dot{V}O_2 \times \text{body weight}$$
$$= 45 \text{ mL} \cdot kg^{-1} \cdot min^{-1} \times 80 \text{ kg}$$
$$= 3,600 \text{ mL} \cdot min^{-1}$$

c. To get $L \cdot min^{-1}$, divide $mL \cdot min^{-1}$ by 1,000

$$3,600 \text{ mL} \cdot min^{-1}/1,000 = 3.60 L \cdot min^{-1}$$

d. Multiply $3.60 \text{ L} \cdot min^{-1}$ by the constant 5.0 to get $kcal \cdot min^{-1}$

$$3.60 L \cdot min^{-1} \times 5.0 = 18.0 \text{ kcal} \cdot min^{-1}$$

e. Multiply $18.0 \text{ kcal} \cdot min^{-1}$ by the total number of minutes that he exercises ($\sim$30 min $\times$ 5 times per week = 150 total minutes) to get the total caloric expenditure

$$18.0 \text{ kcal} \cdot min^{-1} \times 150 \text{ min} = 2,700 \text{ kcal} \cdot wk^{-1}$$

f. Divide by 3,500 to get pounds of fat

$$2,700 \text{ kcal} \cdot wk^{-1}/3,500 \text{ kcal} \cdot lb^{-1} \text{ of fat} = 0.7714 \text{ lb of fat} \cdot wk^{-1}$$

g. Divide 10 lb by 0.7714 to get how many weeks it will take him to lose 10 lb of fat

$$10 \text{ lb of fat}/0.7714 = 12.96 \text{ wk or}$$
approximately 13.0 wk

**3—C.** Echocardiography
In the diagnosis of coronary artery disease, electrocardiography, radionuclide imaging, and echocardiography are commonly used by themselves or with other tests. However, echocardiography uses sound waves to assess heart wall motion, abnormalities, ejection fraction, systolic and diastolic function, and cardiac output. Other important diagnostic studies for coronary artery disease include coronary angiography.

**4—C.** Moderate intensity, 6 d $\cdot$ wk$^{-1}$, large muscle groups, and moderate duration
Patients who have had heart transplant should exercise at an RPE of between 11 and 16 (moderate) and not use a target HR prescription. Duration should include a prolonged warm-up and cool-down. In addition, resistance training can be used in moderation.

**5—C.** Exercising only when temperature and humidity are moderate
Recommended precautions for the exercising patient with diabetes include wearing proper footwear, maintaining adequate hydration, monitoring blood glucose level regularly, always wearing a medical identification bracelet or other form of identification, avoiding injecting insulin into exercising muscles, always exercising with a partner, and avoiding exercise during peak insulin activity. There is no reason why a patient with diabetes cannot exercise at any time if proper precautions are followed.

**6—C.** Asthma
Bronchitis is inflammation of the main air passages to the lungs. Bronchitis can be acute or chronic. Acute bronchitis is characterized by a cough, with or without the production of sputum, and can last several days or weeks. Chronic bronchitis, a type of chronic obstructive pulmonary disease, is characterized by the presence of a productive cough that lasts for 3 mo or more per year for at least 2 yr. Emphysema usually refers to a long-term, progressive disease of the lungs that causes shortness of breath. Emphysema is called an obstructive lung disease because the destruction of lung tissue around the alveoli makes these air sacs unable to hold their functional shape upon exhalation. Pulmonary vascular disease is a category of disorders that affect the blood circulation in the lungs. Examples include pulmonary arterial hypertension and pulmonary edema.

**7—B.** Junctional arrhythmia
A junctional arrhythmia is a supraventricular ectopic rhythm that results from a focus of automaticity located in the bundle of His.

A ventricular arrhythmia could be a premature ventricular complex (PVC) in which one of the ventricles depolarizes first and then spreads to the other ventricle or ventricular fibrillation, which is often triggered by the simultaneous conduction of ischemic ventricular cells within multiple locations of the ventricles. An AV block result when supraventricular impulses are delayed in the AV node. A premature ventricular contraction occurs when the ventricles are prematurely depolarized.

**8—D.** All of the above statements are true.
All of these statements are true regarding contraindications to exercise testing.

**9—A.** P wave
The cardiac impulse originating in the sinoatrial node that spreads to both atria causing atrial depolarization is indicated on the ECG as a P wave. Atrial repolarization usually is not seen on the ECG because it is obscured by the ventricular electrical potentials. Ventricular depolarization is represented on the ECG by the QRS complex. Ventricular repolarization is represented on the ECG by the ST segment, the T wave, and, at times, the U wave.

**10—C.** $150–200 \text{ kcal} \cdot \text{d}^{-1}$
A minimal caloric threshold of 150–200 kcal of physical activity per day is associated with a significant 20%–30% reduction in risk of all-cause mortality and this should be the initial goal for previously sedentary individuals.

**11—D.** Decreased endothelial-mediated vasomotor tone
The mechanisms responsible for a reduction in deaths from coronary artery disease include its effect on other risk factors, reduced myocardial oxygen demand both at rest and at submaximal workloads (resulting in an increased ischemic and anginal threshold), reduced platelet aggregation, and improved endothelial-mediated vasomotor tone.

**12—C.** Rapid weight loss
Rapid weight loss is considered to be $3 \text{ lb} \cdot \text{wk}^{-1}$ for women and $3–5 \text{ lb} \cdot \text{wk}^{-1}$ for men after the first 2 wk of the diet. Long-term maintenance usually is a problem with rapid weight loss; one study reported total recidivism within 3–5 yr. Modifications in diet and exercise generally are associated with more permanent weight loss.

**13—C.** CABG surgery
CABG surgery usually is reserved for patients who have a poor prognosis for survival or are unresponsive to pharmacologic treatment, stents, or PTCA. Such patients include those with angina, left main coronary artery stenosis, multiple vessel disease, and left ventricular dysfunction.

**14—A.** Persons with AICD must be monitored closely during exercise, keeping the HR 10 beats or more below the activation rate for a shock. There are many benefits of chronic exercise for a patient with an AICD. Several precautions need to be taken, however, including monitoring the HR and knowing the rate at which the AICD is set to shock the patient. The rate for activation is preset and varies for each patient.

**15—B.** 55%
The anaerobic threshold is normally expressed as a percentage of an individual's $\dot{V}O_{2max}$. For example, if $\dot{V}O_{2max}$ occurs at 6 mph on a treadmill test and a sharp rise in blood lactate concentration above resting levels is seen at 3 mph, then the anaerobic threshold is said to be 50% $\dot{V}O_{2max}$. In well-trained athletes, anaerobic threshold typically occurs at 70%–80% $\dot{V}O_{2max}$. In untrained individuals, it occurs much sooner at 50%–60% $\dot{V}O_{2max}$. This is because the adaptations from regular aerobic exercise have not occurred (*e.g.*, increased mitochondria and capillary density).

**16—D.** Nitrates
Nitrates relax peripheral venous vessels, which decrease preload, attenuate myocardial oxygen demand, and alleviate ischemia. Nitrates do not reduce the risk of postmyocardial infarction mortality. β-Adrenergic blockers reduce myocardial ischemia by lowering myocardial oxygen demand. These agents lower blood pressure, control ventricular arrhythmias, and significantly reduce first-year mortality rates in patients after myocardial infarction by 20%–35%. Niacin lowers low-density lipids by inhibiting secretion of lipoproteins from the liver. Aspirin is a platelet inhibitor.

**17—B.** 510 cal
The steps are as follows:
a. Choose the American College of Sports Medicine's (ACSM's) leg cycling formula.
b. Write down your knowns and convert the values to the appropriate units.

$110 \text{ lb}/2.2 = 50 \text{ kg}$
$50 \text{ rpm} \times 6 \text{ m} = 300 \text{ m} \cdot \text{min}^{-1}$
$2.5 \text{ kp} = 2.5 \text{ kg}$
$60 \text{ min of cycling}$

c. Write down the ACSM leg cycling formula.

Leg cycling $(mL \cdot kg^{-1} \cdot min^{-1}) =$ $(1.8 \times$ work rate/body weight$) +$ $3.5 + 3.5 \, (mL \cdot kg^{-1} \cdot min^{-1})$

d. Calculate the work rate.

Work rate $= kg \cdot m \cdot min^{-1}$
$= 2.5 \, kg \cdot 300 \, m \cdot min^{-1}$
$= 750 \, kg \cdot m \cdot min^{-1}$

e. Substitute the known values for the variable name.

$mL \cdot kg^{-1} \cdot min^{-1} = (1.8 \times 750/50) + 3.5 + 3.5$

f. Solve for the unknown.

$mL \cdot kg^{-1} \cdot min^{-1} = 27 + 3.5 + 3.5$
Gross leg cycling $\dot{V}O_2 = 34 \, mL \cdot kg^{-1} \cdot min^{-1}$

g. To find out how many calories she expends, we must first convert her oxygen consumption to absolute terms.

Absolute $\dot{V}O_2 =$ relative $\dot{V}O_2 \times$ body weight
$= 34 \, mL \cdot kg^{-1} \cdot min^{-1} \times 50 \, kg$
$= 1,700 \, mL \cdot min^{-1}$

h. Convert $mL \cdot min^{-1}$ to $L \cdot min^{-1}$ by dividing by 1,000.

$1,700 \, mL \cdot min^{-1}/1,000 = 1.7 \, L \cdot min^{-1}$

i. Next, we must see how many calories she expends in 1 min by multiplying her absolute $\dot{V}O_2$ (in $L \cdot min^{-1}$) by the constant 5.0.

$1.7 \, L \cdot min^{-1} \times 5.0 = 8.5 \, kcal \cdot min^{-1}$

j. Finally, multiply the number of calories she expends in 1 min by the number of minutes that she cycles.

$8.5 \, kcal \cdot min^{-1} \times 60 \, min = 510$ total cal

**18—D.** Midclavicular line, fifth intercostal space
The proper anatomic location of $V_4$ is the midclavicular line, fifth intercostal space. Precordial leads $V_1$ and $V_2$ are located at the fourth intercostal space, right and left sternal borders. There is no precordial lead site at the midaxillary line, fifth intercostal space.

**19—A.** Stroke volume
During exercise, stroke volume increases curvilinearly with work rate until it reaches near maximum at a level equivalent to approximately 50% of aerobic capacity, increasing only slightly thereafter. The left ventricle is able to contract with greater force during exercise because of a greater end-diastolic volume and enhanced mechanical ability of muscle fibers to produce force.

**20—A.** Extreme cold
Exposure to cold causes vasoconstriction (higher blood pressure response), lowers the anginal threshold in patients with angina, can provoke angina at rest (variant or Prinzmetal angina), and can induce asthma, general dehydration, and dryness or burning of the mouth and throat.

**21—D.** Bronchitis
Bilateral ankle edema is a characteristic sign of heart failure, whereas unilateral edema of a limb often results from venous thrombosis or lymphatic blockage. Intermittent claudication, a condition caused by an inadequate blood supply, is an aching, crampy, and sometimes burning pain in the legs that typically occurs with exercise and disappears with rest. Orthopnea is characterized by the inability to breathe easily unless sitting up straight or standing erect and is a symptom of heart failure. Bronchitis, a pulmonary disorder, is characterized by inflammation and edema of the trachea and bronchial tubes. Classic symptoms of bronchitis include chronic cough, sputum production, and dyspnea.

**22—C.** Infarction
A thrombosis is a specific clot that may cause a myocardial infarction. Ischemia is insufficient blood flow to the heart muscle. Thrombolysis (thrombolytic therapy) uses a specific clot-dissolving agent administered during acute myocardial infarction to restore blood flow and to limit myocardial necrosis. Myocardial infarction is an irreversible necrosis of the heart muscle resulting from prolonged coronary artery blockage.

**23—D.** Digitalis
Digitalis is used to treat heart failure and certain arrhythmias. Shortening of the QT interval and a "scooping" of the ST–T complex characterize the effects of digitalis on the ECG.

**24—A.** The patient should avoid upper body resistance training because of sternal leg wounds for 4–6 mo. Avoiding tension on the upper body typically is recommended for 8–12 wk, not for 2–4 mo. All of the other precautions are appropriate.

**25—D.** Tobacco smoking
Aging, male gender, and family history of coronary artery disease are risk factors that cannot be controlled. Tobacco smoking can be modified or eliminated.

**26—B.** TGs
TGs are the only substance listed that has been proved to be directly affected by exercise. Lipoprotein (a) has not been shown to change

favorably with exercise. LDL cholesterol and total cholesterol are affected by diet and may be lowered indirectly from weight loss associated with exercise.

**27—D.** High risk
Low-risk individuals are those men younger than 45 yr and women younger than 55 yr who are asymptomatic and meet no more than one risk factor. Moderate-risk individuals are those men ≥45 yr and women ≥55 yr of age or those who meet the threshold for two or more risk factors. High-risk individuals are those with one or more signs and symptoms or known cardiovascular, pulmonary, or metabolic disease.

**28—B.** Mobitz type I
Second-degree AV block is subdivided into two types: Mobitz type I and Mobitz type II. Mobitz type I also is known as the Wenckebach phenomenon. In this condition, the conduction of the impulse through the AV junction becomes increasingly more difficult, resulting in a progressively longer PR interval, until a QRS complex is dropped following a P wave. This indicates that the AV junction failed to conduct the impulse from the atria to the ventricles. This pause allows the AV node to recover, and the following P wave is conducted with a normal or slightly shorter PR interval.

**29—C.** ST segment
ST segments are considered to be sensitive indicators of myocardial ischemia or injury. A Q wave is a negative deflection of a QRS complex preceding an R wave. A "pathologic" Q wave is an indication of an old transmural myocardial infarction. The PR interval is the time that it takes from the initiation of an electrical impulse in the sinoatrial node to the initiation of electrical activity in the ventricles. The T wave indicates ventricular repolarization.

**30—D.** Waist circumference >35 in
The identification and classification of obesity and coronary artery disease risk has been somewhat discretionary, with a multitude of available techniques. BMI ≥30 kg · m$^{-2}$, waist-to-hip ratio >0.95, and body fat levels >25% are all objective measures of obesity for males. Waist circumference levels >35 in is specific to women.

**31—A.** Acute myocardial infarction
An ECG is an excellent tool for detecting cardiac rhythm and conduction abnormalities, chamber enlargements, ischemia, and

infarction. In an ECG recording, ST-segment elevation with an absence of R waves that are replaced by Q waves is a sign of acute myocardial infarction.

**32—C.** 29.76 mL · kg$^{-1}$ · min$^{-1}$
The steps are as follows:
a. Choose the ACSM's walking formula.
b. Write down your knowns and convert the values to the appropriate units.

$$3.5 \text{ mph} \times 26.8 = 93.8 \text{ m} \cdot \text{min}^{-1}$$
$$10\% \text{ grade} = 0.10$$

c. Write down the ACSM's walking formula.

walking (kg$^{-1}$ · min$^{-1}$) = (0.1 × speed) + (1.8 × speed × fractional grade) + 3.5 (mL · kg$^{-1}$ · min$^{-1}$)

d. Substitute the known values for the variable name.

mL · kg$^{-1}$ · min$^{-1}$ = (0.1 × 93.8) + (1.8 × 93.8 × 0.1) + 3.5 mL · kg$^{-1}$ · min$^{-1}$ = 9.38 + 16.884 + 3.5

e. Solve for the unknown.

mL · kg$^{-1}$ · min$^{-1}$ = 9.38 + 16.884 + 3.5
gross walking $\dot{V}O_2$ = 29.76 mL · kg$^{-1}$ · min$^{-1}$

**33—B.** Women <50 yr of age with fewer than two risk factors
The purpose of health screening before engaging in vigorous exercise is to identify clients who require additional medical testing to determine the presence of disease, contraindications for exercise testing or training, or referral to a medically supervised exercise program. Men younger than 40 yr and women younger than 50 yr with fewer than two coronary artery disease risk factors do not require a physician's evaluation before initiating vigorous exercise.

**34—C.** Perform emergency medical procedures
Emergency plans must be created, practiced, and implemented in the event of a medical emergency. Clinical personnel must understand the risks associated with exercise and exercise testing, be able to implement preventive measures, and have knowledge regarding the care of an injury or medical emergency.

**35—D.** Adherence to insurance codes for billing
Program certification of clinical exercise rehabilitation programs, although a new concept, involves many components that have already been established as part of the exercise program such as a clearly articulated mission

CES

statement, a defined organizational chart with methods to measure client health outcomes, a developed, implemented, and well-used policy and procedures manual, and so forth. The certification of a rehabilitation program is about the quality of the program as opposed to the financial operations (*e.g.*, billing practices and use of insurance codes).

**36—A.** Angina
Angina pectoris is the pain associated with myocardial ischemia. The pain often is felt in the chest, neck, cheeks, shoulder, or arms. It can be brought on by physical or psychological stress and is relieved after resting or by removing the stressor. Angina can be either classic (typical) or vasospastic (Prinzmetal).

**37—D.** To evaluate aerobic capacity
The overall goal of health screening before participation in a graded exercise testing or an exercise program is to obtain essential information that will ensure the safety of the participant. Thus, health screening helps to determine the presence of disease, enables one to consider possible contraindications to exercise testing and training, and helps to determine whether referral to a medically supervised exercise program is needed.

**38—B.** Place the patient in the recovery position with the head to the side to prevent airway obstruction. The proper response to a patient who has experienced a cardiac arrest yet is breathing and has a pulse is to call to the emergency medical system immediately; place the patient in the recovery position, with the head to the side to avoid an airway obstruction; and then stay with the patient and continue to monitor his or her vital signs.

**39—B.** $2.17 \text{ L} \cdot \text{min}^{-1}$
The steps are as follows:
a.  Choose the ACSM's walking formula.
b.  Write down your knowns and convert the values to the appropriate units.

   5% grade = 0.05
   4.0 mph = $107.2 \text{ m} \cdot \text{min}^{-1}$
   200 lb = 90.91 kg

c.  Write down the ACSM's walking formula:

   walking $(\text{kg}^{-1} \cdot \text{min}^{-1})$ = $(0.1 \times \text{speed})$ + $(1.8 \times \text{speed} \times \text{fractional grade})$ + $3.5 \text{ (mL} \cdot \text{kg}^{-1} \cdot \text{min}^{-1})$

d.  Substitute knowns

   $\dot{V}O_2 = (0.1 \times 107.2) + (1.8 \times 107.2 \times 0.05) + 3.5$

e.  Solve

   $\dot{V}O_2 = 23.87 \text{ mL} \cdot \text{kg}^{-1} \cdot \text{min}^{-1}$
   $\dot{V}O_2 = 23.83 \times 90.01 \text{ kg}/1{,}000$
   $\dot{V}O_2 = 2.17 \text{ L} \cdot \text{min}^{-1}$

**40—C.** Electrocardiography
Electrocardiography is the least sensitive and specific of all these tests. Directly visualizing the coronary arteries using coronary angiography provides the highest sensitivity and specificity. Radionuclide imaging and echocardiography have about the same sensitivity and specificity.

**41—A.** To effectively breathe through a progressively smaller airway
Flow-resistive training involves breathing through a progressively smaller airway or opening. Paced breathing helps to coordinate breathing with activities of daily living. Respiratory muscle training increases respiratory muscle endurance and strength. Ventilatory threshold is the breakpoint in ventilation during exercise and likely reflects a balance between lactate production and removal.

**42—C.** Family history
Nonmodifiable risk factors include age, male gender, and family history of premature coronary heart disease. Modifiable risk factors include hypertension, dyslipidemia, tobacco use, diabetes mellitus, overweight or obesity, and physical inactivity.

**43—B.** Staff salaries
Staff salaries are not capital expenses but are grouped under variable costs. Capital expense is for large-scale purchases such as renovations, expansions, furniture, and fixtures.

**44—C.** Media
The media contains most of the smooth muscle cells, which maintain arterial tone. The endothelium comprises a single layer of cells that form a tight barrier between blood and the arterial wall to resist thrombosis, promote vasodilation, and inhibit smooth muscle cells from migration and proliferation into the intima. The intima is the very thin, innermost layer of the artery wall and is composed mainly of connective tissue with some smooth muscle cells. The adventitia is the outermost layer of the arterial wall and consists of connective tissue, fibroblasts, and a few smooth muscle cells. Adventitia is highly vascularized and provides the media and intima with oxygen and other nutrients.

CES

**45—B.** $V_2$

$V_2$ electrode is located at the fourth intercostal space just to the left of the sternal border. $V_1$ is at the fourth intercostal space just to the right of the sternal border. $V_3$ is at the midpoint of a straight line between $V_2$ and $V_4$. $V_4$ is at the mid-clavicular line onto the fifth intercostal space.

**46—C.** 444 kcal

First, determine the MET level for each activity.

Warm-up is 2.0 MET × 5 min = 10 MET
Treadmill is 9.0 MET × 20 min = 180 MET
Cycle is 8.0 MET × 20 min = 160 MET
Cool-down is 2.50 MET × 5 min = 12.5 MET

Then, determine the total number of MET for all activities. 10 + 180 + 160 + 12.5 = 362.5 MET. Multiply 362.5 MET by 3.5 (because 1 MET = 3.5 mL · kg$^{-1}$ · min$^{-1}$), which is equal to 1,268.75 mL · kg$^{-1}$.

Multiply 1,268.75 mL · kg$^{-1}$ by body weight (70 kg), which is equal to 88,812.5 mL. Divide that number by 1,000 (because 1,000 mL = 1 L), is equal to 88.81 L. Multiply 88.81 L by 5 (because 5 kcal = 1 L of oxygen consumed), which is equal to 444 kcal.

**47—C.** Decreasing the intensity and decreasing the duration

High ambient temperature or relative humidity increases the risk of heat-related disorders including heat cramps, heat syncope, dehydration, heat exhaustion, and heat stroke. In this type of environment, the exercise prescription should be altered by initially lowering the intensity and the duration of exercise to allow for acclimatation.

**48—C.** All emergency situations must be documented with dates, times, actions, people involved, and outcomes.

The emergency plan must be written down and available in all testing and exercise areas. The plan should list the specific responsibilities of each staff member, required equipment, and pre-determined contacts for an emergency response. All emergencies must be documented with dates, times, actions, people involved, and results. The plan should be practiced with both announced and unannounced drills periodically. All staff members, including nonclinical staff members, should be trained in the emergency plan.

**49—D.** Multiple sclerosis

Osteoarthritis is a degenerative joint disease that generally is localized first on an articular cartilage. Rheumatoid arthritis is an inflammatory disease affecting joints as well as organs.

Osteoporosis involves the loss of bone density. Multiple sclerosis is a chronic inflammatory disorder with demyelination occurring in the central nervous system.

**50—B.** Bronchitis

Signs and symptoms of bronchitis include chronic cough, mucous production, and mucous gland enlargement that involves the large airways. The body attempts to heal by depositing collagen in the airway walls. The effects includes further airway narrowing, an increase in airway resistance decreasing ventilation to the lung, increased perfusion resulting in ventilation–perfusion mismatch, arterial hypoxemia, and pulmonary arterial hypertension. Common clinical symptoms of emphysema are shortness of breath or coughing, sputum production notable in the morning, hypoxemia, and eventual cor pulmonale. Emphysema primarily involves abnormalities of the lung parenchyma and smaller airways. Asthma is an episodic reversible condition that is characterized by increased airway reactivity to various stimuli resulting in widespread reversible narrowing of the airways. Pulmonary hypertension is a mean pulmonary artery pressure at rest >25 mm Hg or >30 mm Hg with exercise.

**51—D.** Prolong both the warm-up and the cool-down.

Warm-up may have preventative value, decreasing the occurrence of ischemic ST-segment depression, decreasing transient global left ventricular dysfunction following sudden strenuous exertion, and decreasing ventricular dysrhythmias. Cool-down provides a gradual recovery from exercising. It allows the return of HR and blood pressure close to resting levels, maintains venous return, prevents postexercise hypotension, and facilitates dissipation of body heat.

**52—C.** Flutter waves at a rate of 250–350 atrial depolarizations per minute

Ventricular tachycardia is characterized by three or more consecutive ventricular beats per minute or faster, a wide QRS complex (≥120 ms), AV dissociation (the P waves and QRS complexes have no relationship) and a QRS complex that does not have the morphology of bundle-branch block. Atrial flutter is characterized by flutter waves at a rate of 250–350 atrial depolarizations per minute.

**53—C.** 40%–60% of one repetition maximum

Rapid strength gains will be achieved at higher resistance or weight (80%–100% of one repetition maximum) and lower repetitions (reps) (6–8). For muscular endurance, a lower weight is used (40%–60% of one repetition maximum) with higher number of reps—usually ≥15.

**54—B.** Second degree, Mobitz type I
Second degree: Mobitz type I (Wenckebach). PR Interval lengthens until a P wave fails to conduct.

**55—C.** Posterior
$V_1$, $V_2$ based on abnormal Q waves except for true posterior myocardial, which is reflected by abnormal R waves.

**56—C.** $<70$ mg $\cdot$ dL$^{-1}$
Since publication of Adult Treatment Panel III, major clinical trials question the treatment thresholds for LDL. In particular, an LDL goal of $<70$ mg $\cdot$ dL$^{-1}$ appears to be appropriate for those in a category of "very high risk."

**57—A.** Cooper 12-min test
The advantages of field tests are that they all potentially could be maximal tests and by their nature are unmonitored for blood pressure and HR. An individual's level of motivation and pacing ability also can have a profound impact on test results. These all-out run tests may be inappropriate for sedentary individuals or individuals at increased risk for cardiovascular and musculoskeletal complications.

**58—D.** Peripheral adaptations are largely responsible for an increase in exercise tolerance.
Physical conditioning in patients with heart failure and moderate-to-severe left ventricular dysfunction results in improved functional capacity and quality of life and reduced symptoms. Peripheral adaptation (increased skeletal muscle oxidative enzymes and improved mitochondrial size and density) are responsible for the increase in exercise tolerance.

**59—A.** Postmenopausal women
A reduction in the risk of osteoporosis, low back pain, hypertension, and diabetes are associated with resistance training. In addition, the benefits of increased muscular strength, bone density, enhanced strength of connective tissue, and the increase or maintenance of lean body mass may also occur. These adaptations are beneficial for all ages, including middle-aged and older adults, and, in particular, post-menopausal women who may experience a more rapid loss of bone mineral density.

**60—C.** Supraventricular aberrant conduction
Supraventricular aberrant conduction — QRS complex is ≥0.11 s; widened QRS usually with unchanged initial vector; P present or absent but with relationship to QRS.

**61—B.** 1 in 2,500
With the physical demands of exercise, emergency situations can occur, especially in a clinical setting where patients with disease are exercising. The incidence of a cardiac arrest during exercise testing is 4 in 10,000 (1/2,500).

**62—A.** Precontemplation
Patients express lack of interest in making change. Moving patients through this stage involves the use of multiple resources to stress the importance of the desired change. This can be achieved through written materials, educational classes, physician and family persuasion, and other means.

**63—A.** LDL cholesterol
Lowering total cholesterol and LDL cholesterol has proved to be effective in reducing and even reversing atherosclerosis. The goal is to reduce the availability of lipids to the injured endothelium. In primary prevention trials, lowering total cholesterol and LDL cholesterol has been shown to reduce the incidence and mortality of coronary artery disease.

**64—A.** ACE inhibitors and angiotensin II blockers
ACE inhibitor and angiotensin II receptor blockers: ⇔ HR (R and E)
Calcium channel blockers: ⇑ or ⇑ or ⇔ HR (R and E)
β-Blockers: ⇓ HR (R and E)
Thyroid medications: ⇑ HR (R and E)

**65—C.** Naughton
The Naughton protocol is appropriate for diseased populations. It is more gradual with increases in intensity and it uses a lower speed than other common protocols (*e.g.*, Bruce protocol). The speed remains constant (2 mph) throughout the test. The grade starts at 0% and increases every 2 min. Small increments in grade allow claudication times to be stratified according to peripheral arterial disease severity.

**66—C.** Digitalis
Digitalis can modify the ST–T contour and slow AV conduction. Digitalis may produce characteristic scooping of the ST–T complex. The ST segment and T wave are fused together, and it can be impossible to tell where one ends and the other begins. This may occur

when digitalis is in the therapeutic range. With digitalis toxicity, digitalis can cause virtually any arrhythmia and all degrees of AV.

**67—C.** A lower HR
Inderal is a β-blocker that diminishes the effect of norepinepherine and epinephrine and lowers HR.

**68—A.** MET
MET is a physiological measure indicating the energy cost of a given physical activity. MET values are used as a means of indicating the intensity of activities in a way comparable among people of different body weight.

**69—D.** Lack of metabolic determination (*i.e.*, $\dot{V}O_{2max}$)
Sufficient physiological stress is needed to reach an ischemic threshold. There can be compensation by collateral circulation with single vessel disease. Sufficient ECG leads (*e.g.*, 12-lead) are required to monitor a complete view of the heart. However, not determining $\dot{V}O_{2max}$ is not a cause for a false negative.

**70—D.** Turbulent blood flow
When measuring blood pressure, blood flows in spurts as the pressure in the artery rises above the pressure in the cuff and then drops back down beyond the cuffed region of the arm. This results in turbulence that produces the audible sounds (Korotkoff sounds).

**71—B.** A systolic blood pressure greater than 200 mm Hg
A systolic blood pressure of >250 mm Hg (not >200 mm Hg) is a relative indication for exercise stress test termination. The other three conditions are reasons for exercise stress test termination.

**72—D.** TG level $\leq 200$ mg $\cdot$ dL$^{-1}$
All of the guidelines listed are correct except the TG level. The 2001 NCEP guidelines list normal TG as <150 mg $\cdot$ dL$^{-1}$.

**73—C.** HR
Myocardial oxygen consumption is increased by a number of variables, including increased HR. A decreased HR at a given intensity (4 MET) would reduce myocardial oxygen consumption. The other three choices do not directly affect myocardial oxygen demand.

**74—B.** Patients with peripheral arterial disease should exercise to leg pain level 3 (on 4-point scale), with intermittent rest periods.
The guidelines recommend patients with peripheral arterial disease achieve 3 (intense pain) on the 4-point claudication scale during exercise. Rest periods should then be allowed until the pain fully resolves before continuing exercise.

**75—D.** Upper middle class
Obese and elderly persons are often less physically active because of various physical or medical limitations (*e.g.*, osteoarthritis, frailty). The less educated are often not aware of the important health and fitness benefits of being physically active on a regular basis.

**76—D.** Subendocardial ischemia
The most common ECG change with subendocardial ischemia is ST-segment depression, NOT ST-segment elevation. ST-segment depression indicates insufficient blood flow (*i.e.*, ischemia) to the heart muscle.

**77—D.** Stroke volume is equal to the ratio of end-diastolic volume to end-systolic volume.
For healthy adults, stroke volume is calculated by subtracting end-systolic volume from end-diastolic volume.

**78—B.** HR
Adaptations to long-term aerobic activity include an increased oxidative capacity of the exercised muscles, increased blood flow through active muscles, and increased venous blood flow return to the heart. These adaptations (*i.e.*, increased aerobic fitness) result in a decreased HR at the same level of submaximal exercise intensity.

**79—C.** Increase maximum coronary blood flow
RPP is an indicator of myocardial oxygen demand. An increase in maximal RPP indicates that there is improved/increased blood flow to the coronary arteries.

**80—A.** Severe coronary artery disease
Severe coronary artery disease will result in less oxygen delivery to the myocardium because of blockage(s), which will reduce or limit oxygenated blood flow to the myocardium.

**81—B.** Increased peripheral resistance
During increasing aerobic activity, there is a volume load on the heart and cardiovascular system, which causes a *decrease* in peripheral vascular resistance. This volume load results in a rise in systolic blood pressure and no change or a slight decrease in diastolic blood pressure. An increase in $\dot{V}O_2$, cardiac output, and mean arterial pressure is typically seen with an increased workload.

**82—D.** Decreased RPP
RPP is a measure of the stress put on the cardiac muscle (myocardial oxygen demand) based on the number of times it needs to beat per minute and the arterial blood pressure that it is pumping against (HR × systolic blood pressure). A

CES

decreased RPP indicates less myocardial oxygen demand. An *increased* RPP can be associated with exercise-induced myocardial ischemia.

**83—D.** Lower stroke volume
Regular aerobic activity typically increases stroke volume at rest. Increased aerobic fitness usually results in a lower resting HR ($HR_{rest}$). The lower HR prolongs diastole (ventricular filling), increasing end-diastolic volume and enables more blood to be ejected with each beat. So physically inactive men will typically have a lower stroke volume compared to physically active men of the same age and weight.

**84—C.** Systolic pressure and HR
HR $\times$ systolic blood pressure = RPP. For example, HR is 80 bpm, systolic pressure is 140; 80 $\times$ 140 = 11,200.

**85—D.** RPP
(HR $\times$ systolic blood pressure) is a measure or indicator of the stress put on the cardiac muscle (myocardial oxygen demand), making it a better indicator of the ischemic threshold compared to HR or blood pressure alone. Oxygen uptake is not a direct measure of ischemia.

**86—C.** Increase HR
HR during maximal exercise will not increase with adaptations from long-term physical activity. HR during maximal exercise is related to age.

**87—D.** All of the above
An increase in any or all of the three choices will increase myocardial oxygen consumption. Likewise, decreasing any or all three choices will decrease myocardial oxygen consumption.

**88—C.** Quadriceps femoris
The quadriceps femoris muscle is the major muscle responsible for knee extension, as dictated by its proximal and distal attachments. The muscle has four heads (quad), three of which originate from the anterior portion of the ilium and one of which originates on the shaft of the femur. All four heads converge and insert on the tibia via a common tendon (patellar). Contraction of the muscle causes the knee to extend. The biceps brachii is found in the upper body and is an elbow flexor. Although the biceps femoris and gastrocnemius muscles cross the knee joint, they do so posteriorly and are primarily active in knee flexion and ankle plantarflexion, respectively.

**89—D.** Increased diastolic blood pressure
Because of the vasodilation associated with exercise-induced stimulation of the sympathetic nervous system, diastolic pressure remains unchanged, or even slightly decreased, during exercise.

**90—B.** Blood pressure elevations are highest during isometric muscular actions.
During isometric contractions, constant — rather than rhythmic — force is generated by the skeletal muscle fibers. This constant force exerts pressure on the blood vessels, which results in occlusion (or blocking) of blood flow through the vessels. Owing to this vascular resistance and the heart's efforts to overcome it, blood pressure is highest during isometric contractions. Because of the associated cardiovascular challenges, isometric contractions should be avoided, particularly among those with known cardiovascular disease.

**91—C.** Exercise training slows down the progression of osteoarthritis.
Little scientific evidence suggests that regular exercise slows down the progression of osteoarthritis. Physical activity can lead to the same benefits observed in the general population. Further, exercise improves strength, balance, and postural stability, which may reduce falls in this at-risk population.

**92—A.** Decreased TG and increased HDL
Chronic exercise training has its greatest benefit on lowering TG and increasing HDL. Changes in total cholesterol or LDL cholesterol are influenced more by dietary habits and body weight than by exercise training.

**93—A.** A coronary artery stent carries a lower rate of revascularization than does PTCA.
Restenosis occurs within 6 mo in approximately 30%–50% of patients who have had a PTCA, whereas a stent has about a 25% failure rate and the drug-eluting stent having a restenosis rate in the low single digits. Atherectomy can be used along with PTCA and is useful when the PTCA catheter cannot pass through the artery, but atherectomy is not a prerequisite for PTCA. Internal mammary artery grafts are preferred over saphenous venous grafts because of superior patency (90% vs. <50% at 10 yr). About 25%–50% of patients will experience a restenosis within 6 mo of laser angioplasty.

**94—B.** An increase in the anginal threshold compared with a test without the medication.
β-Blockers increase the anginal threshold by reducing myocardial oxygen demand at rest and during exercise. This occurs through a reduction in chronotropic (HR) and inotropic (strength of contraction) responses. Blood pressure is also reduced at rest and during

exercise by a reduction in cardiac output (reduced chronotropic and inotropic response) and a reduction in total peripheral resistance. β-Blockers do not produce ST-segment changes on the resting ECG.

**95—A.** Has been physically active on a regular basis for <6 mo.
Stages of motivational readiness describe five categories of readiness to change or maintain behavior. As applied to physical activity or exercise, they are precontemplation (stage 1), contemplation (stage 2), preparation (stage 3), action (stage 4), and maintenance (stage 5). The action stage is when the person is engaged in physical activity or exercise that meets the current ACSM's recommendations for physical activity but has not maintained this program for 6 mo or more.

**96—A.** Monitored immediately, then every 1–2 min for 5 min of recovery or until exercise-induced changes are at baseline.
The 12-lead ECG should be recorded immediately after exercise, then every 1–2 min for 5 min or until exercise-induced ECG changes are at baseline.

**97—D.** MUGA (blood pool imagery) study
MUGA study may be performed to assess resting and exercise cardiac function related to cardiac output, ejection fraction, and wall motion. In this test, technetium-99m is injected into the bloodstream, where it attaches to red blood cells. Areas where the blood pools, such as the ventricles, are visualized by the technetium emissions.

**98—A.** The plan should list the schedule of each staff member so that they can all be accounted for during an emergency.
Accounting for staff in an emergency is not essential. Writing down the plan is essential so that the staff can read it as part of their training as well as have a document to refer to during an emergency. Delineating specific actions by each staff member in an emergency situation and training the staff in these actions obviously are integral parts of any emergency plan.

**99—A.** Limit activities as tolerated to the development of self-care activities, ROM for extremities, and low-resistance activities.
Strenuous and resistive upper body exercises and activity can cause injury to the sternum immediately after CABG surgery. Such exercises should be avoided until the sternum and chest incisions have healed.

**100—C.** Data should be kept on file for at least 1 yr before being discarded.
There is no accepted minimal or maximal amount of time that data should be stored. Clearly, however, data must be stored in a confidential (lock-and-key) manner, and discretion must be used when sharing data.

## CES EXAMINATION QUESTIONS BY DOMAIN

Use the following table as a guide to assist you in your studying process. It is important to note that some questions can be classified as testing multiple domains by the knowledge, skills, and abilities (KSAs).

| Domain Number | I | II | III | IV | V |
|---|---|---|---|---|---|
| Domain Name | Patient/Client Assessment | Exercise Prescription | Program Implementation and Ongoing Support | Leadership and Counseling | Legal and Professional Considerations |
| Percentage of Questions from Domain | 30% | 30% | 20% | 15% | 5% |
| Question Numbers | 3, 7, 8, 9, 16, 18, 19, 20, 21, 22, 25, 27, 28, 29, 30, 31, 33, 37, 42, 44, 45, 52, 54, 55, 56, 57, 60, 61, 65, 66, 67, 68, 69, 70, 71, 72 | 2, 4, 5, 6, 10, 11, 17, 23, 24, 26, 32, 39, 41, 46, 47, 53, 58, 59, 63, 64, 73, 74, 75, 76, 77, 89, 90, 94, 96, 97 | 15, 78, 79, 80, 81, 87, 88, 91, 92, 93, 99 | 12, 13, 14, 49, 50, 82, 83, 84, 85, 86, 95 | 1, 34, 35, 36, 38, 40, 43, 48, 51, 62, 98, 100 |

# Supplementary Figures, Tables, and Boxes from Other ACSM Certification Texts

For your convenience, more than 45 figures, tables, and boxes from other ACSM certification texts are reproduced in this appendix. However, for your full understanding of the concepts presented in these various figures, tables, and boxes, it is strongly recommended that you consult the original source of this material. For instance, a figure may display a concept that is only fully understood when the context that it is presented in is also understood. Thus, you should consider consulting the original sources of these boxes, figures, and tables when studying the concept presented.

# ACSM'S GUIDELINES FOR EXERCISE TESTING AND PRESCRIPTION, 9TH EDITION (GETP9)

The following figures, tables, and boxes come from the indicated chapters of the following source:

Pescatello LS, senior editor. *ACSM's Guidelines for Exercise Testing and Prescription*. 9th ed. Baltimore (MD): Lippincott Williams and Wilkins; 2014.

## GETP9 CHAPTER 1, BENEFITS AND RISKS ASSOCIATED WITH PHYSICAL ACTIVITY

### GETP9 Chapter 1 Boxes

---

**BOX 1.1    Health-Related and Skill-Related Components of Physical Fitness**

**HEALTH-RELATED PHYSICAL FITNESS COMPONENTS**

- Cardiorespiratory endurance: The ability of the circulatory and respiratory system to supply oxygen during sustained physical activity.
- Body composition: The relative amounts of muscle, fat, bone, and other vital parts of the body.
- Muscular strength: The ability of muscle to exert force.
- Muscular endurance: The ability of muscle to continue to perform without fatigue.
- Flexibility: The range of motion available at a joint.

**SKILL-RELATED PHYSICAL FITNESS COMPONENTS**

- Agility: The ability to change the position of the body in space with speed and accuracy.
- Coordination: The ability to use the senses, such as sight and hearing, together with body parts in performing tasks smoothly and accurately.
- Balance: The maintenance of equilibrium while stationary or moving.
- Power: The ability or rate at which one can perform work.
- Reaction time: The time elapsed between stimulation and the beginning of the reaction to it.
- Speed: The ability to perform a movement within a short period of time.

Adapted from The President's Council on Physical Fitness and Sports. *Definitions—Health, Fitness, and Physical Activity* [Internet]. Washington (DC): President's Council on Physical Fitness and Sports; 2000 [cited 2012 Jan 7]. 11 p. Available from: http://purl.access.gpo.gov/GPO/LPS21074 and U.S. Department of Health and Human Services. *Physical Activity and Health: A Report of the Surgeon General*. Atlanta (GA): U.S. Department of Health and Human Services, Public Health Service, Centers for Disease Control and Prevention, National Center for Chronic Disease Prevention and Health Promotion; 1996 [cited 2012 Jan 7]. 278 p. Available from: http://www.fitness.gov/digest_mar2000.htm

---

**BOX 1.2    The ACSM-AHA Primary Physical Activity Recommendations**

- All healthy adults aged 18–65 yr should participate in moderate intensity, aerobic physical activity for a minimum of 30 min on 5 d $\cdot$ wk$^{-1}$ or vigorous intensity, aerobic activity for a minimum of 20 min on 3 d $\cdot$ wk$^{-1}$.
- Combinations of moderate and vigorous intensity exercise can be performed to meet this recommendation.
- Moderate intensity, aerobic activity can be accumulated to total the 30 min minimum by performing bouts each lasting ≥10 min.
- Every adult should perform activities that maintain or increase muscular strength and endurance for a minimum of 2 d $\cdot$ wk$^{-1}$.
- Because of the dose-response relationship between physical activity and health, individuals who wish to further improve their fitness, reduce their risk for chronic diseases and disabilities, and/or prevent unhealthy weight gain may benefit by exceeding the minimum recommended amounts of physical activity.

ACSM, American College of Sports Medicine; AHA, American Heart Association.
Source: Haskell WL, Lee IM, Pate RR, et al. Physical activity and public health: updated recommendation for adults from the American College of Sports Medicine and the American Heart Association. *Med Sci Sports Exerc*. 2007;39(8):1423–34.

## *GETP9* CHAPTER 2, PREPARTICIPATION HEALTH SCREENING

## *GETP9* Chapter 2 Figures

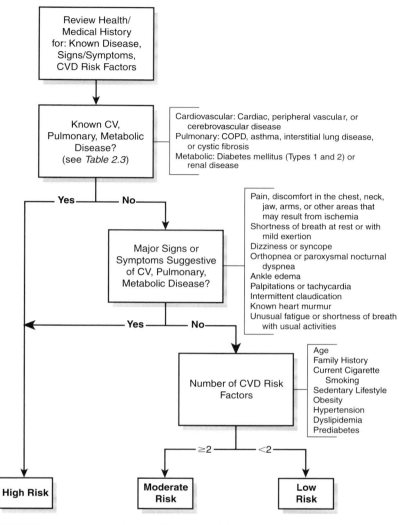

**FIGURE 2.3.** Logic model for classification of risk.

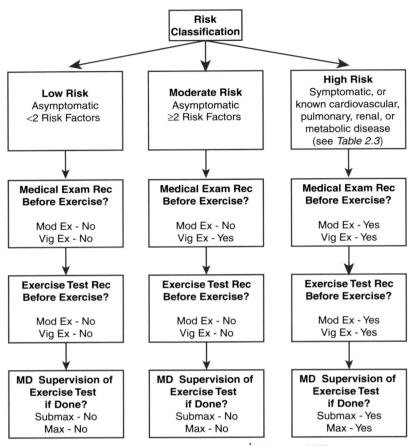

**Mod Ex:**   Moderate intensity exercise; 40%–<60% V̇O₂R; 3–<6 METs
"An intensity that causes noticeable increases in HR and breathing."

**Vig Ex:**   Vigorous intensity exercise; ≥60% V̇O₂R; ≥6 METs
"An intensity that causes substantial increases in HR and breathing."

**Not Rec:**   Reflects the notion a medical examination, exercise test, and physician
supervision of exercise testing are not recommended in the
preparticipation screening; however, they may be considered when there
are concerns about risk, more information is needed for the Ex $R_x$, and/or
are requested by the patient or client.

**Rec:**   Reflects the notion a medical examination, exercise test, and physician
supervision are recommended in the preparticipation health screening
process.

**FIGURE 2.4.** Medical examination, exercise testing, and supervision of exercise
testing preparticipation recommendations based on classification of risk.

## *GETP9* Chapter 2 Tables

| TABLE 2.2.    Atherosclerotic Cardiovascular Disease (CVD) Risk Factors and Defining Criteria | |
|---|---|
| **Risk Factors** | **Defining Criteria** |
| Age | Men ≥45 yr; women ≥55 yr (12) |
| Family history | Myocardial infarction, coronary revascularization, or sudden death before 55 yr in father or other male first-degree relative or before 65 yr in mother or other female first-degree relative |
| Cigarette smoking | Current cigarette smoker or those who quit within the previous 6 mo or exposure to environmental tobacco smoke |
| Sedentary lifestyle | Not participating in at least 30 min of moderate intensity, physical activity (40%–<60% $\dot{V}O_2R$) on at least 3 d of the week for at least 3 mo (22,30) |
| Obesity | Body mass index ≥30 kg · m$^{-2}$ *or* waist girth >102 cm (40 in) for men and >88 cm (35 in) for women (10) |
| Hypertension | Systolic blood pressure ≥140 mm Hg and/or diastolic ≥90 mm Hg, confirmed by measurements on at least two separate occasions, *or* on antihypertensive medication (9) |
| Dyslipidemia | Low-density lipoprotein (LDL) cholesterol ≥130 mg · dL$^{-1}$ (3.37 mmol · L$^{-1}$) *or* high-density lipoprotein[b] (HDL) cholesterol <40 mg · dL$^{-1}$ (1.04 mmol · L$^{-1}$) *or* on lipid-lowering medication. If total serum cholesterol is all that is available, use ≥200 mg · dL$^{-1}$ (5.18 mmol · L$^{-1}$) (21) |
| Prediabetes[a] | Impaired fasting glucose (IFG) = fasting plasma glucose ≥100 mg · dL$^{-1}$ (5.55 mmol · L$^{-1}$) and ≤125 mg · dL$^{-1}$ (6.94 mmol · L$^{-1}$) *or* impaired glucose tolerance (IGT) = 2 h values in oral glucose tolerance test (OGTT) ≥140 mg · dL$^{-1}$ (7.77 mmol · L$^{-1}$) and ≤199 mg · dL$^{-1}$ (11.04 mmol · L$^{-1}$) confirmed by measurements on at least two separate occasions (5) |
| **NEGATIVE RISK FACTOR** | **DEFINING CRITERIA** |
| High-density lipoprotein (HDL) cholesterol | ≥60 mg · dL$^{-1}$ (1.55 mmol · L$^{-1}$) |

[a]If the presence or absence of a CVD risk factor is not disclosed or is not available, that CVD risk factor should be counted as a risk factor except for prediabetes. If the prediabetes criteria are missing or unknown, prediabetes should be counted as a risk factor for those ≥45 yr, especially for those with a body mass index (BMI) ≥25 kg · m$^{-2}$, and those <45 yr with a BMI ≥25 kg · m$^{-2}$ and additional CVD risk factors for prediabetes. The number of positive risk factors is then summed.

[b]High HDL is considered a negative risk factor. For individuals having high HDL ≥60 mg · dL$^{-1}$ (1.55 mmol · L$^{-1}$), for these individuals one positive risk factor is subtracted from the sum of positive risk factors.

$\dot{V}O_2R$, oxygen uptake reserve.

Source: Roger VL, Go AS, Lloyd-Jones DM, et al. Heart Disease and Stroke Statistics—2012 Update: a report from the American Heart Association. *Circulation*. 2012;125(1):e2–220; 31. U.S. Preventive Services Task Force. Screening for coronary heart disease: recommendation statement. *Ann Intern Med*. 2004;140(7):569–72.

**TABLE 2.3. New ACSM Recommendations for Exercise Testing Prior to Exercise-Diagnosed Cardiovascular Disease**

| |
|---|
| Unstable or new or possible symptoms of cardiovascular disease (see *Table 2.2*) |
| Diabetes mellitus and at least one of the following: |
|   Age >35 yr OR |
|   Type 2 diabetes mellitus >10-yr duration OR |
|   Type 1 diabetes mellitus >15-yr duration OR |
|   Hypercholesterolemia (total cholesterol ≥240 mg · L$^{-1}$) (6.62 mmol · L$^{-1}$) OR |
|   Hypertension (systolic blood pressure ≥140 or diastolic ≥90 mm Hg) OR |
|   Smoking OR |
|   Family history of CAD in first-degree relative <60 yr OR |
|   Presence of microvascular disease OR |
|   Peripheral artery disease OR |
|   Autonomic neuropathy |
| End-stage renal disease |
| Patients with symptomatic or diagnosed pulmonary disease including chronic obstructive pulmonary disease (COPD), asthma, interstitial lung disease, or cystic fibrosis. |

ACSM, American College of Sports Medicine; CAD, coronary artery disease.

## *GETP9* CHAPTER 3, PREEXERCISE EVALUATION

## *GETP9* Chapter 3 Figure

---

**Informed Consent for an Exercise Test**

1. **Purpose and Explanation of the Test**
   You will perform an exercise test on a cycle ergometer or a motor-driven treadmill. The exercise intensity will begin at a low level and will be advanced in stages depending on your fitness level. We may stop the test at any time because of signs of fatigue or changes in your heart rate, electrocardiogram, or blood pressure, or symptoms you may experience. It is important for you to realize that you may stop when you wish because of feelings of fatigue or any other discomfort.

2. **Attendant Risks and Discomforts**
   There exists the possibility of certain changes occurring during the test. These include abnormal blood pressure; fainting; irregular, fast, or slow heart rhythm; and, in rare instances, heart attack, stroke, or death. Every effort will be made to minimize these risks by evaluation of preliminary information relating to your health and fitness and by careful observations during testing. Emergency equipment and trained personnel are available to deal with unusual situations that may arise.

3. **Responsibilities of the Participant**
   Information you possess about your health status or previous experiences of heart-related symptoms (*e.g.*, shortness of breath with low-level activity; pain; pressure; tightness; heaviness in the chest, neck, jaw, back, and/or arms) with physical effort may affect the safety of your exercise test. Your prompt reporting of these and any other unusual feelings with effort during the exercise test itself is very important. You are responsible for fully disclosing your medical history as well as symptoms that may occur during the test. You are also expected to report all medications (including nonprescription) taken recently and, in particular, those taken today to the testing staff.

4. **Benefits To Be Expected**
   The results obtained from the exercise test may assist in the diagnosis of your illness, in evaluating the effect of your medications, or in evaluating what type of physical activities you might do with low risk.

5. **Inquiries**
   Any questions about the procedures used in the exercise test or the results of your test are encouraged. If you have any concerns or questions, please ask us for further explanations.

6. **Use of Medical Records**
   The information that is obtained during exercise testing will be treated as privileged and confidential as described in the Health Insurance Portability and Accountability Act of 1996. It is not to be released or revealed to any individual except your referring physician without your written consent. However, the information obtained may be used for statistical analysis or scientific purposes with your right to privacy retained.

7. **Freedom of Consent**
   I hereby consent to voluntarily engage in an exercise test to determine my exercise capacity and state of cardiovascular health. My permission to perform this exercise test is given voluntarily. I understand that I am free to stop the test at any point if I so desire.

   I have read this form, and I understand the test procedures that I will perform and the attendant risks and discomforts. Knowing these risks and discomforts, and having had an opportunity to ask questions that have been answered to my satisfaction, I consent to participate in this test.

   | | |
   |---|---|
   | _____ | _____ |
   | Date | Signature of Patient |
   | _____ | _____ |
   | Date | Signature of Witness |
   | _____ | _____ |
   | Date | Signature of Physician or Authorized Delegate |

---

**FIGURE 3.1.** Sample of informed consent form for a symptom-limited exercise test.

## GETP9 Chapter 3 Box

| BOX 3.5 | Contraindications to Exercise Testing |
| --- | --- |

### ABSOLUTE

- A recent significant change in the resting electrocardiogram (ECG) suggesting significant ischemia, recent myocardial infarction (within 2 d), or other acute cardiac event
- Unstable angina
- Uncontrolled cardiac dysrhythmias causing symptoms or hemodynamic compromise
- Symptomatic severe aortic stenosis
- Uncontrolled symptomatic heart failure
- Acute pulmonary embolus or pulmonary infarction
- Acute myocarditis or pericarditis
- Suspected or known dissecting aneurysm
- Acute systemic infection, accompanied by fever, body aches, or swollen lymph glands

### RELATIVE[a]

- Left main coronary stenosis
- Moderate stenotic valvular heart disease
- Electrolyte abnormalities (*e.g.*, hypokalemia or hypomagnesemia)
- Severe arterial hypertension (*i.e.*, systolic blood pressure [SBP] of >200 mm Hg and/or a diastolic BP [DBP] of >110 mm Hg) at rest
- Tachydysrhythmia or bradydysrhythmia
- Hypertrophic cardiomyopathy and other forms of outflow tract obstruction
- Neuromotor, musculoskeletal, or rheumatoid disorders that are exacerbated by exercise
- High-degree atrioventricular block
- Ventricular aneurysm
- Uncontrolled metabolic disease (*e.g.*, diabetes, thyrotoxicosis, or myxedema)
- Chronic infectious disease (*e.g.*, HIV)
- Mental or physical impairment leading to inability to exercise adequately

[a]Relative contraindications can be superseded if benefits outweigh the risks of exercise. In some instances, these individuals can be exercised with caution and/or using low-level endpoints, especially if they are asymptomatic at rest.

Modified from Gibbons RJ, Balady GJ, Bricker JT, et al. ACC/AHA 2002 guideline update for exercise testing: summary article. A report of the American College of Cardiology/American Heart Association Task Force on Practice Guidelines (Committee to Update the 1997 Exercise Testing Guidelines). *J Am Coll Cardiol.* 2002;40(8):1531–40. [cited 2007 Jun 15]. Available from: http://www.ncbi.nlm.nih.gov/pubmed/12356646

## *GETP9* CHAPTER 4, HEALTH-RELATED PHYSICAL FITNESS TESTING AND INTERPRETATION

### *GETP9* Chapter 4 Table

**TABLE 4.4.  Population-Specific Formulas for Conversion of Body Density to Percent Body Fat**

| | Population | Age | Gender | %BF | FFBd[a] (g · cm$^{-3}$) |
|---|---|---|---|---|---|
| ETHNICITY | African American | 9–17 | Women | $(5.24 / Db) - 4.82$ | 1.088 |
| | | 19–45 | Men | $(4.86 / Db) - 4.39$ | 1.106 |
| | | 24–79 | Women | $(4.86 / Db) - 4.39$ | 1.106 |
| | American Indian | 18–62 | Men | $(4.97 / Db) - 4.52$ | 1.099 |
| | | 18–60 | Women | $(4.81 / Db) - 4.34$ | 1.108 |
| | Asian Japanese Native | 18–48 | Men | $(4.97 / Db) - 4.52$ | 1.099 |
| | | | Women | $(4.76 / Db) - 4.28$ | 1.111 |
| | | 61–78 | Men | $(4.87 / Db) - 4.41$ | 1.105 |
| | | | Women | $(4.95 / Db) - 4.50$ | 1.100 |
| | Singaporean (Chinese, Indian, Malay) | | Men | $(4.94 / Db) - 4.48$ | 1.102 |
| | | | Women | $(4.84 / Db) - 4.37$ | 1.107 |
| | Caucasian | 8–12 | Men | $(5.27 / Db) - 4.85$ | 1.086 |
| | | | Women | $(5.27 / Db) - 4.85$ | 1.086 |
| | | 13–17 | Men | $(5.12 / Db) - 4.69$ | 1.092 |
| | | | Women | $(5.19 / Db) - 4.76$ | 1.090 |
| | | 18–59 | Men | $(4.95 / Db) - 4.50$ | 1.100 |
| | | | Women | $(4.96 / Db) - 4.51$ | 1.101 |
| | | 60–90 | Men | $(4.97 / Db) - 4.52$ | 1.099 |
| | | | Women | $(5.02 / Db) - 4.57$ | 1.098 |
| | Hispanic | | Men | NA | NA |
| | | 20–40 | Women | $(4.87 / Db) - 4.41$ | 1.105 |
| ATHLETES | Resistance trained | 24 ± 4 | Men | $(5.21 / Db) - 4.78$ | 1.089 |
| | | 35 ± 6 | Women | $(4.97 / Db) - 4.52$ | 1.099 |
| | Endurance trained | 21 ± 2 | Men | $(5.03 / Db) - 4.59$ | 1.097 |
| | | 21 ± 4 | Women | $(4.95 / Db) - 4.50$ | 1.100 |
| | All sports | 18–22 | Men | $(5.12 / Db) - 4.68$ | 1.093 |
| | | 18–22 | Women | $(4.97 / Db) - 4.52$ | 1.099 |
| CLINICAL POPULATIONS[b] | Anorexia nervosa | 15–44 | Women | $(4.96 / Db) - 4.51$ | 1.101 |
| | Cirrhosis | | | | |
| | Childs A | | | $(5.33 / Db) - 4.91$ | 1.084 |
| | Childs B | | | $(5.48 / Db) - 5.08$ | 1.078 |
| | Childs C | | | $(5.69 / Db) - 5.32$ | 1.070 |
| | Obesity | 17–62 | Women | $(4.95 / Db) - 4.50$ | 1.100 |
| | Spinal cord injury (paraplegic/quadriplegic) | 18–73 | Men | $(4.67 / Db) - 4.18$ | 1.116 |
| | | 18–73 | Women | $(4.70 / Db) - 4.22$ | 1.114 |

[a]FFBd, fat-free body density based on average values reported in selected research articles.

[b]There are insufficient multicomponent model data to estimate the average FFBd of the following clinical populations: coronary artery disease, heart/lung transplants, chronic obstructive pulmonary disease, cystic fibrosis, diabetes mellitus, thyroid disease, HIV/AIDS, cancer, kidney failure (dialysis), multiple sclerosis, and muscular dystrophy.

%BF, percentage of body fat; Db, body density; NA, no data available for this population subgroup.

Adapted with permission from Heyward VH, Wagner DR. *Applied Body Composition Assessment.* 2nd ed. Champaign (IL): Human Kinetics; 2004. p. 9.

## *GETP9* Chapter 4 Box

| BOX 4.3 | Generalized Skinfold Equations |
|---|---|

### MEN

- **Seven-Site Formula** (chest, midaxillary, triceps, subscapular, abdomen, suprailiac, thigh)
  Body density = 1.112 − 0.00043499 (sum of seven skinfolds)
  + 0.00000055 (sum of seven skinfolds)$^2$ − 0.00028826 (age) *[SEE 0.008 or ~3.5% fat]*

- **Three-Site Formula** (chest, abdomen, thigh)
  Body density = 1.10938 − 0.0008267 (sum of three skinfolds)
  + 0.0000016 (sum of three skinfolds)$^2$ − 0.0002574 (age) *[SEE 0.008 or ~3.4% fat]*

- **Three-Site Formula** (chest, triceps, subscapular)
  Body density = 1.1125025 − 0.0013125 (sum of three skinfolds)
  + 0.0000055 (sum of three skinfolds)$^2$ − 0.000244 (age) *[SEE 0.008 or ~3.6% fat]*

### WOMEN

- **Seven-Site Formula** (chest, midaxillary, triceps, subscapular, abdomen, suprailiac, thigh)
  Body density = 1.097 − 0.00046971 (sum of seven skinfolds)
  + 0.00000056 (sum of seven skinfolds)$^2$ − 0.00012828 (age) *[SEE 0.008 or ~3.8% fat]*

- **Three-Site Formula** (triceps, suprailiac, thigh)
  Body density = 1.099421 − 0.0009929 (sum of three skinfolds)
  + 0.0000023 (sum of three skinfolds)$^2$ − 0.0001392 (age) *[SEE 0.009 or ~3.9% fat]*

- **Three-Site Formula** (triceps, suprailiac, abdominal)
  Body density = 1.089733 − 0.0009245 (sum of three skinfolds)
  + 0.0000025 (sum of three skinfolds)$^2$ − 0.0000979 (age) *[SEE 0.009 or ~3.9% fat]*

SEE, standard error of estimate.
Adapted from Jackson AW, Pollock ML. Practical assessment of body composition. *Phys Sportsmed.* 1985;13(5):76–80, 82–90 and Pollack ML, Schmidt DH, Jackson AS. Measurement of cardiorespiratory fitness and body composition in the clinical setting. *Compr Ther.* 1980;6(9):12–27.

## GETP9 CHAPTER 7, GENERAL PRINCIPLES OF EXERCISE PRESCRIPTION

## GETP9 Chapter 7 Figure

*Heart Rate Reserve (HRR) Method*
  Available test data:
    $HR_{rest}$: 70 beats $\cdot$ min$^{-1}$
    $HR_{max}$: 180 beats $\cdot$ min$^{-1}$
  Desired exercise intensity range: 50%–60%
  Formula: Target Heart Rate (THR) = [($HR_{max} - HR_{rest}$) $\times$ % intensity] + $HR_{rest}$
    1)  Calculation of HRR:
        HRR = ($HR_{max} - HR_{rest}$)
        HRR = (180 beats $\cdot$ min$^{-1}$ − 70 beats $\cdot$ min$^{-1}$) = 110 beats $\cdot$ min$^{-1}$
    2)  Determination of exercise intensity as %HRR:
        Convert desired %HRR into a decimal by dividing by 100
        %HRR = desired intensity $\times$ HRR
        %HRR = 0.5 $\times$ 110 beats $\cdot$ min$^{-1}$ = 55 beats $\cdot$ min$^{-1}$
        %HRR = 0.6 $\times$ 110 beats $\cdot$ min$^{-1}$ = 66 beats $\cdot$ min$^{-1}$
    3)  Determine THR range:
        THR = (%HRR) + $HR_{rest}$
        To determine lower limit of THR range:
          THR = 55 beats $\cdot$ min$^{-1}$ + 70 beats $\cdot$ min$^{-1}$ = 125 beats $\cdot$ min$^{-1}$
        To determine upper limit of THR range:
          THR = 66 beats $\cdot$ min$^{-1}$ + 70 beats $\cdot$ min$^{-1}$ = 136 beats $\cdot$ min$^{-1}$
        THR range: 125 beats $\cdot$ min$^{-1}$ to 136 beats $\cdot$ min$^{-1}$

$\dot{V}O_2$ *Reserve ($\dot{V}O_2R$) Method*
  Available test data:
    $\dot{V}O_{2max}$: 30 mL $\cdot$ kg$^{-1}$ $\cdot$ min$^{-1}$
    $\dot{V}O_{2rest}$: 3.5 mL $\cdot$ kg$^{-1}$ $\cdot$ min$^{-1}$
  Desired exercise intensity range: 50%–60%
  Formula: Target $\dot{V}O_2$ = [($\dot{V}O_{2max} - \dot{V}O_{2rest}$) $\times$ % intensity] + $\dot{V}O_{2rest}$
    1)  Calculation of $\dot{V}O_2R$:
        $\dot{V}O_2R = \dot{V}O_{2max} - \dot{V}O_{2rest}$
        $\dot{V}O_2R$ = 30 mL $\cdot$ kg$^{-1}$ $\cdot$ min$^{-1}$ − 3.5 mL $\cdot$ kg$^{-1}$ $\cdot$ min$^{-1}$
        $\dot{V}O_2R$ = 26.5 mL $\cdot$ kg$^{-1}$ $\cdot$ min$^{-1}$
    2)  Determination of exercise intensity as %$\dot{V}O_2R$:
        Convert desired intensity (%$\dot{V}O_2R$) into a decimal by dividing by 100
        %$\dot{V}O_2R$ = desired intensity $\times$ %$\dot{V}O_2R$
        Calculate %$\dot{V}O_2R$:
        %$\dot{V}O_2R$ = 0.5 $\times$ 26.5 mL $\cdot$ kg$^{-1}$ $\cdot$ min$^{-1}$ = 13.3 mL $\cdot$ kg$^{-1}$ $\cdot$ min$^{-1}$
        %$\dot{V}O_2R$ = 0.6 $\times$ 26.5 mL $\cdot$ kg$^{-1}$ $\cdot$ min$^{-1}$ = 15.9 mL $\cdot$ kg$^{-1}$ $\cdot$ min$^{-1}$
    3)  Determine target $\dot{V}O_2R$ range:
        (%$\dot{V}O_2R$) + $\dot{V}O_{2rest}$
        To determine the lower target $\dot{V}O_2$ range:
          Target $\dot{V}O_2$ = 13.3 mL $\cdot$ kg$^{-1}$ $\cdot$ min$^{-1}$ + 3.5 mL $\cdot$ kg$^{-1}$ $\cdot$ min$^{-1}$ =
          16.8 mL $\cdot$ kg$^{-1}$ $\cdot$ min$^{-1}$
        To determine upper target $\dot{V}O_2$ range:
          Target $\dot{V}O_2$ = 15.9 mL $\cdot$ kg$^{-1}$ $\cdot$ min$^{-1}$ + 3.5 mL $\cdot$ kg$^1$ $\cdot$ min$^{-1}$ =
          19.4 mL $\cdot$ kg$^{-1}$ $\cdot$ min$^{-1}$
        Target $\dot{V}O_2$ range: 16.8 mL $\cdot$ kg$^{-1}$ $\cdot$ min$^{-1}$ to 19.4 mL $\cdot$ kg$^{-1}$ $\cdot$ min$^{-1}$
    4)  Determine MET target range (optional):
        1 MET = 3.5 mL $\cdot$ kg$^{-1}$ $\cdot$ min$^{-1}$
        Calculate lower MET target:
          1 MET/3.5 mL $\cdot$ kg$^{-1}$ $\cdot$ min$^{-1}$ = $\times$ MET/16.8 mL $\cdot$ kg$^{-1}$ $\cdot$ min$^{-1}$
          $\times$ MET = 16.8 mL $\cdot$ min$^{-1}$/3.5 mL $\cdot$ kg$^{-1}$ $\cdot$ min$^{-1}$ = 4.8 METs
        Calculate upper MET target:
          1 MET/3.5 mL $\cdot$ kg$^{-1}$ $\cdot$ min$^{-1}$ = $\times$ MET/19.4 mL $\cdot$ kg$^{-1}$ $\cdot$ min$^{-1}$
          $\times$ MET = 19.4 mL $\cdot$ kg$^{-1}$ $\cdot$ min$^{-1}$/3.5 mL $\cdot$ kg$^{-1}$ $\cdot$ min$^{-1}$ = 5.5 METs
    5)  Identify physical activities requiring EE within the target range from
        compendium of physical activities (1,2) or by using metabolic calcula-
        tions shown in *Table 7.3* or reference (22). Also see the following exam-
        ples of use of metabolic equations.

**FIGURE 7.1.** Examples of the application of various methods for prescribing exercise intensity. $HR_{max}$, maximal heart rate; $HR_{rest}$, resting heart rate; MET, metabolic equivalent; $\dot{V}O_2$, volume of oxygen consumed per unit of time; $\dot{V}O_{2max}$, maximal volume of oxygen consumed per unit of time.

*%HR$_{max}$ (Measured Or Estimated) Method:*
  Available data:
    A man 45 yr of age
  Desired exercise intensity: 70%–80%
  Formula: THR = HR$_{max}$ × desired %
  Calculate estimated HR$_{max}$ (if measured HR$_{max}$ not available):
    HR$_{max}$ = 220 − age
    HR$_{max}$ = 220 − 45 = 175 beats · min$^{-1}$
      1)  Determine THR range:
          THR = Desired % × HR$_{max}$
          Convert desired % HR$_{max}$ into a decimal by dividing by 100
          Determine lower limit of THR range:
            THR = 175 beats · min$^{-1}$ × 0.70 = 123 beats · min$^{-1}$
          Determine upper limit of THR range:
            THR = 175 beats · min$^{-1}$ × 0.80 = 140 beats · min$^{-1}$
          THR range: 123 beats · min$^{-1}$ to 140 beats · min$^{-1}$

*%V̇O$_2$ (Measured or Estimated) Method*
  Available data:
    A woman 45 yr of age
    Estimated V̇O$_{2max}$: 30 mL · kg$^{-1}$ · min$^{-1}$
  Desired V̇O$_2$ range: 50%–60%
  Formula: V̇O$_{2max}$ × desired %
  Determine target V̇O$_2$ range:
    Target V̇O$_2$ = Desired % × V̇O$_{2max}$
      Convert desired intensity (%V̇O$_2$) into a decimal by dividing by 100
      Determine lower limit of target V̇O$_2$ range:
        Target V̇O$_2$ = 0.50 × 30 mL · kg$^{-1}$ · min$^{-1}$ = 15 mL · kg$^{-1}$ · min$^{-1}$
  Determine upper limit of target V̇O$_{2max}$ range:
    Target V̇O$_2$ = 0.60 × 30 mL · kg$^{-1}$ · min$^{-1}$ = 18 mL · kg$^{-1}$ · min$^{-1}$
    Target V̇O$_2$ range: 15 mL · kg$^{-1}$ · min$^{-1}$ to 18 mL · kg$^{-1}$ · min$^{-1}$
      1)  Determine MET target range (optional):
          1 MET = 3.5 mL · kg$^{-1}$ · min$^{-1}$
          Calculate lower MET target:
            1 MET/3.5 mL · kg$^{-1}$ · min$^{-1}$ = × MET/15.0 mL · kg$^{-1}$ · min$^{-1}$
            × MET = 15.0 mL · kg$^{-1}$ · min$^{-1}$/3.5 mL · kg$^{-1}$ · min$^{-1}$ = 4.3 METs
          Calculate upper MET target:
            1 MET/3.5 mL · kg$^{-1}$ · min$^{-1}$ = × MET/18.0 mL · kg$^{-1}$ · min$^{-1}$
            × MET = 18.0 mL · kg$^{-1}$ · min$^{-1}$/3.5 mL · kg$^{-1}$ · min$^{-1}$ = 5.1 METs
      2)  Identify physical activities requiring EE within the target range from
          compendium of physical activities (1,2) or by using metabolic calcula-
          tions shown in *Table 7.3* and reference (22). See the following examples
          of use of metabolic equations.

*Using metabolic calculations (22) or (Table 7.3) to determine running speed on a treadmill*
  Available data:
    A man 32 yr of age
    Weight: 130 lb (59 kg)
    Height: 70 in (177.8 cm)
    V̇O$_{2max}$: 54 mL · kg$^{-1}$ · min$^{-1}$
  Desired treadmill grade: 2.5%
  Desired exercise intensity: 80%
  Formula: V̇O$_2$ = 3.5 + (0.2 × speed) + (0.9 × speed × % grade)
      1.  Determine target V̇O$_2$:
          Target V̇O$_2$ = desired % × V̇O$_{2max}$
          Target V̇O$_2$ = 0.80 × 54 mL · kg$^{-1}$ · min$^{-1}$ = 43.2 mL · kg$^{-1}$ · min$^{-1}$
      2.  Determine treadmill speed:
          V̇O$_2$ = 3.5 + (0.2 × speed) + (0.9 × speed × % grade)
            43.2 mL · kg$^{-1}$ · min$^{-1}$ = 3.5 + (0.2 × speed) + (0.9 × speed × 0.025)
            39.7 = (0.2 × speed) + (0.9 × speed × 0.025)
            39.7 = (0.2 × speed) + (0.0225 × speed)
            39.7 = 0.2225 × speed
            178.4 m · min$^{-1}$ = speed
          Speed on treadmill: 10.7 km · h$^{-1}$ (6.7 mi · h$^1$)

**FIGURE 7.1.** (*Continued*)

*Using metabolic calculations* (22) *(Table 7.2) to determine % grade during walking on a treadmill*

    Available data:

        A man 54 yr of age who is moderately physically active

        Weight: 190 lb (86.4 kg)

        Height: 70 in (177.8 cm)

    Desired walking speed: 2.5 mi $\cdot$ h$^{-1}$ (4 km $\cdot$ h$^{-1}$; 67 m $\cdot$ min$^{-1}$)

    Desired MET: 5 METs

    Formula: $\dot{V}O_2$ = 3.5 + (0.1 × speed) + (1.8 × speed × % grade)

        1.   Determine target $\dot{V}O_2$:

             Target $\dot{V}O_2$ = MET × 3.5 mL $\cdot$ kg$^{-1}$ $\cdot$ min$^{-1}$

             Target $\dot{V}O_2$ = 5 × 3.5 mL $\cdot$ kg$^{-1}$ $\cdot$ min$^{-1}$ = 17.5 mL $\cdot$ kg$^{-1}$ $\cdot$ min$^{-1}$

        2.   Determine treadmill grade:

           $\dot{V}O_2$ = 3.5 + (0.1 × speed) + (1.8 × speed × % grade)

             17.5 mL $\cdot$ kg$^{-1}$ $\cdot$ min$^{-1}$ = 3.5 + (0.1 × 67 m $\cdot$ s$^{-1}$) +

             (1.8 × 67 m $\cdot$ s$^{-1}$ × % grade)

             14 = (0.1 × 67 m $\cdot$ s$^{-1}$) + (1.8 × 67 m $\cdot$ s$^{-1}$ × % grade)

             14 = 6.7 + (120.6 × % grade)

             7.3 = 120.6 × % grade

             0.06 = % grade

             % grade = 6%

*Using metabolic calculations* (22) *(Table 7.3) to determine target work rate (kg $\cdot$ m $\cdot$ min$^{-1}$) on a Monarch leg cycle ergometer*

    Available data:

        A woman 42 yr of age

        Weight: 190 lb (86.4 kg)

        Height: 70 in (177.8 cm)

    Desired $\dot{V}O_2$: 18 kg $\cdot$ m $\cdot$ min$^{-1}$

    Formula: $\dot{V}O_2$ = 7.0 + (1.8 × work rate)/body mass

        1.   Calculate work rate on cycle ergometer:

           $\dot{V}O_2$ = 7.0 + (1.8 × work rate)/body mass)

             18 mL $\cdot$ kg$^{-1}$ $\cdot$ min$^{-1}$ = 7.0 + (1.8 × work rate)/86.4 kg

             11 = (1.8 × work rate)/86.4

             950.4 = 1.8 × work rate

             528 = work rate

           Work rate = 528 kg $\cdot$ m $\cdot$ min$^{-1}$ = 86.6 W

**FIGURE 7.1.** (*Continued*)

## GETP9 Chapter 7 Tables

**TABLE 7.1. Methods of Estimating Intensity of Cardiorespiratory and Resistance Exercise**

| | Cardiorespiratory Endurance Exercise | | | | | | | | | | | Resistance Exercise |
| | Relative Intensity | | | | Intensity (%VO$_{2max}$) Relative to Maximal Exercise Capacity in MET | | | Absolute Intensity | Absolute Intensity (MET) by Age | | | Relative Intensity |
| Intensity | %HRR or %VO$_2$R | %HR$_{max}$ | %VO$_{2max}$ | Perceived Exertion (Rating on 6–20 RPE Scale) | 20 METs %VO$_{2max}$ | 10 METs %VO$_{2max}$ | 5 METs %VO$_{2max}$ | MET | Young (20–39 yr) | Middle Age (40–64 yr) | Older (≥65 yr) | % One Repetition Maximum |
|---|---|---|---|---|---|---|---|---|---|---|---|---|
| Very light | <30 | <57 | <37 | Very light (RPE ≤9) | <34 | <37 | <44 | <2 | <2.4 | <2.0 | <1.6 | <30 |
| Light | 30–<40 | 57–<64 | 37–<45 | Very light to fairly light (RPE 9–11) | 34–<43 | 37–<46 | 44–<52 | 2.0–<3 | <4.8 | <4.0 | <3.2 | 30–<50 |
| Moderate | 40–<60 | 64–<76 | 46–<64 | Fairly light to somewhat hard (RPE 12–13) | 43–<62 | 46–<64 | 52–<68 | 3.0–<6 | 4.8–<7.2 | 4.0–<6.0 | 3.2–<4.8 | 50–<70 |
| Vigorous | 60–<90 | 76–<96 | 64–<91 | Somewhat hard to very hard (RPE 14–17) | 62–<91 | 64–<91 | 68–<92 | 6.0–<8.8 | 7.2–<10.2 | 6.0–<8.5 | 4.8–<6.8 | 70–<85 |
| Near maximal to maximal | ≥90 | ≥96 | ≥91 | ≥ Very hard (RPE ≥18) | ≥91 | ≥91 | ≥92 | ≥8.8 | ≥10.2 | ≥8.5 | ≥6.8 | ≥85 |

HR$_{max}$, maximal heart rate; HRR, heart rate reserve; MET, metabolic equivalent; RPE, rating of perceived exertion; VO$_{2max}$, maximum oxygen consumption; VO$_2$R, oxygen uptake reserve.

Adapted from Garber CE, Blissmer B, Deschenes MR, et al. American College of Sports Medicine position stand. The quantity and quality of exercise for developing and maintaining cardiorespiratory, musculoskeletal, and neuromotor fitness in apparently healthy adults: guidance for prescribing exercise. Med Sci Sports Exerc. 2011;43(7):1334–559.

## TABLE 7.3. Metabolic Calculations for the Estimation of Energy Expenditure ($\dot{V}O_{2max}$ [mL · kg$^{-1}$ · min$^{-1}$]) During Common Physical Activities

| Activity | Resting Component | Horizontal Component | Vertical Component/ Resistance Component | Limitations |
|---|---|---|---|---|
| | **Sum of Resting + Horizontal + Vertical/Resistance Components** | | | |
| Walking | 3.5 | 0.1 × speed[a] | 1.8 × speed[a] × grade[b] | Most accurate for speeds of 1.9–3.7 mi · h$^{-1}$ (50–100 m · min$^{-1}$) |
| Running | 3.5 | 0.2 × speed[a] | 0.9 × speed[a] × grade[b] | Most accurate for speeds >5 mi · h$^{-1}$ (134 m · min$^{-1}$) |
| Stepping | 3.5 | 0.2 × steps · min$^{-1}$ | 1.33 × (1.8 × step height[c] × steps · min$^{-1}$) | Most accurate for stepping rates of 12–30 steps · min$^{-1}$ |
| Leg cycling | 3.5 | 3.5 | (1.8 × work rate[d])/ body mass[e] | Most accurate for work rates of 300–1,200 kg · m · min$^{-1}$ (50–200 W) |
| Arm cycling | 3.5 | | (3 × work rate[d])/ body mass[e] | Most accurate for work rates between 150–750 kg · m · min$^{-1}$ (25–125 W) |

[a]Speed in m · min$^{-1}$.

[b]Grade is percent grade expressed in decimal format (*e.g.*, 10% = 0.10).

[c]Step height in m.

*Multiply by the following conversion factors:*

  lb to kg: 0.454; in to cm: 2.54; ft to m: 0.3048; mi to km: 1.609; mi ? h$^{-1}$ to m · min$^{-1}$: 26.8; kg · m · min$^{-1}$ to W: 0.164; W to kg · m · min$^{-1}$: 6.12; $\dot{V}O_{2max}$ L · min$^{-1}$ to kcal · min$^{-1}$: 4.9; $\dot{V}O_2$ MET to mL · kg$^{-1}$ · min$^{-1}$: 3.5.

[d]Work rate in kilogram meters per minute (kg · m · min$^{-1}$) is calculated as resistance (kg) × distance per revolution of flywheel × pedal frequency per minute. Note: Distance per revolution is 6 m for Monark leg ergometer, 3 m for the Tunturi and BodyGuard ergometers, and 2.4 m for Monark arm ergometer.

[e]Body mass in kg

$\dot{V}O_{2max}$, maximal volume of oxygen consumed per unit of time.

Adapted from Armstrong LE, Brubaker PH, Whaley MH, Otto RM, American College of Sports Medicine. *ACSM's Guidelines for Exercise Testing and Prescription.* 7th ed. Baltimore (MD): Lippincott Williams & Wilkins; 2005. 366 p.

| TABLE 7.5. | Aerobic (Cardiovascular Endurance) Exercise Evidence-Based Recommendations |
|---|---|
| **FITT-VP** | **Evidence-Based Recommendation** |
| *F*requency | • ≥5 d · wk⁻¹ of moderate exercise, or ≥3 d · wk⁻¹ of vigorous exercise, or a combination of moderate and vigorous exercise on ≥3–5 d · wk⁻¹ is recommended. |
| *I*ntensity | • Moderate and/or vigorous intensity is recommended for most adults.<br>• Light-to-moderate intensity exercise may be beneficial in deconditioned persons. |
| *T*ime | • 30–60 min · d⁻¹ of purposeful moderate exercise, or 20–60 min · d⁻¹ of vigorous exercise, or a combination of moderate and vigorous exercise per day is recommended for most adults.<br>• <20 min of exercise per day can be beneficial, especially in previously sedentary persons. |
| *T*ype | • Regular, purposeful exercise that involves major muscle groups and is continuous and rhythmic in nature is recommended. |
| *V*olume | • A target volume of ≥500–1,000 MET-min · wk⁻¹ is recommended.<br>• Increasing pedometer step counts by ≥2,000 steps · d⁻¹ to reach a daily step count ≥7,000 steps · d⁻¹ steps is beneficial.<br>• Exercising below these volumes may still be beneficial for persons unable or unwilling to reach this amount of exercise. |
| *P*attern | • Exercise may be performed in one (continuous) session per day or in multiple sessions of ≥10 min to accumulate the desired duration and volume of exercise per day.<br>• Exercise bouts of <10 min may yield favorable adaptations in very deconditioned individuals. |
| *P*rogression | • A gradual progression of exercise volume by adjusting exercise duration, frequency, and/or intensity is reasonable until the desired exercise goal (maintenance) is attained.<br>• This approach may enhance adherence and reduce risks of musculoskeletal injury and adverse cardiac events. |

Adapted from Garber CE, Blissmer B, Deschenes MR, et al. American College of Sports Medicine position stand. The quantity and quality of exercise for developing and maintaining cardiorespiratory, musculoskeletal, and neuromotor fitness in apparently healthy adults: guidance for prescribing exercise. *Med Sci Sports Exerc.* 2011;43(7):1334–559.

## TABLE 7.6.  Resistance Exercise Evidence-Based Recommendations

| FITT-VP | Evidence-Based Recommendation |
|---|---|
| **F**requency | • Each major muscle group should be trained on 2–3 d · wk$^{-1}$. |
| **I**ntensity | • 60%–70% 1-RM (moderate-to-vigorous intensity) for novice to intermediate exercisers to improve strength<br>• ≥80% 1-RM (vigorous-to-very vigorous intensity) for experienced strength trainers to improve strength<br>• 40%–50% RM (very light-to-light intensity) for older individuals beginning exercise to improve strength<br>• 40%–50% 1-RM (very light-to-light intensity) may be beneficial for improving strength in sedentary individuals beginning a resistance training program<br>• <50% 1-RM (light-to-moderate intensity) to improve muscular endurance<br>• 20%–50% 1-RM in older adults to improve power |
| **T**ime | • No specific duration of training has been identified for effectiveness. |
| **T**ype | • Resistance exercises involving each major muscle group are recommended.<br>• Multijoint exercises affecting more than one muscle group and targeting agonist and antagonist muscle groups are recommended for all adults.<br>• Single joint exercises targeting major muscle groups may also be included in a resistance training program, typically after performing multijoint exercise(s) for that particular muscle group.<br>• A variety of exercise equipment and/or body weight can be used to perform these exercises. |
| **R**epetitions | • 8–12 repetitions is recommended to improve strength and power in most adults.<br>• 10–15 repetitions is effective in improving strength in middle-aged and older individuals starting exercise.<br>• 15–20 repetitions are recommended to improve muscular endurance. |
| **S**ets | • 2–4 sets are recommended for most adults to improve strength and power.<br>• A single set of resistance exercise can be effective especially among older and novice exercisers.<br>• ≤2 sets are effective in improving muscular endurance. |
| **P**attern | • Rest intervals of 2–3 min between each set of repetitions are effective.<br>• A rest of ≥48 h between sessions for any single muscle group is recommended. |
| **P**rogression | • A gradual progression of greater resistance, and/or more repetitions per set, and/or increasing frequency is recommended. |

1-RM, one repetition maximum.

Adapted from Garber CE, Blissmer B, Deschenes MR, et al. American College of Sports Medicine position stand. The quantity and quality of exercise for developing and maintaining cardiorespiratory, musculoskeletal, and neuromotor fitness in apparently healthy adults: guidance for prescribing exercise. *Med Sci Sports Exerc.* 2011;43(7):1334–559.

## TABLE 7.7. Flexibility Exercise Evidence-Based Recommendations

| FITT-VP | Evidence-Based Recommendation |
|---------|-------------------------------|
| **F**requency | • ≥2–3 d · wk$^{-1}$ with daily being most effective |
| **I**ntensity | • Stretch to the point of feeling tightness or slight discomfort |
| **T**ime | • Holding a static stretch for 10–30 s is recommended for most adults.<br>• In older individuals, holding a stretch for 30–60 s may confer greater benefit.<br>• For proprioceptive neuromuscular facilitation (PNF) stretching, a 3–6 s light-to-moderate contraction (*e.g.*, 20%–75% of maximum voluntary contraction) followed by a 10–30 s assisted stretch is desirable. |
| **T**ype | • A series of flexibility exercises for each of the major muscle-tendon units is recommended.<br>• Static flexibility (*i.e.*, active or passive), dynamic flexibility, ballistic flexibility, and PNF are each effective. |
| **V**olume | • A reasonable target is to perform 60 s of total stretching time for each flexibility exercise. |
| **P**attern | • Repetition of each flexibility exercise 2–4 times is recommended.<br>• Flexibility exercise is most effective when the muscle is warmed through light-to-moderate aerobic activity or passively through external methods such as moist heat packs or hot baths. |
| **P**rogression | • Methods for optimal progression are unknown. |

PNF, proprioceptive neuromuscular facilitation.

## *GETP9* Chapter 7 Box

---

**BOX 7.2**    **Summary of Methods for Prescribing Exercise Intensity Using Heart Rate (HR), Oxygen Uptake ($\dot{V}O_2$), and Metabolic Equivalents (METs)**

- HRR method: Target HR (THR) = [(HR$_{max/peak}$[a] − HR$_{rest}$) × % intensity desired] + HR$_{rest}$
- $\dot{V}O_2$R method: Target $\dot{V}O_2$R[c] = [($\dot{V}O_{2max/peak}$[b] − $\dot{V}O_{2rest}$) × % intensity desired] + $\dot{V}O_{2rest}$
- HR method: Target HR = HR$_{max/peak}$[a] × % intensity desired
- $\dot{V}O_2$ method: Target $\dot{V}O_2$[c] = $\dot{V}O_{2max/peak}$[b] × % intensity desired
- MET method: Target MET[c] = [($\dot{V}O_{2max/peak}$[b])/3.5 mL · kg$^{-1}$ · min$^{-1}$] × % intensity desired

[a]HR$_{max/peak}$ is the highest value obtained during maximal/peak exercise or it can be estimated by 220 − age or some other prediction equation (see *Table 7.2*).
[b]$\dot{V}O_{2max/peak}$ is the highest value obtained during maximal/peak exercise or it can be estimated from a submaximal exercise test. Please see The Concept of Maximal Oxygen Uptake in *Chapter 4* for the distinction between $\dot{V}O_{2max}$ and $\dot{V}O_{2peak}$.
[c]Activities at the target $\dot{V}O_2$ and MET can be determined using a compendium of physical activity (1, 2) or metabolic calculations (22) (*Table 7.3*).
HR$_{max/peak}$, maximal or peak heart rate; HR$_{rest}$, resting heart rate; HRR, heart rate reserve; $\dot{V}O_2$R, oxygen uptake reserve.

# ACSM'S RESOURCE MANUAL FOR GUIDELINES FOR EXERCISE TESTING AND PRESCRIPTION, 7TH EDITION (RM7)

The following figures, tables, and boxes come from the indicated chapters of the following source:

Swain P, senior editor. *ACSM's Resource Manual Guidelines for Exercise Testing and Prescription*. 7th ed. Baltimore (MD): Lippincott Williams and Wilkins; 2014.

## *RM7* CHAPTER 1, FUNCTIONAL ANATOMY

### *RM7* Chapter 1 Figures

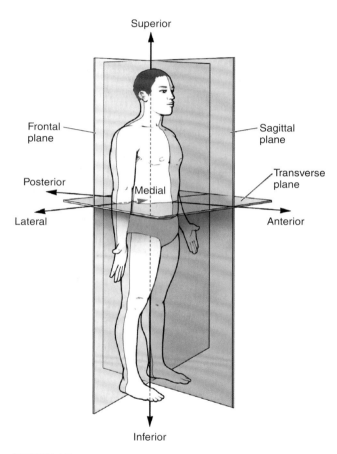

**FIGURE 1.2.** Anatomical planes of the body.

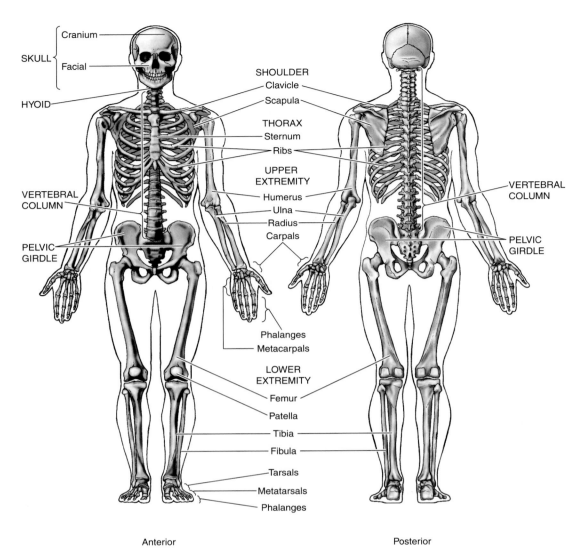

Anterior                                    Posterior

**FIGURE 1.23.** Divisions of the skeletal system.

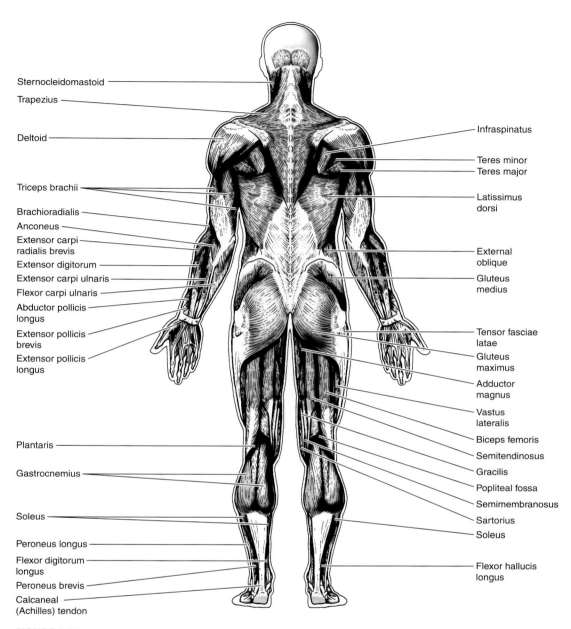

**FIGURE 1.29.** Posterior view of superficial muscles.

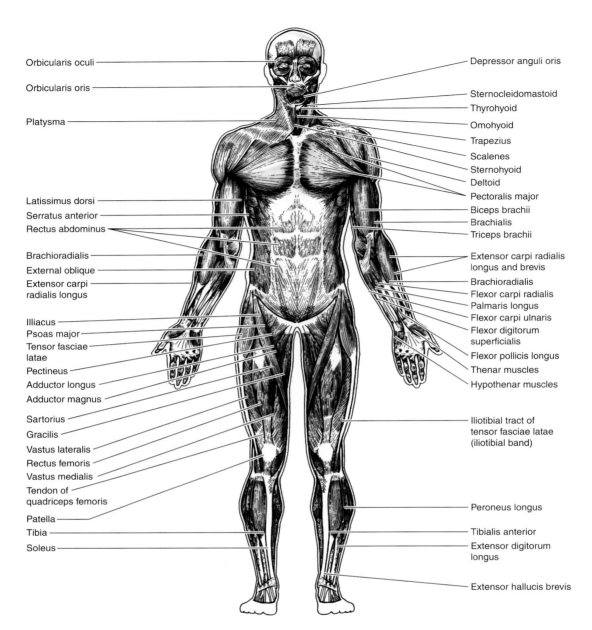

Orbicularis oculi

Orbicularis oris

Platysma

Latissimus dorsi

Serratus anterior

Rectus abdominus

Brachioradialis

External oblique

Extensor carpi
radialis longus

Illiacus

Psoas major

Tensor fasciae
latae

Pectineus

Adductor longus

Adductor magnus

Sartorius

Gracilis

Vastus lateralis

Rectus femoris

Vastus medialis

Tendon of
quadriceps femoris

Patella

Tibia

Soleus

Depressor anguli oris

Sternocleidomastoid

Thyrohyoid

Omohyoid

Trapezius

Scalenes

Sternohyoid

Deltoid

Pectoralis major

Biceps brachii

Brachialis

Triceps brachii

Extensor carpi radialis
longus and brevis

Brachioradialis

Flexor carpi radialis

Palmaris longus

Flexor carpi ulnaris

Flexor digitorum
superficialis

Flexor pollicis longus

Thenar muscles

Hypothenar muscles

Iliotibial tract of
tensor fasciae latae
(iliotibial band)

Peroneus longus

Tibialis anterior

Extensor digitorum
longus

Extensor hallucis brevis

**FIGURE 1.30.** Anterior view of superficial muscles.

## *RM7* CHAPTER 3, EXERCISE PHYSIOLOGY
### *RM7* Chapter 3 Table

| TABLE 3.2.   Comparison of the Relative Hemodynamic Responses to Dynamic and Static Exertion | | |
|---|---|---|
| | **Dynamic (Isotonic)** | **Static (Isometric)** |
| Cardiac output | + + + + | + |
| Heart rate | + + | + |
| Stroke volume | + + | 0 |
| Peripheral resistance | − | + + + |
| Systolic blood pressure | + + + | + + + + |
| Diastolic blood pressure | 0− | + + + + |
| Mean arterial pressure | 0+ | + + + + |
| Left ventricular work | Volume load | Pressure load |

+, increase; −, decrease; 0, unchanged.

## *RM7* CHAPTER 5, LIFESPAN EFFECTS OF AGING AND DECONDITIONING
### *RM7* Chapter 5 Table

| TABLE 5.2.   System Changes | | | | | |
|---|---|---|---|---|---|
| | **Neonatal Infancy** | **Childhood** | **Adolescence** | **Adulthood** | **Senescence** |
| **Cardiovascular System** | | | | | |
| Cardiac output | | ↑ | ↑ | ↔ | ↔ |
| Stroke volume | | ↑ | ↑ | ↔ | ↓ |
| $HR_{max}$ | | ↑ | ↔ | ↓ | ↓ |
| $\dot{V}O_{2max}$ | | ↑ | ↑ | ↓ | ↓ |
| **Pulmonary System** | | | | | |
| Vital capacity | ↑ | ↑ | ↑ | ↓ | ↓ |
| **Musculoskeletal System** | | | | | |
| Bone mineral density | ↑ | ↑ | ↑ | ↔ | ↓ |
| Fat-free body mass | ↑ | ↑ | ↑ | ↑ | ↓ |
| Anaerobic capacity | | ↑ | ↑ | ↑ | ↓ |
| Flexibility | | ↑ | ↑ | ↓ | ↓ |
| % Body fat | | ↑ | ↑ | ↑ | ↑ |
| **Nervous System** | | | | | |
| Motor control | ↑ | ↑ | ↑ | ↔ | ↓ |
| **Immune System** | | | | | |
| Immune system function | | ↑ | ↑ | ↔ | ↓ |

↑ = increases; ↔ = no change; ↓ = decreases.

## *RM7* CHAPTER 10, LEGAL CONSIDERATIONS FOR EXERCISE PROGRAMMING

### *RM7* Chapter 10 Box

| BOX 10.1 | Tips for Exercise Professionals |
|---|---|

Some tips for exercise professionals regarding legal matters include the following:

1. Know and apply in practice the most rigorous and current peer-developed guidelines applicable to your services, clients, and organization or environment.
2. Maintain credentials relevant to your service (e.g., personal certification or public licensure) and professional liability insurance coverage.
3. Use appropriate informed consent for all services in which such consent is relevant (consult with qualified attorney and risk manager).
4. Instruct clients in techniques of participation and limitations relevant to their health and physical capabilities, observe their related participation, correct problems, and follow up to verify that they manage their own participation safely and effectively.
5. Document fulfillment of your service in a manner consistent with standard of care and your written program policies and procedures.
6. Communicate critical information in a timely way to authorized parties.
7. Develop emergency response plans, rehearse for emergencies, document and upgrade procedures based on rehearsal experiences, and institute automated external defibrillation programs as applicable.
8. Report incidents and follow up to continuously improve emergency readiness and performance.
9. Maintain equipment and inspect facilities on a frequent and regular basis.

## *RM7* CHAPTER 19, EXERCISE PROGRAM SAFETY AND EMERGENCY PROCEDURES

### *RM7* Chapter 19 Tables

| TABLE 19.2. Acute Responses for Cardiopulmonary and Metabolic Conditions/Emergencies | | |
|---|---|---|
| **Condition** | **Definition/Signs and Symptoms** | **Acute Care** |
| Dizziness/fainting Syncope | Disoriented; confused; skin color — pale; rapid, irregular pulse; weak Temporary loss of consciousness | Determine responsiveness, place supine with legs elevated, administer oral fluids if conscious, begin emergency breathing or compressions as needed, and check blood sugar if patient does not respond immediately. Activate EMS. |
| Hypoglycemia | Low blood sugar. Profuse sweating, tachycardia, hunger, blurred or double vision, tremors, headache, confusion, seizure, unconsciousness, sudden moodiness | Check blood sugar, administer 5–20 g (6) of CHO (4 oz or ½ cup regular soda or orange juice or three glucose tablets) if conscious. Repeat in 15 min if continued hypoglycemia. Consume meal or snack to prevent recurrence. If unconscious, use glucagon emergency kit if trained, if not, activate EMS. |
| Hyperglycemia | Abnormally high blood sugar. Nausea, polyuria, blurred vision, lethargy, sweet fruity breath, vomiting, hyperventilation | Postpone exercise if an individual is not feeling well or tests positive for urinary ketones (4). Stop activity if symptoms persist, turn head to side if vomiting, check blood sugar, and administer large amounts of noncaloric or low-calorie fluids orally if conscious. Continue to monitor blood glucose. Trained professionals may give insulin to lower blood sugar; activate EMS. |
| Angina | Pain/pressure in the chest, neck, jaw, arm and/or back; sweating; denial of medical problem; nausea; shortness of breath | Stop activity; place in seated or supine position (whichever is most comfortable); check pulse, blood pressure, and rhythm if possible; give nitroglycerin and oxygen per ACLS protocol if known history of CAD. Activate EMS or physician evaluation (unless patient is diagnosed with chronic stable angina, which is relieved with rest and/or medication). Get 12-lead EKG. |
| Sudden cardiac arrest | An abnormal heart rhythm usually caused by lack of oxygen to the heart; victim may be unresponsive without breathing or pulse. | Activate EMS, CAB (chest compressions, airway, rescue breathing); when AED/manual defibrillator is available, defibrillate shockable rhythms; continue CPR as indicated. |
| Dyspnea | Labored breathing. Hyperventilation, dizziness, wheezing, coughing, loss of coordination | Stop activity. Maintain open airway, assist with administration of bronchodilator if prescribed (18). Try pursed-lip breathing; move into a more relaxed position; if no relief, activate EMS and transport. |
| Tachypnea | Abnormally rapid respiration rate. Hyperventilation | Stop activity. Maintain open airway; treat cause if known; if signs/symptoms persist, activate EMS. |
| Stroke or TIA | Lack of oxygen to the brain. May cause symptoms such as drowsiness, confusion, severe headache with no known cause, nausea, or loss of vision and voluntary movement, muscle weakness, slurred speech, loss of coordination, or facial droop | Activate EMS; note time symptoms started. Start CPR if needed; check glucose if possible. Monitor vitals and signs/symptoms; give oxygen if hypoxic. |

*(continued)*

## TABLE 19.2. Acute Responses for Cardiopulmonary and Metabolic Conditions/Emergencies *(Continued)*

| Condition | Definition/Signs and Symptoms | Acute Care |
|---|---|---|
| Hypertension | High blood pressure — if resting SBP >200 or DBP >110. SBP >250 or DBP >115 without symptoms of stroke or TIA during exercise test or SBP >200 and/or DBP >105 during exercise bout | Do not exercise. Alert provider or take to ER. Stop activity; monitor vitals and signs/symptoms. If BP does not drop quickly, alert physician or take to ER. |
| Hypotension | Low BP that causes symptoms such as syncope, dizziness, and fatigue. | Stop activity. Place in a supine position, elevate legs, assess vital signs, and give oral fluids if conscious. Activate EMS if symptoms do not resolve and BP does not improve. Treat the cause. |
| Tachycardia | Resting HR ≥100 bpm or abnormally high HR given the condition (anxiety, exercise, etc.). Other signs and symptoms such as dyspnea or angina may be present. | Stop activity. Assess vital signs, secure airway, give oxygen, and identify the rhythm. Activate EMS or obtain physician evaluation, follow ACLS guidelines for tachycardia, and treat contributing factors. |
| Bradycardia | Resting HR <60 bpm with symptoms; it is not unusual for patients on β-blockers or athletic individuals to have slow resting HRs without symptoms. | Stop activity. Maintain airway, check vital signs, give oxygen, and identify rhythm. Check for signs of poor perfusion; activate EMS. |
| Exertional rhabdomyolysis | Muscle pain, swelling and weakness, dark urine | Activate EMS and transport to hospital immediately, cool, and administer oral fluids if conscious. |
| Hyperthermia | Heat injury | |
| Heat cramps | Painful, involuntary, isolated muscle spasms most commonly affecting calves, arms, abdominal, and back muscles | Stop activity. Administer chilled oral electrolyte-carbohydrate fluids; application of ice and massage followed by gentle stretching; monitor vitals and hydration status. |
| Heat exhaustion | Heavy sweating, pale, muscle spasms, headache, nausea, loss of consciousness, dizziness, tachycardia, hypotension, headache, fatigue | Stop activity and move to cool area; remove clothes; cool with cool spray; encourage cool electrolyte-carbohydrate drinks but avoid chilling the victim. Monitor core temperature, refer for physician evaluation, or activate EMS if no rapid improvement. |
| Heat stroke | Hot, dry skin but can be sweating; dyspnea; tachycardia; confusion; dizziness; syncope; seizure; often unconscious with core body temperature >40° C (104° F) | Activate EMS and immediately move to cool area, remove clothing, dowse with cool water (ice water bath to chin preferred), or wrap in cool wet sheets. Administer fluids if conscious; monitor core temperature and vitals. |
| Hypothermia | Body temperature falls below 35° C or 95° F, shivering, loss of coordination, muscle stiffness, and lethargy, decrease in mental function, disorientation | Activate EMS and move to a warm place. Remove any wet clothing and replace with dry, warm clothing and cover with blankets or warm water to rewarm gradually. Monitor vital signs; give hot liquids. |

CHO, carbohydrate; CAD, coronary artery disease; EKG, electrocardiogram; TIA, transient ischemic attack; SBP, systolic blood pressure; DBP, diastolic blood pressure; ER, emergency room; BP, blood pressure; HR, heart rate; bpm, beats per minute.

Adapted from Markenson D, Ferguson JD, Chameides L, et al. Part 17: first aid: 2010 American Heart Association and American Red Cross Guidelines for First Aid. *Circulation.* 2010;122(18 Suppl 3):S934–46.

| TABLE 19.3. | Acute Responses for Common Musculoskeletal Injuries/Emergencies | | |
|---|---|---|---|
| **Injury** | **Description** | **Signs/Symptoms** | **Acute Care** |
| Blisters/ corns | Closed skin wounds | Pain, swelling, infection | Clean with antiseptic soap. Apply sterile dressing, antibiotic ointment. |
| Lacerations/ abrasions | Open skin wounds | Pain, redness, bleeding, swelling, mild fever | Follow universal precautions to prevent the transfer of blood-borne pathogens. Apply direct pressure to stop bleeding. Irrigate with large volumes of water to remove debris. Clean with soap or sterile saline; apply antibiotic ointment and sterile dressing for abrasions and superficial injuries. Refer to physician for stitches/tetanus. Wash your hands immediately after providing care. |
| Strain[a] | A stretch or tear in a muscle, tendon, and/or fascia | | |
| Grade I | Affects only a few fibers | Mild discomfort, pain, tightness, possible localized spasms | RICE (see *Table 19-4* for definitions and protocol) |
| Grade II | More extensive damage to more fibers | Loss of function, swelling, bruising, and localized tenderness | RICE; refer for physician evaluation |
| Grade III | Severe tear or complete rupture | Palpable defect, complete loss of function, severe pain, swelling, and bruising | Immobilization, RICE, prompt physician evaluation as surgery may be required. |
| Sprain[a] | A stretch or tear to the ligaments and stabilizing connective tissues of a joint | | |
| Grade I | Slight tear or stretch without joint instability | Minimal pain, swelling, little or no loss of function, slight or no bruising | RICE |
| Grade II | Partial tear | Bruising, moderate pain, swelling, difficulty with weight bearing, and some loss of function | RICE, physician evaluation |
| Grade III | Complete tear | Severe pain, swelling, bruising, unable to bear weight on the joint | Immobilization, RICE, prompt physician evaluation |
| Stress fracture | Microscopic damage to the bone due to repetitive stress | Insidious onset of pain that persists when attempting activity, point-specific tenderness | Physician evaluation, rest, non–weight-bearing activities |
| Simple acute fracture | Sudden break of a bone | Swelling, bruising, disability, pain | Immobilize joint with padded splint in position found if warranted, physician evaluation, X-rays |

[a]Signs and symptoms for each grade include those for the grade below the one listed (*i.e.*, grade II includes those of grades I and II; grade III includes signs and symptoms listed under grades I, II, and III).

## TABLE 19.4.    RICE Protocol for Acute Injuries

| Treatment | Purpose | Application |
|---|---|---|
| Rest | Pain control, prevention of reinjury | Complete rest, immobilization, or reduction in training intensity, duration, frequency, or use of non–weight-bearing activities, depending on severity of injury |
| Ice | Reduction of pain, swelling, inflammation, spasms, and bleeding | Immediately post injury, 10–20 min, two to three times per day; use plastic bag, ice and water mixture; place a thin towel between skin and ice bag |
| Compression | Reduction of swelling | Elastic wrap/compression sleeve |
| Elevation | Reduction of swelling | Elevate extremity above heart level |

Adapted from Markenson D, Ferguson JD, Chameides L, et al. Part 17: first aid: 2010 American Heart Association and American Red Cross Guidelines for First Aid. *Circulation.* 2010;122(18 Suppl 3):S934–46; and Prentice WE, Arnheim DD. *Arnheim's Principles of Athletic Training: A Competency-Based Approach.* 14th ed. New York (NY): McGraw-Hill Higher Education; 2011. 940 p.

*RM7* **Chapter 19 Box**

| BOX 19.1 | **Strategies for Developing an Emergency Care Plan** |

- Who is the staff member in charge of the facility's emergency plan and programming and is there physician oversight (medical director)?
- Is an outline of the entire emergency care plan displayed and accessible at a central staff location?
- Are different emergency procedures developed and posted for various areas within the facility (testing areas, pool, weight room, outdoor areas, and gymnasium)?
- What care will be provided?
- Who will render care?
- Are all staff and supervisors certified in first aid, CPR, AED, and/or ACLS as appropriate?
- Is there a plan for public access defibrillation (PAD)?
- Is staff training documented in personnel files or the emergency procedure plan?
- Have all staff received training for OSHA's blood-borne pathogen guidelines and procedures?
- Are the responsibilities of individual staff members identified (e.g., team leader, captain, medical liaison)?
- Is there a manager/team leader available during all hours of operation to oversee a medical emergency?
- Who will activate EMS? Are telephone numbers for emergency procedures clearly posted?
- Are all staff members familiar with the information to be provided to EMS over the telephone, and is this information posted next to the phone?
    Type of emergency (injury, illness)
    Current status of involved or injured individuals
    Type of assistance being given
    Exact location of the facility and the afflicted individual within the facility
    Specific point of entry into the facility
    Telephone number being used
- Who will supervise the other activity areas if supervisors must leave to assist at an accident scene?
- Who will help with crowd control?
- Who has access to keys for locked areas or doors?
- Who will direct ambulance, EMS, or the code team to the emergency scene?
- Have the facility administrators invited representatives from EMS to become familiar with the floor plan and activities of the facility?
- Are emergency response training sessions conducted regularly (at least once every 3 mo) and documented?
- Does emergency training consists of both announced and unannounced mock drills?
- Are emergency drills and training documented and evaluated with recommendations for necessary changes?

- Is EMS involved in the training and conduction of drills?
- Do all staff members know the location and have easy access to first-aid kits, latex or similar gloves, AED, splints, stretchers, fire extinguishers, and other emergency equipment?
- Are emergency equipment and supplies clearly labeled and routinely checked, and do they receive routine maintenance?
- Is the facility conducting and documenting cardiovascular risk screening of all new members, guests, and patients?
- Are persons at high risk directed to seek facilities providing appropriate levels of care and staff supervision?
- Are appropriate documents (health appraisal, physician permission to participate, assumption of risk or waiver, informed consent, emergency information, and advanced directives) completed and accessible to staff in the event of an emergency?
- Have staff members been appropriately informed of orthopedic or other health problems, including cognitive problems such as dementia or Alzheimer disease, that might affect participation?
- Are emergency notification cards on file for each participant that include telephone numbers of family members, physician names, telephone numbers with special instructions, and alternative telephone numbers if primary contacts are unavailable? Patients/members should be encouraged to update this information on a regular basis.
- Are properly documented injury and accident reports including statements by the injured and witnesses and their contact information completed and stored in an appropriate secure location for review and follow-up by administration?
- Is there a plan for collecting facts and data after the accident including interviewing witnesses, retention of any broken equipment parts, and taking photographs if appropriate (*e.g.,* if exercise equipment malfunction were a potential concern)?
- Was the accident/injury report submitted to the facility's insurance administrator and legal counsel in a timely manner (within 24 h of the accident) and marked as "privileged and confidential" when appropriate?
- Are employees given appropriate protocols for handling inquiries made by media and other representatives regarding the incident?

Adapted from Peterson JA, Tharrett SJ, American College of Sports Medicine. *ACSM's Health/Fitness Facility Standards and Guidelines.* 4th ed. Champaign (IL): Human Kinetics; 2011. 211 p.

## *RM7* CHAPTER 46, COUNSELING PHYSICAL ACTIVITY BEHAVIOR CHANGE

## *RM7* Chapter 46 Box

| BOX 46.5 | Assessing Physical Activity Stages of Change |
| --- | --- |

**PHYSICAL ACTIVITY STAGES OF CHANGE**

**INSTRUCTIONS:** For each question below, please circle Yes (Y) or No (N). Please be sure to follow the instructions carefully.

|  | Yes | No |
| --- | --- | --- |
| 1. I am currently physically active. | Y | N |
| 2. I intend to become more physically active in the next 6 mo. | Y | N |

For activity to be regular, it must add up to a total of 30 or more minutes per day and be done at least 5 d ? wk21. For example, you could take one 30-min walk or three 10-min walks each day.

|  | Yes | No |
| --- | --- | --- |
| 3. I currently engage in regular physical activity. | Y | N |
| 4. I have been regularly physically active for the past 6 mo. | Y | N |

| Stage | ITEM | | | |
| --- | --- | --- | --- | --- |
|  | 1 | 2 | 3 | 4 |
| Precontemplation | No | No | — | — |
| Contemplation | No | Yes | — | — |
| Preparation | Yes | — | No | — |
| Action | Yes | — | Yes | No |
| Maintenance | Yes | — | Yes | Yes |

Modified with permission from Marcus B, Forsyth L. *Motivating People to be Physically Active.* 2nd ed. Champaign (IL): Human Kinetics; 2009. 200 p.

## *RM7* CHAPTER 48, PLANNING, IMPLEMENTING, AND EVALUATING PHYSICAL ACTIVITY PROGRAMS

### *RM7* Chapter 48 Figure

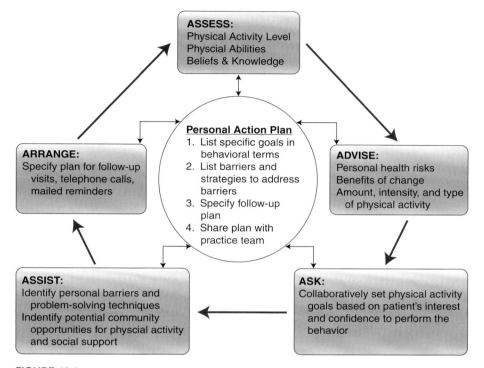

**FIGURE 48.1.** The five A's model applied to physical activity promotion in clinical settings.

## *ACSM'S RESOURCES FOR THE PERSONAL TRAINER,* 4TH EDITION (*RPT4*)

The following figures, tables, and boxes come from the indicated chapters of the following source:

Bushman BA, senior editor. *ACSM's Resources for the Personal Trainer.* 4th ed. Baltimore (MD): Lippincott Williams and Wilkins; 2014.

## *RPT4* CHAPTER 3, ANATOMY AND KINESIOLOGY

## *RPT4* Chapter 3 Figures

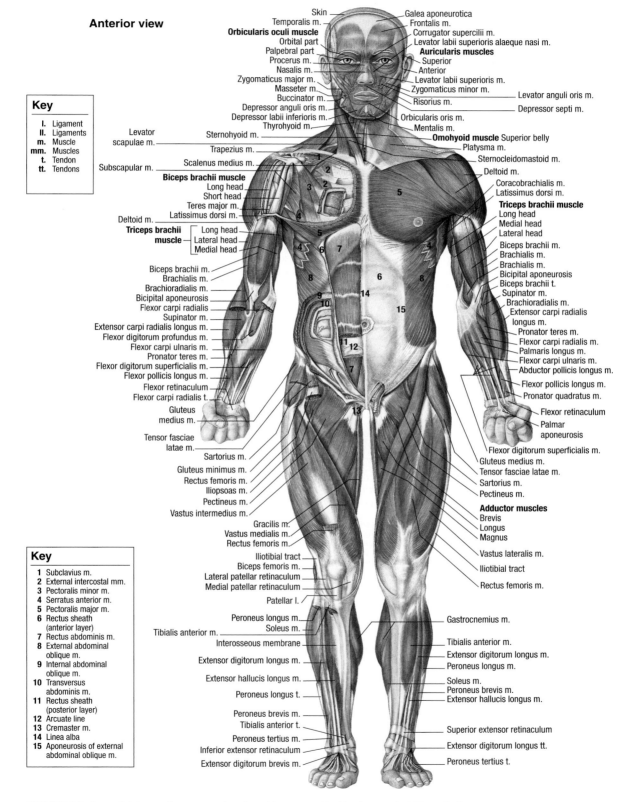

**Anterior view**

**Key**

| | |
|---|---|
| **l.** | Ligament |
| **ll.** | Ligaments |
| **m.** | Muscle |
| **mm.** | Muscles |
| **t.** | Tendon |
| **tt.** | Tendons |

**Key**

1 Subclavius m.
2 External intercostal mm.
3 Pectoralis minor m.
4 Serratus anterior m.
5 Pectoralis major m.
6 Rectus sheath
  (anterior layer)
7 Rectus abdominis m.
8 External abdominal
  oblique m.
9 Internal abdominal
  oblique m.
10 Transversus
  abdominis m.
11 Rectus sheath
  (posterior layer)
12 Arcuate line
13 Cremaster m.
14 Linea alba
15 Aponeurosis of external
  abdominal oblique m.

**FIGURE 3.8.** Superficial muscles — anterior view. (Asset provided by Anatomical Chart Co.)

**Posterior view**

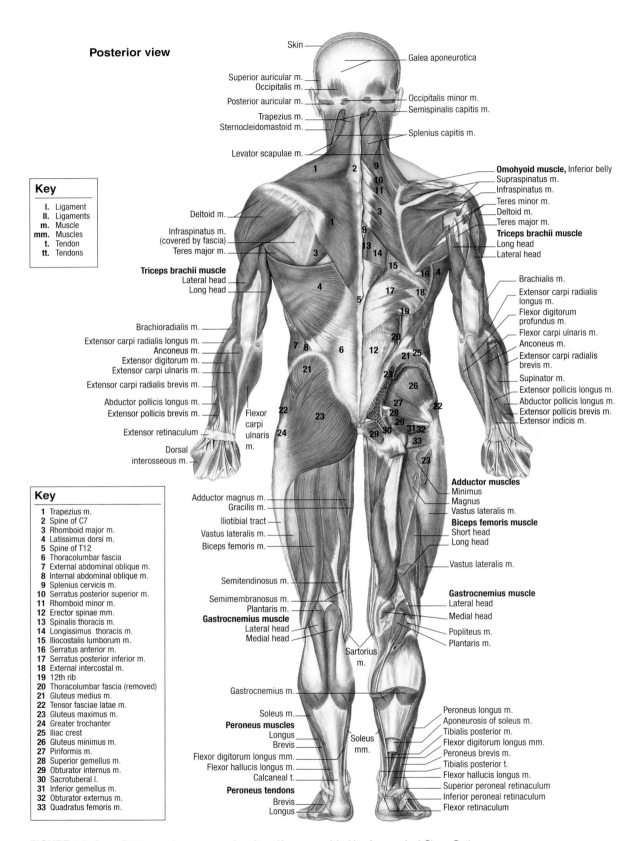

Skin
Galea aponeurotica
Superior auricular m.
Occipitalis m.
Posterior auricular m.
Occipitalis minor m.
Semispinalis capitis m.
Trapezius m.
Sternocleidomastoid m.
Splenius capitis m.
Levator scapulae m.

**Key**

| | |
|---|---|
| **l.** | Ligament |
| **ll.** | Ligaments |
| **m.** | Muscle |
| **mm.** | Muscles |
| **t.** | Tendon |
| **tt.** | Tendons |

Deltoid m.
Infraspinatus m. (covered by fascia)
Teres major m.

**Triceps brachii muscle**
Lateral head
Long head

Brachioradialis m.
Extensor carpi radialis longus m.
Anconeus m.
Extensor digitorum m.
Extensor carpi ulnaris m.
Extensor carpi radialis brevis m.
Abductor pollicis longus m.
Extensor pollicis brevis m.
Extensor retinaculum
Dorsal interosseous m.

Flexor carpi ulnaris m.

**Omohyoid muscle,** Inferior belly
Supraspinatus m.
Infraspinatus m.
Teres minor m.
Deltoid m.
Teres major m.
**Triceps brachii muscle**
Long head
Lateral head

Brachialis m.
Extensor carpi radialis longus m.
Flexor digitorum profundus m.
Flexor carpi ulnaris m.
Anconeus m.
Extensor carpi radialis brevis m.
Supinator m.
Extensor pollicis longus m.
Abductor pollicis longus m.
Extensor pollicis brevis m.
Extensor indicis m.

Adductor magnus m.
Gracilis m.
Iliotibial tract
Vastus lateralis m.
Biceps femoris m.

**Adductor muscles**
Minimus
Magnus
Vastus lateralis m.
**Biceps femoris muscle**
Short head
Long head
Vastus lateralis m.

Semitendinosus m.
Semimembranosus m.
Plantaris m.
**Gastrocnemius muscle**
Lateral head
Medial head

**Gastrocnemius muscle**
Lateral head
Medial head
Popliteus m.
Plantaris m.

Sartorius m.

Gastrocnemius m.
Soleus m.
**Peroneus muscles**
Longus
Brevis
Flexor digitorum longus mm.
Flexor hallucis longus m.
Calcaneal t.
**Peroneus tendons**
Brevis
Longus

Soleus mm.

Peroneus longus m.
Aponeurosis of soleus m.
Tibialis posterior m.
Flexor digitorum longus mm.
Peroneus brevis m.
Tibialis posterior t.
Flexor hallucis longus m.
Superior peroneal retinaculum
Inferior peroneal retinaculum
Flexor retinaculum

**Key**

1 Trapezius m.
2 Spine of C7
3 Rhomboid major m.
4 Latissimus dorsi m.
5 Spine of T12
6 Thoracolumbar fascia
7 External abdominal oblique m.
8 Internal abdominal oblique m.
9 Splenius cervicis m.
10 Serratus posterior superior m.
11 Rhomboid minor m.
12 Erector spinae mm.
13 Spinalis thoracis m.
14 Longissimus thoracis m.
15 Iliocostalis lumborum m.
16 Serratus anterior m.
17 Serratus posterior inferior m.
18 External intercostal m.
19 12th rib
20 Thoracolumbar fascia (removed)
21 Gluteus medius m.
22 Tensor fasciae latae m.
23 Gluteus maximus m.
24 Greater trochanter
25 Iliac crest
26 Gluteus minimus m.
27 Piriformis m.
28 Superior gemellus m.
29 Obturator internus m.
30 Sacrotuberal l.
31 Inferior gemellus m.
32 Obturator externus m.
33 Quadratus femoris m.

**FIGURE 3.9.** Superficial muscles — posterior view. (Asset provided by Anatomical Chart Co.)

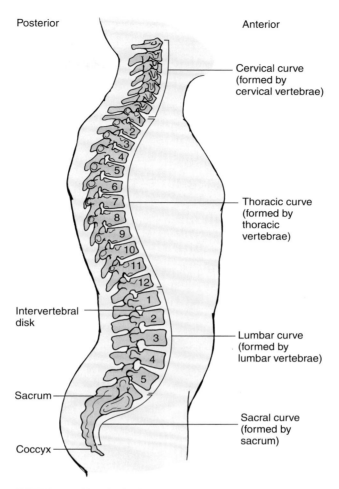

**FIGURE 3.48.** Vertebral column — lateral view showing the four normal curves and regions. (From Oatis CA. *Kinesiology: The Mechanics and Pathomechanics of Human Movement.* Baltimore [MD]: Lippincott Williams & Wilkins; 2003.)

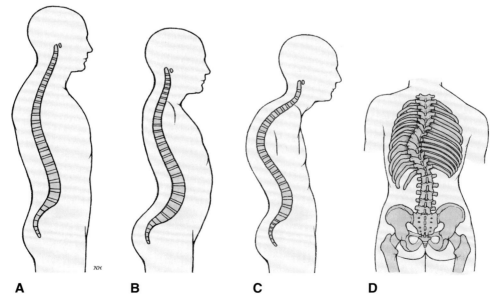

**FIGURE 3.49.** Normal and abnormal curves of the vertebral column. **A.** Normal. **B.** Hyperlordosis. **C.** Hyperkyphosis. **D.** Scoliosis. (Courtesy of Neil O. Hardy, Westpoint, CT.)

## *RPT4* Chapter 3 Table

| TABLE 3.3.    Major Joint Motions and Planes of Motion | | | |
|---|---|---|---|
| **Major Joints** | **Type of Joints** | **Joint Movements** | **Planes** |
| Scapulothoracic | Not a true joint ("physiological" or "functional" joint) | Elevation–depression<br>Upward–downward rotation<br>Protraction–retraction<br>Medial–Lateral rotation<br>Anterior–Posterior Tilting | Frontal<br>Frontal<br>Frontal<br>Transitional<br>Sagittal |
| Glenohumeral | Synovial: ball-and-socket | Flexion–extension<br>Abduction–adduction<br>Internal–external rotation<br>Horizontal abduction–adduction<br>Circumduction | Sagittal<br>Frontal<br>Transverse<br>Transverse<br>Multiple |
| Elbow | Synovial: hinge | Flexion–extension | Sagittal |
| Proximal radioulnar | Synovial: pivot | Pronation–supination | Transverse |
| Wrist | Synovial: ellipsoidal | Flexion–extension<br>Abduction–adduction | Sagittal<br>Frontal |
| Metacarpophalangeal | Synovial: ellipsoidal | Flexion–extension<br>Abduction–adduction | Sagittal<br>Frontal |
| Proximal and distal interphalangeal | Synovial: hinge | Flexion–extension | Sagittal |
| Intervertebral | Cartilaginous | Flexion–extension<br>Lateral flexion<br>Rotation | Sagittal<br>Frontal<br>Transverse |
| Hip | Synovial: ball-and-socket | Flexion–extension<br>Abduction–adduction<br>Internal–external rotation<br>Circumduction | Sagittal<br>Frontal<br>Transverse<br>Multiple |
| Knee | Synovial: bicondylar | Flexion–extension<br>Internal/external rotation | Sagittal<br>Transverse |
| Ankle: talocrural | Synovial: hinge | Dorsiflexion–plantarflexion | Sagittal |
| Ankle: subtalar | Synovial: gliding | Inversion–eversion | Frontal |

## *RPT4* CHAPTER 4, BIOMECHANICAL PRINCIPLES OF TRAINING

### *RPT4* Chapter 4 Figure

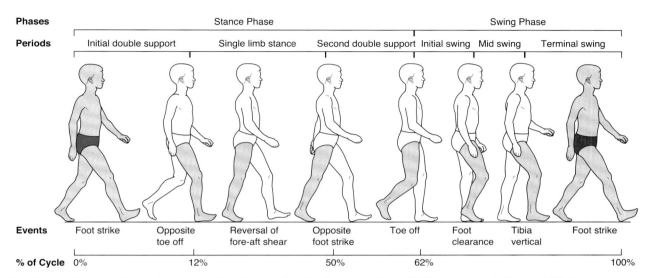

**FIGURE 4.16.** Normal walking gait. (Adapted from Rose J, Gamble JG, editor. *Human Walking.* 2nd ed. Baltimore [MD]: Lippincott Williams & Wilkins; 1994, p. 26.)

## *RPT4* CHAPTER 5, EXERCISE PHYSIOLOGY

### *RPT4* Chapter 5 Figure

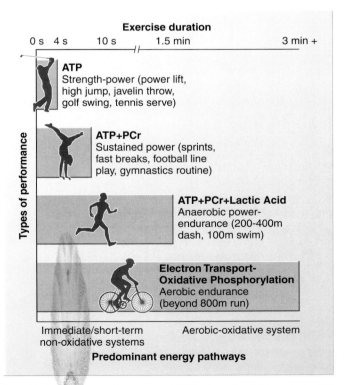

**FIGURE 5.4.** Comparison of activity with the energy pathways used ATP, adenosine triphosphate; PCr, creatine phosphate; ATP + PCr + lactic acid, anaerobic glycolysis; electron transport-oxidative phosphorylation, aerobic oxidation. (Reprinted with permission from Premkumar K. *The Massage Connection, Anatomy and Physiology.* 2nd ed. Baltimore [MD]: Lippincott Williams & Wilkins; 2004.)

## *RPT4* Chapter 5 Table

| TABLE 5.2.   Benefits of Increasing Cardiorespiratory Activities and/or Improving Cardiorespiratory Fitness[a] | |
|---|---|
| Improved cardiorespiratory function:<br>• Increased maximal oxygen uptake<br>• Increased maximal Q and SV<br>• Increased capillary density in skeletal muscle<br>• Increased mitochondrial density<br>• Increased lactate threshold<br>• Lower HR and BP at a fixed submaximal work rate<br>• Lower myocardial oxygen demand at a fixed submaximal work rate<br>• Lower minute ventilation at a fixed submaximal work rate | Decreased risk of the following:<br>• Mortality from all causes<br>• Coronary artery disease<br>• Cancer (colon, perhaps breast and prostate)<br>• Hypertension<br>• Noninsulin-dependent diabetes mellitus<br>• Osteoporosis<br>• Anxiety<br>• Depression |
| Improved immune function:<br>Improved glucose tolerance and insulin sensitivity | Improved blood lipid profile:<br>• Decreased triglycerides<br>• Increased high-density lipoprotein cholesterol<br>• Decreased postprandial lipemia |
| Improved work, recreational, and sports performance | Improved body composition |
| Decreased fatigue in daily activities | Enhanced sense of well-being |

[a]Many of the health benefits accrue from physical activity may have relatively little effect on increasing cardiorespiratory fitness (U.S. Dept. of Health and Human Services. *Physical Activity Guidelines Advisory Committee Report 2008*).

## *RPT4* CHAPTER 10, THE INITIAL CLIENT CONSULTATION

## *RPT4* Chapter 10 Figures

### New Client Intake Form

**Contact Information**

Date: _____ _____ Phone _____ In-Person

Name:

_____

Address:

_____

Preferred method of contact:

_____ Phone (home): _____

_____ Phone (cell): _____

_____ Email: _____

Training Schedule Interest (circle all that apply):

Sunday Monday Tuesday Wednesday Thursday Friday Saturday Sunday

am        am        am        am              am          am       am        am

midday midday midday midday   midday   midday midday  midday

pm        pm        pm        pm            pm          pm       pm        pm

**Health and Fitness Information**

General Health and Fitness Goals (check all that apply):

_____ strength _____ disease management

_____ endurance _____ stress management

_____ sport performance _____ weight management

_____ physical appearance _____ energy/vitality

Health or other Fitness Professional(s) treating client:

_____

_____

Medical Considerations/Limitations:

_____

_____

MD Release Form Needed: _____ Yes _____ No

MD Name/Phone Contact (if necessary):

_____

Action Items

Referral to Health of Fitness Professional: _____ Yes _____ No

Referral:

_____

If compatible:

MD Release Form (if necessary) Date Sent: _____ Rec'd: _____

Initial Client Consultation Date: _____

Service Introduction Packet Delivered: _____ In-Person _____ Email _____ Mail

Comments:

_____

_____

**FIGURE 10.3.** Example of a new client intake form.

## Personal Training Client Agreement

I, _____, have read and agree to the following:
(Client's Name-Please Print)

- Appointments will be scheduled directly through my assigned Personal Trainer and can be scheduled on days and times that are mutually agreed upon.

- I have exchanged contact information with my Personal Traininer and have indicated my preference for being contacted. I understand that the facility staff is not authorized to give out my Personal Trainer's personal contact information.

- I may not bring an outside Personal Trainer into the facility to train with me.

- Private personal training sessions are one hour.

- I understand that I am expected to arrive for my appointments on time, dressed and ready to train. If I arrive late for my appointment, I understand that my training session will end at the previously scheduled time.

- Cancellation Policy: I understand that appointments must be cancelled by contacting my Personal Trainer directly, within 24 hours of my scheduled time, in order to avoid being charged for the full session.

- No Show Policy: I understand that if I do not show up for my scheduled training session, I will be charged for the full session.

- In the event that my Personal Trainer fails to contact me within 24 hours of our scheduled session, or does not show up, he/she will schedule an additional session at no cost to me.

- I understand that I may communicate any customer service issue and/or acknowledge excellent performance to the Facility Manager.


Client Signature: _____    Date: _____

Personal Trainer (Print): _____    Date: _____

**FIGURE 10.4**. Example of personal training client agreement. (Adapted with permission from Plus One Health Management, Inc., New York, New York, 2008.)

## *RPT4* CHAPTER 11, SCREENING AND RISK CLASSIFICATION

## *RPT4* Chapter 11 Figure

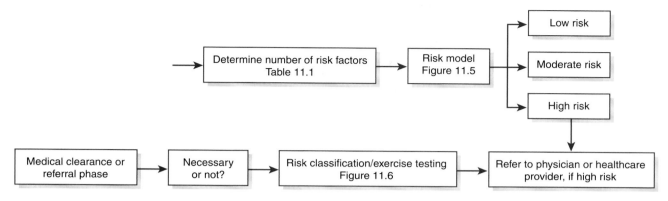

**Screening Process**

## *RPT4* CHAPTER 13, COMPREHENSIVE PROGRAM DESIGN

### *RPT4* Chapter 13 Table

| TABLE 13.5. | Sample Progressive Balance Program | | | |
|---|---|---|---|---|
| | **Level 1** | **Level 2** | **Level 3** | **Challenge** |
| Seated balance activities | Seated chair lean | Add arm movements:<br>• Raise one arm at a time to the front and then to the sides<br>• Raise both arms to the front and then to the sides<br>Add leg movements:<br>• Raise one knee at a time<br>• Raise one leg (straightened) at a time | Combine arm and leg movements | • Sit on a pillow<br>• Sit on a stability ball<br>• Close one eye<br>• Close both eyes<br>• Turn head to the right and then to the left |
| Standing balance activities | Upright stance (variations including wide stance, narrow stance, semi-tandem, and tandem) | In all four variations, add:<br>• Forward and back-ward sway<br>• Lateral sway (side to side) | Add arm movements to sway:<br>• Raise one arm at a time to the front and then to the sides<br>• Raise both arms to the front and then to the sides | • Close one eye<br>• Close both eyes<br>• Turn head to the right and then to the left<br>• Hold an item, such as a book |
| Movement balance activities | Walk forward and backward | • Wide stance walk<br>• Narrow stance walk<br>• Walk on heels<br>• Walk on toes | • Tandem walk forward and backward<br>• Walk while carrying an item<br>• Walk with head turns | • Barefoot<br>• One eye closed<br>• Surface change (mat, sand, etc.)<br>• Obstacles |
| | Walk side to side | • Sidestep on heels<br>• Sidestep on toes<br>• Turn in a circle | • Sidestep while carrying an item<br>• Sidestep with head turns<br>• Crossover walk: cross one foot over the other foot | |

Adapted with permission from Bushman B, ed. *ACSM's Complete Guide to Fitness & Health*. Champaign (IL): Human Kinetics; 2011. 396 p.

## *RPT4* CHAPTER 14, RESISTANCE TRAINING PROGRAMS

### *RPT4* Chapter 14 Box

| BOX 14.1 | Likert-Type Chart to Determine Muscle Soreness |
|---|---|

| | |
|---|---|
| 0 | |
| 1 | Minor soreness |
| 2 | |
| 3 | Moderate soreness |
| 4 | |
| 5 | Extreme soreness |
| 6 | |

## *RPT4* CHAPTER 15, CARDIORESPIRATORY TRAINING PROGRAMS

## *RPT4* Chapter 15 Box

### BOX 15.1    Benefits of Regular Physical Activity/Exercise

#### IMPROVEMENT IN CARDIOVASCULAR AND RESPIRATORY FUNCTION

Increased maximal oxygen uptake resulting from both central and peripheral adaptations

Decreased minute ventilation at a given absolute submaximal intensity

Decreased myocardial oxygen cost for a given absolute submaximal intensity

Decreased heart rate and blood pressure at a given submaximal intensity

Increased capillary density in skeletal muscle

Increased exercise threshold for the accumulation of lactate in the blood

Increased exercise threshold for the onset of disease signs or symptoms (*e.g.*, angina pectoris, ischemic ST-segment depression, claudication)

#### REDUCTION IN CORONARY ARTERY DISEASE RISK FACTORS

Reduced resting systolic/diastolic pressures

Increased serum high-density lipoprotein cholesterol and decreased serum triglycerides

Reduced total body fat and reduced intraabdominal fat

Reduced insulin needs and improved glucose tolerance

Reduced blood platelet adhesiveness and aggregation

#### DECREASED MORBIDITY AND MORTALITY

Primary prevention (*i.e.*, interventions to prevent the initial occurrence)

Higher activity and/or fitness levels are associated with lower death rates from coronary artery disease.

Higher activity and/or fitness levels are associated with lower incidence rates for combined cardiovascular diseases, coronary artery disease, stroke, Type 2 diabetes, osteoporotic fractures, cancer of the colon and breast, and gallbladder disease.

Secondary prevention (*i.e.*, interventions after a cardiac event [to prevent another])

Based on meta-analyses (pooled data across studies), cardiovascular and all-cause mortality are reduced in patients with postmyocardial infarction who participate in cardiac rehabilitation exercise training, especially as a component of multifactorial risk factor reduction.

Randomized controlled trials of cardiac rehabilitation exercise training involving patients with postmyocardial infarction do not support a reduction in the rate of nonfatal reinfarction.

#### OTHER BENEFITS

Decreased anxiety and depression

Enhanced physical function and independent living in older persons

Enhanced feelings of well-being

Enhanced performance of work, recreational, and sport activities

Reduced risk of falls and injuries from falls in older persons

Prevention or mitigation of functional limitations in older adults

Effective therapy for many chronic diseases in older adults

Source: Pescatello LS, senior editor. *ACSM's Guidelines for Exercise Testing and Prescription.* 9th ed. Baltimore (MD): Lippincott Williams & Wilkins; 2014; Nelson ME, Rejeski WJ, Blair SN, et al. Physical activity and public health in older adults: recommendations from the American College of Sports Medicine and the American Heart Association. *Med Sci Sports Exerc.* 2007;39(8):1435–45; and U.S. Department of Health and Human Services. *Physical Activity and Health: A Report of the Surgeon General.* Atlanta (GA): U.S. Department of Health and Human Services, Public Health Service, Centers for Disease Control, National Center for Chronic Disease Prevention and Health Promotion; 1996. 278 p.

## *RPT4* CHAPTER 16, GUIDELINES FOR DESIGNING FLEXIBILITY PROGRAMS

## *RPT4* Chapter 16 Table

| TABLE 16.1.  Overview of Stretching Technique and Appropriate Use | | | |
|---|---|---|---|
| **Technique** | **Definition** | **Exercise Design** | **Appropriate Use** |
| Static stretching | This is the most common method used to improve flexibility. Static stretching consists of slowly moving to minor discomfort and then holding that stretch. | All major muscle groups should be targeted at least 2–3 d · wk⁻¹. Hold each static stretches for 10–30 s, 30–60 s for older adults. ACSM recommends stretches be repeated two to four times to accumulate a total of 60 s for each flexibility exercise. | Appropriate for use following a thorough warm-up (a thorough warm-up consists of 5–10 min of light-to-moderate multijoint, large muscle group movements) or during the cool-down period. |
| Dynamic stretching | Dynamic stretching involves moving parts of your body through a full range of motion while gradually increasing the reach and/or speed of movement in a controlled manner. These exercises are very rhythmic in nature. Dynamic stretching is often incorporated in the "active" phase of the group exercise warm-up due to their similarity to the movements or patterns that will be used during the conditioning period. | Begin gradually with a small range of motion progressing to larger range of motion, repeating each activity 5–12 times. | Appropriate for use during the warm-up or as part of the cool-down. |
| Proprioceptive neuromuscular facilitation (PNF) | PNF stretching involves both the stretching and contraction of the targeted muscle group. Although there are several ways to employ PNF, the most common technique is termed "contract-relax." Following the preliminary passive stretch, the muscle is isometrically contracted for 6 s, relaxed for 2–3 s, then passively moved into the final stretch, which is held for 10–30 s. This method is most effective with the use of a trainer to assist the client through the stretch. | All major muscle groups should be targeted at least 2–3 d · wk⁻¹. A 3–6 s of muscle contraction at 20%–75% maximum intensity is followed by 10–30 s of assisted stretching. A total of 60 s of stretching time should be achieved per targeted muscle group. | Appropriate for use following a thorough warm-up or during the cool-down period. Appropriate for certified fitness professionals to use with clients if properly educated on the technique. |
| Passive stretching | The client is not actively involved in this type of stretching. The client assumes a position and then either holds it with some other part of the body (*i.e.*, arm), or with the assistance of a partner or some other apparatus (*i.e.*, stretching strap). The goal is to slowly move the client into the stretch in order to prevent a forceful action and possible injury. | Exercise design would follow the static stretching protocol. | Appropriate for use following a thorough warm-up or during the cool-down period. Appropriate for certified fitness professionals to use with clients if properly educated on the technique. |
| Ballistic stretching | This approach involves a bouncing or jerky type movement to reach the muscle's range of motion limits. This bouncing motion may produce a powerful stretch reflex that counteracts the muscle lengthening and could possibly lead to tissue injury. Although ballistic stretch is not common practice for the general population, its use in training and rehabilitation of athletes where explosive movements are critical, it may have a justifiable role. | Exercise design would be determined by activity-specific needs on an individual basis. | Not appropriate for the general population. May be suitable for athletes involved in ballistic sport skills. |

## *RPT4* CHAPTER 17, PERSONAL TRAINING SESSION COMPONENTS

## *RPT4* Chapter 17 Figure

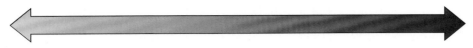

| Least skill | Most skill |
|---|---|
| Easiest, most stable | Hardest, least stable |
| Appropriate for almost everyone | Appropriate only for the very fit |
| Very safe, foundational | Less safe, controversial |

**FIGURE 17.1.** Exercise session continuum.

# B

## Editors for the Previous Two Editions

### EDITORS FOR THE 3RD EDITION

#### SENIOR EDITORS

**Khalid W. Bibi, PhD**
Professor and Chair, Department of Sports Medicine,
Health & Human Performance
Professor, Graduate School of Education
Canisius College
Buffalo, New York

**Michael G. Niederpruem, MS**
Vice President of Certification
American Health Information Management Association
Chicago, Illinois

### EDITORS FOR THE 2ND EDITION

#### SENIOR EDITORS

**Jeffrey L. Roitman, EdD, FACSM**
Director of Cardiac Rehabilitation
Research Medical Center
Kansas City, Missouri

**Khalid W. Bibi, PhD**
Professor, Sports Medicine, Health and Human
Performance
Director, Health and Human Performance Center
Canisius College
Buffalo, New York

#### ASSOCIATE EDITOR

**Walter R. Thompson, PhD, FACSM, FAACVPR**
Professor of Kinesiology and Health (College of
Education)
Professor of Nutrition (College of Health and
Human Services)
Georgia State University
Atlanta, Georgia

## CONTRIBUTORS TO THE 3RD EDITION

### CHAPTER AUTHORS

### Chapter 1

**Jeffrey J. Betts, PhD**
Health Sciences Department
Central Michigan University
Mt. Pleasant, Michigan

**Elaine Filusch Betts, PhD, PT, FACSM**
Physical Therapy
Central Michigan University
Mt. Pleasant, Michigan

**Chad Harris, PhD**
Department of Kinesiology
Boise State University
Boise, Idaho

### Chapter 2

**Michael Deschenes, PhD, FACSM**
Kinesiology Department
College of William & Mary
Willamsburg, Virginia

### Chapter 3

**Deborah Riebe, PhD, FACSM**
Department of Kinesiology
University of Rhode Island
Kingston, Rhode Island

**Robert S. Mazzeo, PhD, FACSM**
Department of Integrative Physiology
University of Colorado
Boulder, Colorado

**David S. Criswell, PhD**
Department of Applied Physiology and Kinesiology
University of Florida
Gainesville, Florida

### Chapter 4

**Carol Ewing Garber, PhD, FFAHA, ACSM**
Department of Biobehavioral Sciences
Teachers College
Columbia University
New York, New York

### Chapter 5

**Andrea Dunn, PhD, FACSM**
Klein Buendel Inc.
Golden, Colorado

**Bess H. Marcus, PhD**
Community Health and Psychiatry and Human Behavior
Brown University
Providence, Rhode Island

**David E. Verrill, MS, FAACVPR**
Presbyterian Hospital
Presbyterian Center for Preventive Cardiology
Charlotte, North Carolina

### Chapter 6

**Stephen C. Glass, PhD, FACSM**
Department of Movement Science
Grand Valley State University
Allendale, Michigan

### Chapter 7

**Frederick S. Daniels, MS, MBA**
CPTE Health Group
Nashua, New Hampshire

**Nancy J. Belli, MA**
Physical Activity Department
Plus One Holdings, Inc.
New York, New York

**Kathy Donofrio**
Swedish Covenant Hospital
Chicago, Illinois

## Chapter 8

**Kathleen M. Cahill, MS, ATC**
Sugar Land, Texas

**John W. Wygand, MA**
Adelphi University
Human Performance Laboratory
Garden City, New York

**Julie J. Downing, PhD, FACSM**
Central Oregon Community College
Health and Human Performance
Bend, Oregon

## Chapter 9

**Janet R. Wojcik, PhD**
Department of Health and Physical Education
Winthrop University
Rock Hill, South Carolina

**R. Carlton Bessinger, PhD, RD**
Department of Human Nutrition
Winthrop University
S. Rock Hill, South Carolina

## Chapter 10

**Frederick S. Daniels, MS**
CPTE Health Group
Nashua, New Hampshire

**Gregory B. Dwyer, PhD, FACSM**
Department of Exercise Science
East Stroudsburg University
East Stroudsburg, Pennsylvania

## Chapter 11

**Khalid W. Bibi, PhD**
Sports Medicine, Health and Human Performance
Canisius College
Buffalo, New York

**Dennis W. Koch, PhD**
Human Performance Center
Canisius College
Buffalo, New York

## Chapter 12

**Theodore J. Angelopoulos, PHD, MPH**
Center for Lifestyle Medicine
University of Central Florida
Orlando, Florida

**Joshua Lowndes, MA**
Center for Lifestyle Medicine
University of Central Florida
Orlando, Florida

## CHAPTER CONTRIBUTORS

### Chapter 1

**John Mayer, PhD, DC**
Spine and Sport Foundation
San Diego, California

**Brian Undermann, PhD, ATC, FACSM**
Department of Exercise and Sports Science
University of Wisconsin-La Crosse
La Crosse, Wisconsin

### Chapter 10

**Neal I. Pire, MA**
Plus One Fitness
New York, New York

**Kathy Donofrio**
Swedish Covenant Hospital
Chicago, Illinois

### Chapter 11

**Stephen C. Glass, PhD, FACSM**
Department of Movement Science
Grand Valley State University
Allendale, Michigan

## CONTRIBUTORS TO THE 2ND EDITION

**Theodore J. Angelopoulos, PhD, MPH, FACSM**
Department of Child, Family, and Community Sciences
University of Central Florida
Orlando, Florida
*Chapter 12, Electrocardiography*

**Elaine Filusch Betts, PhD, FACSM**
Central Michigan University
Mount Pleasant, Michigan
*Chapter 1, Anatomy and Biomechanics*

**Jeffery J. Betts, PhD**
Central Michigan University
Mount Pleasant, Michigan
*Chapter 1, Anatomy and Biomechanics*

**Khalid W. Bibi, PhD**
The Health and Human Performance Center
Canisius College
Buffalo, New York
*Chapter 11, Metabolic Calculations*

**Kathleen M. Cahill, MS, ATC, RCEP**
Sugar Land, Texas
*Chapter 8, Exercise Programming*

**David S. Criswell, PhD**
Department of Exercise and Sport Sciences
University of Florida
Gainesville, Florida
*Chapter 3, Human Development and Aging*

**Frederick S. Daniels, MS**
CPTE Health Group
Nashua, New Hampshire
*Chapter 7, Safety, Injury Prevention, and Emergency Care*
*Chapter 10, Program and Administration/Management*

**Brenda M. Davy**
Virginia Tech University
Blacksburg, Virginia
*Chapter 9, Nutrition and Weight Management*

**Michael R. Deschenes, PhD, FACSM**
Department of Kinesiology
The College of William and Mary
Williamsburg, Virginia
*Chapter 2, Exercise Physiology*

**Andrea L. Dunn, PhD, FACSM**
Cooper Institute for Aerobics Research
Denver, Colorado
*Chapter 5, Human Behavior and Psychology*

**Gregory B. Dwyer, PhD, FACSM**
Department of Exercise Science
East Stroudsburg University
East Stroudsburg, Pennsylvania
*Chapter 10, Program and Administration/Management*

**Stephen C. Glass, PhD, FACSM**
Department of Movement Science
Grand Valley State University
Allendale, Michigan
*Chapter 6, Health Appraisal and Fitness Testing*

**Chad Harris, PhD**
Department of Kinesiology
Boise State University
Boise, Idaho
*Chapter 1, Anatomy and Biomechanics*

**Mark J. Kasper, EdD**
Department of Kinesiology and Physical Education
Valdosta State University
Valdosta, Georgia
*Chapter 4, Pathophysiology and Risk Factors*

**Diana LaHue, RN, MSN**
Electrophysiology Clinic
Research Medical Center
Kansas City, Missouri
*Chapter 12, Electrocardiography*

**Bess H. Marcus, PhD**
Department of Psychiatry and Human Behavior
Brown University
Providence, Rhode Island
*Chapter 5, Human Behavior and Psychology*

**Robert S. Mazzeo, PhD, FACSM**
Department of Integrative Physiology
University of Colorado
Boulder, Colorado
*Chapter 3, Human Development and Aging*

**Susan M. Puhl, PhD**
Associate Professor of Kinesiology
Department of Physical Education and Kinesiology
California Polytechnic State University
San Luis Obispo, California
*Chapter 4, Pathophysiology/Risk Factors*

**Robert Tung, MD, FACC**
Electrophysiology Clinic
Research Medical Center
Kansas City, Missouri
*Chapter 12, Electrocardiography*

**Janet R. Wojcik, PhD**
Department of Psychology
Virginia Tech University
Blacksburg, Virginia
*Chapter 9, Nutrition and Weight Management*

**John W. Wygand, MA**
Department of Health, Physical Education, and Human Performance Science
Adelphi University
Garden City, New York
*Chapter 8, Exercise Programming*

ACSM Certified Clinical Exercise Specialist. *See* CES
ACSM Certified Health Fitness Specialist. *See* HFS
ACSM Certified Personal Trainer. *See* CPT
CES
    case studies, 153–178
        answers, explanations, 179–190
    domains
        Domain I (patient/client assessment)
            case study related to, 153–154
            job task analysis information and resources,
                195–199
        Domain II (exercise prescription)
            case studies related to, 154–163
            job task analysis information and resources,
                200–205
        Domain III (program implementation, ongoing support)
            case study related to, 163–165
            job task analysis information and resources,
                205–211
        Domain IV (leadership, counseling)
            case study related to, 165
            job task analysis information and resources,
                211–214
        Domain V (legal, professional considerations)
            case studies related to, 166–171
            communicating hazards to employees, 169
            engineering controls, 169
            exposure incident defined, 170
            job task analysis information and resources,
                215–217
            labels, 169–170
        examination questions by domain, 237
    ECG case studies, 171–178
        answers, explanations, 190–193
    examination, 219–227
        answers and explanations, 228–237
        questions by domain, 237
    job task analysis, 195–217
        exercise prescription (Domain II)
            clinically appropriate prescription development,
                200–201
            prescription, program review with participant,
                202–203
            safe, effective use of exercise modalities, 204–205
        leadership, counseling (Domain IV)
            collaboration with health care professionals,
                referrals, 214
            disease management, risk factor reduction, 213
            participant performance and progress education,
                211–212

legal, professional considerations (Domain V)
    continuing education programs, 218
    emergency equipment, procedures, 216
    exercise environment evaluation, inspection
        procedures, 216
    Health Insurance Portability and Accountability Act
        (HIPAA), 217
    healthy lifestyle practices, 218
    participant safety procedures, self-monitoring, 217
patient/client assessment (Domain I)
    baseline intake, 196–198
    participant's risk evaluation, monitoring,
        supervision, 198–199
    physician referral, medical records, 195
program implementation, ongoing support (Domain III)
    participant feedback assessment, 207–208
    participant records, progress, clinical status, 211
    program implementation, 205–206
    program reassessment, updates, 208–210
CPT
    case studies, 3–10
        answers, explanations, 10–14
    domains
        Domain I (initial client consultation, assessment)
            case study related to, 3–4
            job task analysis information and resources, 15–23
        Domain II (exercise programming, implementation)
            case study related to, 4–5
            job task analysis information and resources, 24–35
        Domain III (leadership, education implementation)
            case study related to, 6–7
            job task analysis information and resources, 35–40
        Domain IV (legal, professional, business, and
            marketing)
            case studies related to, 8–9
            job task analysis information and resources, 40–51
        examination questions by domain, 74
    examination, 55–62
        answers and explanations, 63–74
        questions by domain, 74
    job task analysis, 15–52
        exercise programming, implementation (Domain II)
            client feedback, satisfaction, enjoyment, 35
            client technique monitoring, exercise response, 33
            exercise frequency, intensity duration determination,
                27–29
            exercise modalities selection, 25–27
            frequency, intensity, duration modification, 34
            program review with client, 30–32
            training program determination, 24–25

CPT (*Continued*)
    initial client consultation, assessment (Domain I)
        behavioral readiness evaluation, exercise adherence, 17
        client data, risk stratification, action plan, physical assessment, 16–17
        client instructions, initial documents, 15
        client interview, 16
        fitness assessments, goal setting, program development baseline, 18–23
        reassessment plan/timeline development, 23
    leadership, education implementation (Domain III)
        client education, knowledge base, fitness-related information, 37–40
        positive exercise experience creation, 35–37
    legal, professional, business, and marketing (Domain IV)
        American College of Sports Medicine's (ACSM's) Code of Ethics, 46
        business plan development, 47–48
        confidentiality, privacy, 51
        continuing education program participation, 45–56
        copyrights, 50
        health care professionals, organizations collaboration, 41–42
        insurance, standards of practice, 49
        lifestyle practices, client role model, 49–50
        marketing, client base, 48
        medical clearance, 40–41
        risk management program, 42–45
HFS
    case studies, 77–85
        answers, explanations, 86–93
    domains
        Domain I (health and fitness assessment)
            case study related to, 77–79
            job task analysis information and resources, 93–101
        Domain II (exercise prescription and implementation)
            case study related to, 79–80
            job task analysis information and resources, 101–116
        Domain III (counseling and behavioral strategies)
            case study related to, 80–82
            job task analysis information and resources, 117–121
        Domain IV (legal/professional)
            case study related to, 82–83
            job task analysis information and resources, 122–125

Domain V (management)
        case study related to, 83–85
        job task analysis information and resources, 126–129
    examination questions by domain, 150
examination, 131–138
    answers and explanations, 139–149
    questions by domain, 150
job task analysis, 93–129
    counseling and behavioral strategies (Domain III)
        behavioral and motivational strategies, 118–119
        communication techniques, 117
        educational resources, 120–121
        support within scope of practice, 121
    exercise prescription and implementation (Domain II)
        cardiorespiratory exercise prescriptions, FITT principle, 103–105
        clinical populations with physician clearance, 113–114
        environmental conditions, 116
        healthy special populations, 114–116
        muscular strength, endurance, flexibility, FITT principle, 106–109
        preactive screening, health appraisal, exercise history, fitness assessments review, 101
        program to achieve outcomes and goals determination, 101–103
        resistance, cardiovascular, flexibility-based activities, 109
        weight management programs, 110–112
    health and fitness assessment (Domain I)
        anthropometric and body composition, 100–101
        assessment protocols, preexercise screening, 93
        cardiovascular fitness assessments, 97–98
        muscular strength, endurance, flexibility, 99–100
        participant's readiness, 93–95
        selection and preparation, healthy participants and with controlled disease, 96
    legal/professional (Domain IV)
        injury prevention program, emergency policies and procedures, 124–125
        risk management guidelines, 122–124
    management (Domain V)
        communication techniques, professional relationships, 129
        fiscal resources, 126–127
        health/fitness facilities management, 127–128
        human resources, 126